Perinatal
Pharmacology
and Therapeutics

Contributors

Mont R. Juchau
G. Carolyn Marlowe
Bernard L. Mirkin
Kenneth E. Moore
Sharanjeet Singh
Leo Stern
John E. Thornburg
William J. Waddell
Sumner J. Yaffe

Perinatal Pharmacology and Therapeutics

EDITED BY

Bernard L. Mirkin Ph.D., M.D.
Division of Clinical Pharmacology
Departments of Pediatrics and Pharmacology
University of Minnesota
Minneapolis, Minnesota

ACADEMIC PRESS New York San Francisco London 1976

A Subsidiary of Harcourt Brace Jovanovich, Publishers

ACADEMIC PRESS, INC.
111 Fifth Avenue, New York, New York 10003

United Kingdom Edition published by
ACADEMIC PRESS, INC. (LONDON) LTD.
24/28 Oval Road, London NW1

Library of Congress Cataloging in Publication Data

Main entry under title:

Perinatal pharmacology and therapeutics.

  Includes bibliographies and index.
    1.   Fetus, Effect of drugs on the.   2.   Maternal-
fetal exchange.   3.   Drug metabolism.   4.   Developmental neurology.   I.   Mirkin, Bernard L.   [DNLM:
1.   Fetus–Drug effects.   2.   Placenta–Drug effects.
WQ210 P4425]
RG600.P418   618.3'2   75-16880
ISBN 0–12–498350–2

D
618.32
PER

Contents

5   Clinical Implications of Perinatal Pharmacology
Sumner J. Yaffe and Leo Stern

List of Contributors

Numbers in parentheses indicate the pages on which the authors' contributions begin.

Mont R. Juchau, Ph.D. (71), Department of Pharmacology, School of Medicine, University of Washington, Seattle, Washington

G. Carolyn Marlowe (119), Department of Pharmacology, College of Medicine, University of Kentucky, Lexington, Kentucky

Bernard L. Mirkin, Ph.D., M.D. (1), Division of Clinical Pharmacology, Departments of Pediatrics and Pharmacology, University of Minnesota, Minneapolis, Minnesota

Kenneth E. Moore, Ph.D. (269), Department of Pharmacology, Michigan State University, East Lansing, Michigan

Sharanjeet Singh, M.D. (1), Division of Clinical Pharmacology, Departments of Pediatrics and Pharmacology, University of Minnesota, Minneapolis, Minnesota

Leo Stern, M.D. (355), Section of Reproductive and Developmental Medicine, Brown University, Providence, Rhode Island

John E. Thornburg, Ph.D. (269), Department of Pharmacology, Michigan State University, East Lansing, Michigan

William J. Waddell, M.D. (119), Department of Pharmacology, College of Medicine, University of Kentucky, Lexington, Kentucky

Sumner J. Yaffe, M.D.* (355), Division of Pharmacology, Department of Pediatrics, Children's Hospital, School of Medicine, State University of New York at Buffalo, Buffalo, New York

---

* Present address: Department of Pediatrics, University of Pennsylvania, Philadelphia, Pennsylvania and Division of Clinical Pharmacology, Children's Hospital of Philadelphia, Philadelphia, Pennsylvania.

Preface

Perinatal pharmacology is devoted to the study of pharmacologically active molecules and the effects they produce on developing organisms. The subject matter presented in this book has been arbitrarily divided into sections dealing with the prenatal (fetal pharmacology) and the postnatal (pediatric pharmacology) consequences of drugs administered during different phases of mammalian development. This organizational format was selected to emphasize the fact that xenobiotic chemical substances may influence development in myriad ways over a broad time span, covering the periods from conception to parturition, through neonatal and childhood existence, and even into early adult life. The essential processes influencing drug disposition and pharmacodynamic action during different stages of biological maturation have been considered in a detailed and critical manner.

The broad perspective of perinatal pharmacology has necessitated that the scope of this book be restricted to allow in-depth discussions of areas currently under active investigation. Omission of apparently significant areas have occurred, not because they were deemed unimportant, but primarily because the data available was considered insufficient (at this point in time) to allow substantive conclusions to be presented. This probably is more a reflection of one's inability to assimilate the vast amount of data which has been recently generated in this area, and for this I must ask the indulgence of my many colleagues in the field.

I wish to acknowledge an indebtedness to my primary collaborators who suffered through several revisions and unforseen setbacks during which it appeared that I had placed unnecessarily stringent demands upon them. It is indeed a commentary on their overall excellence, commitment, and insight that we have come forth with a relatively integrated viewpoint which hopefully will stimulate and enlighten all readers regardless of their specific disciplinary concerns.

I am also grateful to the many individuals who knowingly and unknowingly participated as sounding boards for a variety of the concepts presented in the different chapters. In particular, I am deeply appreciative of the unseen contribution of Drs. John A. Anderson and Frederick E. Shideman who collectively shared my vision of establishing developmental and pediatric clinical pharmacology as a viable discipline at the University of Minnesota. I also extend my thanks to Dr. Geoffrey S. Dawes and Paul S. Johnson for their hospitality and intellectual stimulation during my sabbatical leave at the University of Oxford. Finally, the patience and goodwill displayed by the staff of Academic Press must not go unrecognized since, together with the forebearance of my family, it is probably the single factor which "carried the day."

Bernard L. Mirkin

Perinatal
Pharmacology
and Therapeutics

1

Placental Transfer of Pharmacologically Active Molecules

Bernard L. Mirkin

Sharanjeet Singh

I. Introduction

Chemical substances entering the body in the form of food additives, environmental pollutants, or therapeutic agents are commonly disseminated via the systemic circulation to undergo widespread tissue distribution. These compounds may also be transferred into the luminal secretions of the fallopian tube and uterine cavity through which the ovum and blastocyst must pass during the early stages of embryogenesis.

1

Numerous investigations have demonstrated the transplacental passage of many different types of pharmacologically active compounds as well as the untoward and capricious effects such agents may exert upon mammalian development (Wilson, 1973).

While it has proved extremely difficult to identify categorically which characteristic(s) of the host or drug molecule is (are) most influential in the causation of adverse effects upon the fetus, the following factors appear to be of great importance: stage of fetal development at the time of drug exposure; duration of exposure; amount of drug administered; quantitative rates of drug transfer to and from the fetus; distribution of drug in the fetus; and the physicochemical properties and pharmacodynamic actions of the drug molecule.

This chapter presents a comprehensive discussion of the basic mechanisms regulating placental drug transfer, fetal drug distribution, and the pharmacokinetic patterns of different classes of drugs in the maternal–placental–fetal unit.

II. Morphological and Comparative Physiology of the Placenta

Shortly after fertilization, probably within the initial 24 hours, the ovum undergoes cleavage to produce blastomeres which are approximately equal in size. This process is initiated in the segment of the fallopian tube most proximal to the ovary and continues as the fertilized ovum proceeds toward the uterine cavity.

Blastocyst formation, characterized by the development of a cavity within the morula,* appears to be associated with the transfer of substances from the luminal fluid of the uterus into the blastocyst as well as from endogenous secretions of cells comprising the morula (Martin, 1968). At the time of implantation which generally occurs about 6 to 7 days after fertilization, formation of the placenta begins and the different histological components of this organ can be distinguished. The placenta undergoes maturational changes which may significantly influence the transfer of xenobiotic and endogenously formed molecules across the complex biological membranes contained within this organ.

The early studies of Flexner and Gellhorn (1942) suggested that the ease with which substances passed across the placental membranes was directly proportional to the number of membrane layers separating the fetal and maternal bloodstreams, i.e., the fewer the membrane layers the more rapid the transfer. The statement was based on the apparent corre-

---

* The mass of blastomeres resulting from the early cleavage divisions of the fertilized ovum (zygote).

lation between morphological changes in the villi of late third trimester placentas and the increased placental transfer rate of sodium observed at this gestational stage.

However, even for molecules which cross the placenta by simple diffusion, the anatomic thickness of this organ cannot be consistently related to the number of membrane layers which are either morphologically discernible or functionally operational. Placentas of all types have regions in which the membranes overlying the fetal and maternal capillaries are virtually absent or markedly attenuated. Consequently, the distance separating the maternal and fetal circulations in such areas may be no greater in a six-layered epitheliochorial placenta than in a hemochorial placenta consisting of three membrane layers (Wimsatt, 1962). The depth of the tissue layers interposed between the fetal capillaries and the maternal blood supply have been estimated to vary from 1 to 100 μm in different animal species (Metcalfe et al., 1967). At term, the mean thickness of the trophoblastic membranes in the human placenta has been reported to be 3.5 μm (Aherne and Dunhill, 1966). As the placenta matures, a marked change in these structures occurs and they decrease from a thickness of 25 μm early in gestation to 2 μm at parturition (Strauss et al., 1965). Recent data suggest that the relative permeability of the rat placenta to diphenylhydantoin is biphasic in nature; transfer appears to be at a maximum in the early and late stages of gestation, decreasing significantly during midgestation (Stevens and Harbison, 1974).

Histological analyses of the major types of placentas have demonstrated that the number and thickness of tissue layers interposed between the fetal and maternal vascular systems are species dependent (see Table I; Amoroso, 1952; Dawes, 1968). Anatomic classifications explicitly define the morphological distinctions existing between most mammalian placentas but do not provide additional insight regarding the functional significance of these differences. Comparative studies on the placental transfer of drugs in different species are meager and at present it can only be assumed that placentas of the hemochorial and nonhemochorial type respond similarly with respect to drug transfer. The lack of detailed information makes it virtually impossible to assess how variations in the number, composition, and characteristics of placental membranes may influence the placental passage of different drugs.

Some indication of the complexity of this problem can be obtained from studies in which the trophoblastic ultrastructure of different types of hemochorial placentas has been histologically defined. These data demonstrate that the labyrinthine hemomonochorial placentas contain spaces in which the maternal plasma is relatively stagnant due to the presence of numerous and extensive microvilli (Enders, 1967). Stasis of maternal

TABLE I   Anatomic Classification of Placentas[a]

Histological type	Tissues separating fetal and maternal circulatory systems						Typical species
	Maternal (Uterine mucous membrane)			Fetal (Allantochorion)			
	Endothelium	Connective	Epithelium	Trophoblast	Connective	Endothelium	
Epitheliochorial	+	+	+	+	+	+	Pig, horse, donkey
Syndesmochorial	+	+	−	+	+	+	Sheep, goat, cow
Endotheliochorial	+	−	−	+	+	+	Cat, dog, ferret
Hemochorial	−	−	−	+	+	+	Man, rhesus monkey
Hemoendothelial	−	−	−	−	±	+	Rabbit, guinea pig, rat, mouse

[a] Adapted from Amoroso (1952) and Dawes (1968).

blood within the intervillous space may cause delayed and nonhomogeneous mixing of drug in the maternal placental circulation. Consequently,
the diffusion of drugs into the fetal circulation of species possessing a
hemomonochorial placenta (guinea pig, chipmunk) may be retarded even
though it contains fewer tissue layers than the hemotrichorial placenta
(rat, mouse), in which physical impediments to maternal blood flow are
minimal.

Differences in transplacental electrical potentials have been observed
among closely related rodent species. Potentials of 15 mV (fetus positive)
were recorded in the rat, 0 mV in the rabbit, and 18 mV (fetus negative)
in the guinea pig at equivalent stages in gestation (Mellor, 1969). These
biogenic potentials in some manner provide an index of fetal maturity
in each species, since at birth the rat is developmentally immature, the
rabbit intermediate, and the guinea pig most advanced. The trophoblastic
layering of the hemochorial placenta in these rodents differs* (Enders,
1967) so that a causal relationship between transplacental electrical potential, placental transfer rate, and anatomic constitution may exist.

While the nature of the relationship between structure and function
in biological membranes has not been clearly elucidated, all functional
membranes appear to be composed primarily of lipids and proteins. The
proportion of lipid (and its constituent fatty acids) to protein differs

* The rat has a three-layered trophoblast, the rabbit two layers, and the guinea
pig only one layer.

significantly in each type of membrane. Data derived from experiments using myelin sheaths as models have generally been extrapolated to, and considered relevant for, the plasma membranes of different tissues with little consideration given to the significance of differences in their respective biochemical characteristics or molecular organization.

Myelin is low in protein with a protein/lipid ratio of approximately 0.5, and contrasts markedly with other membranes in which the ratio is 2.0 or greater. Additionally, myelin's phospholipid composition differs from that of most basement membranes (Dowben, 1969; Van Bruggen, 1971). Myelin appears to be relatively inactive metabolically, in contrast to other membranes which are capable of synthesizing and degrading numerous types of cellular substrates. The placental membranes are probably best identified with the latter group because of their capacity for carrying out numerous enzymatic reactions which may be related to normal fetal development. Over 85 enzymes involving the metabolism of steroids, carbohydrates, proteins, and lipids have been identified in placental extracts (Hagerman, 1970). The biotransformation of drugs has been demonstrated in homogenates prepared from placental tissue (Juchau, 1972), however, the *in vivo* significance of this process remains unclear at present (see Chapter 2).

The structural organization of most membranes and their constituents is generally considered to be in a dynamic rather than static state of existence (Sjöstrand, 1963; Dowben, 1969). The membranes are conceived to be planar aggregates of micellar subunits (either spherical or lamellar, with an internal liquid crystalline phase) which are neither constant in their physical state nor collectively arranged in a fixed pattern (Tien and James, 1971). These subunits undergo reversible structural changes probably corresponding to phase transitions and functional needs. The rapid structural and functional modification of the placenta throughout gestation suggests that it may possess characteristics which are unique among the biomembranes. Consequently, it appears that generalizations regarding drug transfer across the placenta which are based upon data derived from investigations carried out in other nonplacental membrane systems may not be valid (Oh and Mirkin, 1971; Oh, 1973; Mirkin and Oh, 1974).

III. Transfer of Drugs into the Preimplantation Blastocyst and Luminal Secretions of the Oviduct and Uterus

Therapeutic agents and other chemical substances may interact with the developing ovum at many different sites during its passage through the oviduct and fallopian tubes. The penetration of drugs into most portions of the mammalian reproductive system has been shown to occur prior to the development of a functional placenta (see Table II).

Studies performed in a variety of species have demonstrated that the composition of fluids in the oviduct varies in accordance with the stage of the menstrual cycle, the nature of the steroid hormone present in the circulation, and the presence or absence of pregnancy (Hamner and Fox, 1969; Mastroiani et al., 1961). Amino acids (Jaszczak et al., 1970) and chloride ions (Brunton and Brinster, 1971) are actively secreted into the luminal fluids of the fallopian tube so that the blastocyst is exposed to high concentrations of these substances during the interval between fertilization and implantation. Since active secretory mechanisms appear to exert an important regulatory influence on the composition of fluids in the uterine and fallopian lumen, drugs affecting these processes may alter the chemical nature of such secretions and significantly influence drug distribution patterns as well as their rates of penetration into the blastocyst.

The oviductal and uterine secretions of rabbits possess a higher pH than that of plasma (McLachlan et al., 1970; Vishwakrama, 1962). Thus, basic drugs would generally be anticipated to achieve lower concentrations and acidic drugs higher concentrations in these fluids if their respective pH values exceeded that of plasma. Deviations from this distribution pattern might occur via the active transport of drug or active reabsorption of water from the oviduct. Currently, little is known about either of these processes which potentially can alter drug distribution in the

TABLE II   Potential Sites at Which Drugs May Affect Ontogenesis

Developmental stage	Anatomic location	Primary source of drug
Ovum	Ovary	Maternal circulation
Preimplantation blastocyst	Oviduct	Luminal secretions
	Fallopian tube	Luminal secretions
Postimplantation blastocyst	Uterus	Luminal secretions
		Maternal circulation (at nidation)
Embryo	Uterus	Maternal circulation via placental transfer
Fetus	Uterus	Administration directly to the fetus or indirectly via instillation into the amniotic fluid

luminal fluids of the uterus or fallopian tubes (see Chapter 3 for a detailed discussion of drug distribution in the mammalian reproductive system).

The extent to which exogenously administered drugs can or will accumulate in the luminal secretions of the uterus appears to be primarily determined by specific physicochemical properties of each drug and possibly by the active secretory mechanisms mentioned previously. Some compounds achieve uterine fluid concentrations which are about 50% greater than those of plasma if measurements are made 6 hours after drug administration. Xenobiotic agents which exhibit this distribution pattern are nicotine, thiopental, isoniazid, DDT, and caffeine (Sieber and Fabro, 1971). It is of considerable interest to note that these compounds can be detected in the uterine secretions of pregnant animals but not in the secretions of nonpregnant animals evaluated under similar experimental conditions.

In contrast to the data of Sieber and Fabro (1971), it has been quite convincingly demonstrated that inulin, oubain, tetraethylammonium (TEA), and α-aminoisobutyric acid (AIB), if administered systemically to the nonpregnant ovariectomized rat, will appear slowly, and in low concentrations, in the uterine luminal fluid; whereas, barbital, dimethyloxazolidinedione (DMO), antipyrine, and tritiated water are distributed into these secretions much more rapidly (Conner and Miller, 1973). The compounds investigated can be grouped into the following categories based on equilibration half-times calculated from their respective rates of penetration into luminal fluid: inulin, TEA, and AIB do not establish equilibrium with uterine luminal fluids during an experimental period of 90 minutes; barbital and DMO have equilibration half-times of 90 minutes; antipyrine and tritiated water have equilibration half-times of less than 10 minutes. These data suggest that the rate of transfer of chemical compounds into the luminal secretions of reproductive organs is closely correlated with their lipid solubility at physiological pH (7.4) and that no specific active transport system appears to be essential for this process (Table III).

The blastocyst migrating toward its eventual site of implantation in the uterus is exposed to the effects of chemical compounds which are present in secretions of the fallopian and uterine lumen. The rabbit blastocyst which has been frequently utilized as an experimental model can regulate its internal concentrations of lactic acid, bicarbonate, and glucose to a remarkable degree. Pretreatment of impregnated rabbits with a variety of drugs does not appear to alter the ability of the blastocyst to modulate these processes (Lutwak-Mann and Hay, 1962).

TABLE III   **Relationship between Partition Coefficient, Uterine Fluid/Plasma Concentration Ratio, and Equilibration Half-Time**[a]

Compound[b]	Partition coefficient[b,c]	Uterine fluid/plasma conc. ratio[d]	Equilibration half-time (minutes)[e]
Inulin	9.4	0.004	Not established
TEA	22.0[f]	0.04	Not established
AIB	3.9	0.03	Not established
Oubain	2.9	0.21	Not established
DMO	29.0	0.55	90
Barbital	45.0	0.95	90
Antipyrine	400.0	1.06	<5

[a] Data derived from Conner and Miller, 1973.

[b] Abbreviations: TEA = tetraethylammonium bromide; AIB = α-aminoisobutyric acid; DMO = dimethyloxazolidinedione.

[c] Partition coefficient = n-heptane/phosphate buffer, pH 7.4.

[d] Concentration ratio obtained 60 minutes after i.v. administration to animal.

[e] Equilibration half-time represents the time (minutes) required for the uterine fluid drug concentration to reach 50% of the plasma concentration.

[f] Partition coefficient = 6.0 when H_2O used in place of phosphate buffer.

While the teratogenic potential of many different chemical agents has been assessed in the rabbit blastocyst model, there is a paucity of data relating to the transfer of drugs into this structure under systematically controlled experimental conditions. Pharmacologically active substances, such as caffeine, nicotine, DDT, barbital, thiopental, and isoniazid, can be detected in the preimplantation blastocyst from 1 to 6 hours after administering these compounds to the pregnant rabbit (Fabro and Sieber, 1969). Incubation of the 6-day-old rabbit blastocyst with drugs, under *in vitro* conditions, has shown that the rate of uptake of salicylic acid, sulfanilamide, antipyrine, and hexamethonium by the blastocyst correlates closely with the lipid solubility and extent of ionization of each compound (Table IV). The influence of molecular weight on drug penetration has also been evaluated, and dextrans possessing molecular weights between 15,000 and 17,000 can penetrate the blastocyst, whereas dextrans with molecular weights in the range of 60,000 to 90,000 cannot.

These data clearly illustrate that the physiocochemical characteristics of drug molecules are important in determining their pattern of distribution as well as rates of penetration into the luminal secretions and the developing blastocyst. Whether these properties have any significant relationship to the teratogenetic or embryotoxic potential of a given chemical agent still remains a moot point at this juncture.

TABLE IV   **Relationship between Ionization, Lipid Solubility, and Rate of Drug Uptake by the Preimplantation Rabbit Blastocyst**[a]

Compound	% Ionized (pH 7.2)	Partition coefficient[b]	Equilibration half-time (minutes)[c]
Thiopental	28.5	38.0	1.5
Antipyrine	<0.01	23.0	1.7
Caffeine	<0.01	23.0	2.5
Thalidomide	0.01	32.0	44.7
Sulfanilamide	0.06	0.02	6.7
Barbital	20.1	0.30	9.5
Isoniazid	99.9	0.04	10.4
Salicylic acid	99.9	0.01	15.6
Uric acid	99.8	0.06	20.0
Hexamethonium	>99.9	0.33	66.6

[a] Data derived from Sieber and Fabro, 1971.

[b] Partition coefficient = $CHCl_3$/Ringer phosphate; pH 7.2.

[c] Time required for incubated compound to achieve concentration in blastocyst equal to half that occurring at equilibrium.

IV. Mechanisms of Drug Transfer across Biological Membranes*

Different types of processes regulate the movement of small molecules through biological membranes. Their respective influence on the passage of drugs across the placenta and into the fetal environment is considered in the ensuing discussion.

A. Simple Diffusion

A substantial body of evidence has shown that most xenobiotic substances probably cross the placental membranes by simple diffusion. A multiplicity of factors may modulate this process.

Estimating the rate of diffusion of a drug is complex and at a minimum requires the following information†: differences in drug concentration between the membrane bound compartments, the surface area available for transfer, the thickness of the membrane, and the specific physicochemical characteristics of the drug. The mathematical expression of

* This section was written in collaboration with Dr. Y. Oh, Department of Pharmacology, Ewha Medical College, Seoul, South Korea.

† Simple diffusion is dependent upon the kinetic motion of the drug molecule. The net movement of a given molecular species is proportional to the concentration gradient established (Fick's differential equation for passive diffusion, see Davson, 1970).

these interrelationships and their application to placental transfer is described in Eq. (1).

$$\text{Rate of diffusion} = K \frac{A(C_\mathrm{m} - C_\mathrm{f})}{X} \tag{1}$$

where

A = surface area available for transfer
C_m = maternal blood concentration
C_f = fetal blood concentration
X = thickness of placental membranes
K = diffusion constant of drug

The diffusion constant of a drug appears to be primarily determined by its molecular weight, spatial configuration, degree of ionization, and lipid solubility. If the thickness and surface area of the membrane remain constant for a given tissue, they may be incorporated into the diffusion constant K, to give the permeability rate constant P [see Eq. (2)], where S represents the drug concentration on the maternal side of the placenta.

$$dS/dt = P(C_\mathrm{m} - C_\mathrm{f}) \tag{2}$$

Most drugs behave chemically, like weak electrolytes. The ionized form of the drug molecule is generally water soluble and its molecular size frequently too large to permit ready diffusion through the pores of the plasma membrane. The nonionized form of the drug is usually lipid soluble, permitting this moiety to permeate with little resistance, when compared to ionized particles which penetrate with difficulty. Weak acids and weak bases are transferred rapidly, whereas highly ionized strong acids and bases penetrate membranes slowly. This broadly applied concept appears to have some validity in predicting drug transfer across the placenta (see Section V).

Foreign organic substances penetrate most membranes as though the cell boundary has the characteristics of a lipoid barrier. Therefore, the rate of diffusion of any given molecule through a lipoid membrane is proportional to its lipid/water partition coefficient. Unfortunately, there is no way to predict which organic solvent constitutes the best model of a biological cell membrane. When lipid/water partition coefficients for a chemically heterogenous group of drugs are ranked, considerable discrepancy may be observed depending on the solvent used, between the partition coefficient ranking and the amount of drug penetrating the plasma membrane (Danielli, 1970; Goldstein *et al.*, 1968; Hogben and Adrian, 1971). The best empirical correlation between partition coefficient and drug diffusion rate across a biological membrane has been obtained with nonpolar solvents such as n-heptane, benzene, or 1-octanol (Goldstein *et al.*, 1968; Hansch, 1968).

The relationship of partition coefficient (P) and log P (octanol/water),[*] to biological response is not categorically linear. When compounds possessing very high or very low partition coefficients are investigated, the correlation can be expressed in terms of either a linear or parabolic function. A theoretical explanation for this phenomenon has been offered but it still seems to lack precise experimental verification. It has been proposed that the higher the partition coefficient or log P (octanol/water), the tighter will be the binding between the drug and the first protein or lipid phase with which it makes contact. As lipid solubility approaches infinity, binding of the drug to the lipid phase becomes so firm that it cannot readily cross into an aqueous phase from the lipid phase. Consequently, such compounds tend to localize the initial lipophilic phase encountered (Danielli, 1970). In contrast, a drug with a partition coefficient approximating zero is so water soluble that it tends to remain almost exclusively in the first aqueous phase entered.

Hansch (1968) defined log P_0 (octanol/water) as the "ideal" log P. That is, one which would allow a drug to have the least hindrance in its movement through macromolecules to a specific receptor or site of action. Lien (1970) utilized the data of Brodie (1964) to calculate the "ideal" log P_0 for drug absorption from the gastrointestinal tract. He obtained a value of 1.97 which was very close to the log P_0 of 2.0 which had been determined as optimal for other biological systems. Penniston et al. (1969) showed that the value of log P_0 is, in fact, a function of the number of barriers a drug has to cross prior to reaching its site of action. As the number of barriers is increased, log P_0 approaches zero (i.e., $P = 1$); this represents the point where the free energy change in moving from one phase to another is zero. Members of a set of congeners having this "ideal" partition coefficient will be least retarded in their movement through both the hydro- and lipophilic phases of biological membranes. Although the pharmacological activity of a drug does not completely depend upon its lipid/water partition coefficient, there is general agreement that most pharmacokinetic parameters are strongly influ-

---

[*] Log P represents another mode of expressing the partition coefficient of a drug. It incorporates the degree of ionization of the molecule at a given pH, since lipid solubility is greater for the un-ionized than ionized molecular species. The general equation is as follows:

$$\log P = \frac{C_{(\text{octanol})}}{C_{\text{H}_2\text{O}}(1 - \alpha)}$$

where $C_{(\text{octanol})}$ = drug concentration in octanol, $C_{\text{H}_2\text{O}}$ = drug concentration in water, and α = degree of ionization (expressed as fraction of initial drug concentration) (Hansch, 1968).

enced by the lipid–water equilibrium (i.e., log P) of any given compound (Seydel, 1971). Therefore, it would appear to be of great pharmacological significance if the ideal log P_0 necessary for optimum passage of drugs across the placenta could be determined.

The use of penetration rate constants to express the extent of drug diffusion across a biological membrane by the uncritical application of Fick's law has been criticized by several investigators (Hogben and Adrian, 1971; Hansch, 1971). The limitations of such extrapolations are well described in the following statement: "In any real situation it is frequently difficult to define the boundary condition necessary for the solution of the differential equation; secondly, the Fick's equation assumes that the permeation coefficient across a complex and unknown membrane is a constant, which is not necessarily true" (Hogben and Adrian, 1971). Since the structural composition of most biological membranes is dynamic and labile rather than static, a membrane may shift between different structural states each possessing rather distinct functional characteristics (Sjöstrand, 1963; Kavanau, 1963). The spatial orientation of lipids in the membrane, as either ordered lipid bilayers or random micellar configurations, appears to constitute the essential distinction between these structural states (Tien and James, 1971).

The electropotential difference between the two sides of a membrane also seems to be an important factor affecting simple diffusion, especially that of charged molecules. Hogben and Adrian (1971) have suggested that the flux ratio equation developed by Ussing (1963) would be most accurate in predicting molecular transfer rates regulated only by simple passive diffusion. This equation expresses the unidirectional flux ratio in the following manner:

$$\frac{M_{in}}{M_{out}} = \frac{C_o}{C_i} \frac{zFE}{e^{RT}} \tag{3}$$

where
M_{in} = inward flux of substance
M_{out} = outward flux of substance
C_o = concentration of substance in the outside solution
C_i = concentration of substance in the inside solution
E = potential difference between the outside and the inside solution
z = charge borne by the substance
F = Faraday constant
R = gas constant
T = absolute temperature

Situations in which the resting potential of the cell is zero or where the transported molecular species is uncharged and therefore uninfluenced by the electrical field, allows reduction of Eq. (3) to flux Eq. (4). It describes the simple diffusion of an uncharged substance in the absence of solvent drag (Ussing, 1963):

$$M_{in}/M_{out} = C_o/C_i \qquad (4)$$

A major difficulty encountered in applying the Ussing equation to the analysis of drug transfer has been the necessity of knowing the electrochemical activity rather than simple molar concentration, of the transported species on each side of the membrane (Ussing, 1949; Davis, 1969; Hogben and Adrian, 1971). In many physiological investigations, including those involving the kinetics of placental drug transfer, it is impossible to determine these parameters precisely.

Interactions (e.g., hydrogen bonding or adsorption) between diffusing molecules and cell water localized near the structural proteins of biological membranes and their water channels are of great significance. They determine the rotational freedom of the diffusing ion and indirectly its rate of permeation (selective permeability). Intracellular water appears to exist in a different physical state from "normal" extracellular water. Solutes such as hydrated ions and nonelectrolytes have a low-distribution ratio in cell water because they are restricted in their rotational motion by the hydrogen bonds formed in cell water which is also highly polarized by charged structural proteins present in the cell membranes. It has been stated that some apparent deficiencies in the Ussing equation may be due to uncertainty concerning the electrochemical activity coefficients of the solute species (Ling, 1965).

A primary requisite for the application of both the Fick's and Ussing's equations is that the membrane must be in a steady state with respect to solute concentration so that the penetration or flux in any given direction remains constant. Penniston *et al.* (1969) have developed a non-steady-state kinetic model based on the multicompartment concept, which may be somewhat more relevant for the non-steady-state pharmacokinetics frequently observed *in vivo*.

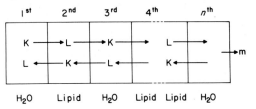

FIG. 1. Multicompartmental model illustrating lipid barrier between aqueous compartments. (After Penniston *et al.*, 1969.) The rate constant for passage from the aqueous to the lipid phase is K, and that for the reverse passage is L.

This model consists of a series of equivolume compartments sequentially arranged into alternating lipid and aqueous phases designed to simulate the multiple interactions of a solute (e.g., drug molecule) with plasma protein or other membranes prior to reaching its primary site of action (Fig. 1). Binding of the solute in the final phase or primary site of action occurs via an irreversible first-order chemical reaction possessing a rate constant, m. Since the paradigm proposed is strictly theoretical in origin, its validity must still be established by appropriate experimental studies.

B. Facilitated Diffusion

Situations in which the transfer rate of a molecule is greater than would be predicted by diffusion alone or where it appears to be influenced by the structural and spatial characteristics of the molecule, constitute examples of facilitated diffusion. This type of transfer process not only deviates from Fick's law but is also saturable at high substrate concentrations. In addition, compounds which are structurally related to the agent under investigation may compete for the active transfer sites. Placental transfer occurring via pure diffusion occurs down an electrochemical gradient whereas, substances transferred by facilitated diffusion must combine with carrier mechanisms within the cell membrane.

Some examples of facilitated diffusion are presented below.

1. The kinetics of glucose transfer in the perfused guinea pig placenta are altered at high substrate concentrations which saturate the active transfer system. Furthermore, the transplacental passage of glucose is inhibited by competition with fructose or galactose but not by phlorrhizin (Ely, 1966).

2. Maternal iron-transferrin complexes have been shown to concentrate in the allantoic placenta of the rabbit. This is followed by the subsequent release of iron into the placental cells after which the desaturated transferrin returns to the maternal circulation. These data suggest that some constituent of the rabbit placenta, possessing a molecular weight between 4100 and 4700, has the capacity to bind iron. It may represent an iron transport or carrier protein with characteristics similar to those thought to be involved in the process of facilitated diffusion (Larkin et al., 1970).

C. Active Transport

Molecular transfers requiring an expenditure of metabolic energy or which exhibit substrate saturability and are able to flow against an electrochemical gradient, fulfill the primary criteria of active transport processes. Metabolic inhibitors such as oubain, dinitrophenol, fluoride, or arsenate can block the energy production required for active transport and significantly depress substrate movement across the placenta.

While relatively few xenobiotic substances are transferred via this mechanism, the transplacental movement of compounds such as creatinine, vitamin B_{12}, amino acids, and specific ions appear to be primarily dependent upon active transport. The passage of sodium from the fetal to the maternal circulation of the pig (Crawford and McCance, 1960) and its movement in the opposite direction (i.e., maternal to fetal) across the rat placenta represents such a process (Mellor, 1969). There are some data suggesting that the placental transfer of triamterene also requires an energy-dependent mechanism (McNay and Dayton, 1970).

D. Metabolic Conversion of Transferred Substrate

Some molecules are transferred by mechanisms that involve their metabolic conversion from one substance into another. The passage of riboflavin from maternal to fetal plasma seems dependent upon the uptake of flavin adenine dinucleotide by the placenta. This subsequently undergoes cleavage to free riboflavin which is then released into the fetal bloodstream (Lust et al., 1953).

Dehydroascorbic acid passes by diffusion from the maternal to the fetal circulation and is then reduced to ascorbic acid in the fetus, since the latter does not readily pass through the placenta (Räihä, 1958).

E. Physical Disruption of the Placental Membranes

Physical defects between the cells separating the maternal and fetal circulations are known to occur and the passage of red cells from one to another probably results from such imperfections. Pores large enough to permit the passage of intact red cells would of course allow the passage of virtually any type of pharmacologically active molecule. There seems to be no clear evidence that such breaks exert an important role in the placental transfer of drugs, however.

V. Factors Influencing the Placental Transfer of Pharmacologically Active Molecules

A. Hemodynamic Characteristics of the Placental Circulations

The anatomic and functional interrelationships of the maternal, placental, and fetal circulations constitute one of the most exquisite examples of adaptive biological design. This sophisticated life support system provides a maximum surface area for exchange of substrates in the absence of any significant anatomic connections between the two vascular systems. Alterations in the maternal or fetal contributions to placental blood flow can significantly influence the transfer of substrates across this organ.

1. MATERNAL CIRCULATION

Estimates of total uterine blood flow* near parturition have been obtained in many species utilizing a variety of experimental techniques. The intrinsic deficiencies of the procedures used to determine blood flow have been lucidly analyzed by Dawes (1968). Despite the limitations he has described, the following values for total uterine blood flow in different species have generally been accepted:

(a) *Human:* 94–127 ml/minute/kg at 10–28 weeks gestation (Assali *et al.*, 1960), 124 ml/minute/kg (Metcalf *et al.*, 1955) and 150 ml/minute/kg (Assali *et al.*, 1953) at term

(b) *Goats:* 280 ml/minute/kg (Huckabee *et al.*, 1961)

(c) *Sheep:* 110 ml/minute/kg (Campbell *et al.*, 1966) and 201 ml/minute/kg (Dilts, 1970)

(d) *Rhesus monkey:* 94 ml/minute/kg (Lees *et al.*, 1971) and 121 ml/minute/kg (Peterson and Behrman, 1969).

The precise measurement of maternal placental blood flow has proved to be a most vexing problem because of the difficulty in isolating its myometrial, vaginal, and ovarian components.

The estimation of cardiac output and its tissue distribution by radionuclide-labeled microspheres has provided significant information on regional blood flow in the maternal and fetal circulations (Rudolph and Heymann, 1967). A detailed analysis of cardiac output and specific tissue blood flow in pregnant rabbits under eucapnic conditions has been carried out by Duncan (1969) using this technique. Regional blood flows to the primary reproductive organs in this species were as follows (flow expressed as ml/minute and percent of total uterine flow)*: placenta, 20 ml/minute (59%); myometrium, 6.7 ml/minute (19.7%); ovary, 4.6 ml/minute (13%); vagina, 2.2 ml/minute (6.3%); and fallopian tube, 1.0 ml/minute (2.9%). Conversion of these data into blood flow per unit tissue weight (ml/minute/kg) suggests a quite different partitioning of

---

* Total uterine blood flow includes the uterus, placenta, and fetus.

uterine blood flow than does the former mode of expression.* The relative rankings in decreasing order are ovaries, 4500 ml/minute/kg; fallopian tube, 1400 ml/minute/kg; placenta, 380 ml/minute/kg; vagina, 170 ml/minute/kg, and myometrium, 134 ml/minute/kg.

The unusually high flow to the ovaries is quite striking and somewhat unanticipated. It is of interest to note that total blood flow to the rabbit ovary increases during pregnancy, peaking at the sixteenth day of gestation (30-day cycle) to achieve a flow tenfold greater than that observed during the nonpregnant state (Abdul-Karim and Bruce, 1973). The intraovarian distribution of blood flow is nonhomogeneous, since the corpus luteum receives 88% of the total ovarian flow (20,000 ml/minute/kg) at this gestational age.

These observations on regional blood flow may explain why certain pharmacological agents, e.g., diphenylhydantoin (Waddell and Mirkin, 1972), phenobarbital (Waddell, 1971), and tetrahydrocannabinol (Kennedy and Waddell, 1972) have tissue distribution patterns which are characterized by exceedingly high concentrations in the corpora lutea of the ovary. While other factors such as lipid solubility of the drug and lipid content of the tissue also influence the selective uptake of pharmacological agents, regional blood flow appears to be one of the most important determinants.

The homogeneity of uterine and umbilical blood flows has been elegantly studied in the pregnant ewe (Rankin et al., 1970). Data provided by these investigations strongly suggest that the macroscopic distribution of blood flow to the placental cotyledons is extremely even and uniform. Consequently, differences noted between umbilical and uterine venous concentrations of highly diffusible molecules (about 20% in the report by Meschia et al., 1967) are probably not attributable to the nonhomogeneous distribution of placental blood flow.

Many factors can directly influence maternal hemodynamics and indirectly thereby, the maternal distribution and placental transfer of pharmacological agents. Physical obstruction of blood flow may occur during uterine contractions induced by spontaneous labor (Martin et al., 1964; Borrell et al., 1965), by oxytoxic drugs (Greiss, 1965), or the removal of amniotic fluid (Lees et al., 1971). A reduction in maternal uteroplacental perfusion (from 85% of total uterine flow to 75%) can be produced by occlusion of myometrial arterioles or by obstruction of the uterine venous outflow due to compression associated with uterine contraction.

It is probable that each of these causes of transient hypoperfusion affects drug transfer across the placenta quite differently. If blood flow

* Based on data provided in Table 1, page 424 (Duncan, 1969).

is reduced as the result of arterial or arteriolar compression, less blood will reach the placenta per unit time with a concomitant decrease in perfusion. The placental passage of maternally administered drugs, particularly when given as single intravenous pulse injections, will be modified. The quantity of drug transferred across the placenta will be determined by the temporal relationship established between the onset of obstruction of maternal placental blood flow and the exponential decay in plasma drug concentration. If a decrease in maternal placental blood flow occurs during the initial drug redistribution phase, a larger proportion of the compound will be taken up by maternal tissues, reducing the maternal-to-fetal concentration gradient and the amount of drug transferred into the fetal circulation. Drugs whose transfer is flow limited and directly proportional to tissue perfusion (e.g., thiobarbiturates) would probably be most significantly affected by such alterations in the distribution of maternal cardiac output. In contrast, uterine venous obstruction more likely would tend to produce sequestration of maternal blood in the placenta allowing a longer period for diffusion and equlibrium between the maternal and fetal circulations. A greater extraction of drug from the maternal circulation might therefore result.

Vasoactive substances such as catecholamines (Adams *et al.*, 1961; Adamson *et al.*, 1971; Leduc, 1972) or angiotensin II (Behrman and Kittinger, 1968), released endogenously (Romney *et al.*, 1963) or administered directly to the mother also decrease maternal uteroplacental blood flow. While hypoxemia (Duncan, 1969), catecholamines, and hypocapnia induced by hyperventiliation (Leduc, 1972) may all cause a reduction in maternal placental blood flow their effects on maternal systemic arterial pressure, distribution of cardiac output, and probably drug transfer differ markedly. Pathophysiological conditions such as pre-eclampsia (mild and severe) or hypertension (McClure-Browne, 1959), which are associated with impaired uteroplacental flow, would also be expected to decrease drug transfer across the placenta. Hypoproteinemia (hypoalbuminemia) secondary to the nephrotic syndrome or nephritis may lead to an increased maternal ratio of free-to-bound drug. Since it is the free form of drug which diffused across a semipermeable membrane, this circumstance may potentially allow more drug to traverse the placenta.

2. FETAL CIRCULATION

An intriguing relationship exists between the fetal cardiovascular system and the pharmacodynamic actions of drugs entering the fetal circulation. While drug disposition is modified by the unique characteristics of the fetal circulation, in turn, pharmacologically active substances can affect the fetal cardiovascular system and significantly alter its functional reactivity.

Following their transfer across the placental membranes, drugs enter the umbilical vein and must pass through the liver prior to reaching the inferior vena cava or fetal right heart. Umbilical venous blood flow to the fetal liver is diverted into the portal vein to perfuse the hepatic parenchyma or it may bypass the liver via the ductus venosus.* The relative distribution of umbilical venous blood flow between these two circuits may be of major significance in determining the quantity of unmetabolized drug reaching the fetal right heart. This mechanism would appear to be of particular importance during the initial passage of a drug through the fetal circulation and probably less so when steady-state conditions had been established. If a large proportion of the umbilical venous flow shunted through the ductus venosus the concentration of pharmacologically active material presented directly to the fetal heart and central nervous system would be greatly elevated. Since the movement of most drugs into tissue is diffusion limited, increasing the concentration of drug in the blood will create a higher blood to tissue gradient and generally produce higher tissue levels.†

While hepatic drug metabolism is virtually negligible in the fetuses of most subhuman species (Fouts and Adamson, 1959; Hart et al., 1962) the human fetal liver is able to oxidize numerous substrates by the sixteenth week of gestation (Yaffe et al., 1970; Pelkonnen et al., 1971; Rane and Ackermann, 1972). The selective partitioning of blood flow into the ductus venous would probably decrease the proportion of drug normally metabolized immediately after its placental transfer and entry into the fetal circulation. Drugs which undergo biotransformation and inactivation by the fetal liver during a single pass are now able to directly enter the systemic circulation in their active form. Conversely, a disproportionate diversion of umbilical venous flow into the portal vein may cause exceedingly high drug concentrations in the fetal liver and correspondingly low levels in fetal blood, prior to the establishment of equilibrium.

Some insight regarding the complex nature of the relationship between fetal drug distribution, regional blood flow and the specific physicochemi-

---

* Vascular communications in the fetal liver, other than the ductus venosus, have been observed between the umbilical vein and the inferior vena cava (P. Johnson, unpublished observations, 1973).

† This generalization precludes specific circumstances where active drug transport is essential for tissue penetration, e.g., renal tubule, choroid plexus. Other factors such as tissue permeability and affinity for specific drug molecules must also be taken into consideration.

cal characteristics of each drug may be obtained from the following illustrations.

a. *Distribution of Digoxin in the Pregnant Rat* (Mirkin and Singh, 1973; Singh and Mirkin, 1975). Digoxin concentrations were determined in fetal and maternal tissues following the administration of digoxin (0.1 mg/kg i.v.) to pregnant rats on the twentieth gestational day. After equilibrium between the maternal and fetal circulations had been established, digoxin concentrations in maternal and fetal tissues were as follows (expressed as ng/ml or ng/gm wet weight): maternal serum, 28; maternal liver (ML), 254; maternal heart (MH), 73; ML/MH = 3.5; fetal serum, 14; fetal liver (FL), 19, fetal heart (FH), 86; FL/FH = 0.22.

This distribution pattern may be explained on the basis of poor extraction by fetal liver or by substantial hepatic bypass of umbilical venous blood resulting in very low fetal liver concentrations and elevated myocardial levels of digoxin. In contrast, the digoxin concentrations of maternal liver and heart illustrate the converse situation.

An equally important aspect of this study was the observation that maternal-to-fetal tissue concentration ratios had the same relationship, prior to equilibrium, i.e., 2 minutes after injection, as they did at equilibrium. Since the early tissue distribution pattern of a drug probably has a greater dependence upon and more directly reflects blood flow than those obtained at equilibrium, these data reinforce the view that a major portion of the umbilical venous blood flow in the pregnant rat had been diverted through the ductus venosus.

b. *Distribution of Thiopental in the Human and Guinea Pig Fetus* (Finster *et al.*, 1972). Tissues obtained from anencephalic fetuses following routine hysterotomy under thiopental were analyzed and thiopental concentrations expressed as μg/gm wet weight or μg/ml. Case A delivered $1\frac{1}{2}$ hour after thiopental; Case B delivered $2\frac{1}{2}$ hour after thiopental: subcutaneous fat (88; 43); liver, left lobe (65; 43); liver, right lobe (58; 38); lung (25; 14); kidney (16; 11); heart (10; 10); maternal vein (19; 19); umbilical vein (11; 14); and umbilical artery (10; 12).

Comparable studies performed in the pregnant guinea pig demonstrated the accumulation of very high thiopental concentrations in the middle lobe of the fetal liver after the drug had been injected directly into the umbilical vein. The quantity of thiopental in the middle lobe was equivalent to about one-half of the administered dose and was approximately four times greater than that observed in the left lobe. These observations suggested that the fetal liver may shield other fetal tissues, particularly the central nervous system, from exposure to high concentration gradients and the potentially toxic effects of pharmacological agents by the uptake of large quantities of placentally transferred drug.

In harmony with this proposal were the early studies of Barclay *et al.* (1944) which indicated that about 90% of the total umbilical venous blood flow perfused the hepatic parenchyma prior to entering the fetal systemic circulation. If this were the sole determinant of fetal drug distribution, the fetal liver should always exhibit a significantly greater drug concentration relative to other fetal organs. Pharmacokinetic studies carried out in the pregnant rat with diphenylhydantoin (Mirkin, 1971) and aminopyrine (Oh, 1973) have shown that the fetal brain concentration is approximately equivalent to that of the fetal liver. It appears that factors such as lipid solubility, affinity for hepatic microsomal binding sites or other cellular constituents, and permeability of specialized membranes must also influence the fetal distribution of drugs.

c. Interfetal Transfusion Syndrome (Naey, 1963; Corney and Aherne, 1965; Klebe and Ingomar, 1972). The shunting of blood between twins can occur and several studies have shown that the blood volumes of monochorionic twins may differ markedly. This phenomena could lead to an unequal perfusion of one twin in preference to the other with larger amounts of drug being delivered to the twin receiving the higher blood flow, the end result being localization of significantly different concentrations of maternally administered drug in each fetus. A distribution pattern of this type has been reported to occur in animal models (see Chapter 3).

Each of these examples illustrates how the fetal umbilical circulation and fetal liver may regulate the amount of drug entering the fetal right heart and ultimately the fetal systemic circulation. Unfortunately, neither of the investigations cited clearly defined whether selective distribution of umbilical venous blood flow, physicochemical characteristics of the drug (e.g., pK_a, lipid solubility, protein binding), or special properties of the organ itself, constitute the critical determinants modulating drug uptake by the fetal liver.

The quantitative estimation of blood flow to the fetal liver under near-physiological conditions, in particular its lobular distribution pattern, has proven to be a most vexing experimental problem. Radiological studies performed in the fetal lamb (Barclay *et al.*,1944; Peltonen and Hirronen, 1965), the neonatal lamb (Shibata *et al.*, 1969), and in human infants (Meyer and Lind, 1966; Ogawa, 1966) have clearly demonstrated that radioopaque contrast media readily passes from the umbilical vein to the inferior vena cava via the ductus venosus. While such observations provide a very poor quantitative index of ductus venosus blood flow, Franklin *et al.* (1940) used this technique and concluded that the internal caliber of the ductus venosus in the fetal lamb was one-third that of the umbilical vein. Assuming both vessels to be circular, the cross-sectional area of the ductus venosus was estimated as being nine times less than that of the umbilical vein. Calculations based on these observations have been inappropriately interpreted as providing a reliable index of hepatic blood flow. They have led to the highly questionable assumption that only 11% of the umbilical flow reaches the inferior vena cava through the ductus venosus, the remaining 89% entering directly into the hepatic sinusoids and veins (Finster and Mark, 1971; Bonica, 1969).

The studies of Rudolph and Heymann (1967) are in striking disagreement with the previously described data (vide supra). Utilizing a quantitative radiolabeled microsphere technique, their observations in the fetal lamb indicate that 34 to 91% of umbilical venous flow is shunted through the ductus venosus and that the proportion of umbilical blood flow entering the ductus is directly proportional to flow, i.e., the higher the umbilical venous flow the greater the percentage shunted. A similar study performed in the baboon fetus has demonstrated that $55.4 \pm 16.5\%$ of umbilical flow passes through the ductus venosus (Paton *et al.*, 1973).

Some major differences in the proportion of fetal cardiac output entering the ductus venosus exists between species. In the rhesus monkey, which has a high umbilical blood flow, 40% of the fetal cardiac output was shunted via the ductus venosus (Behrman *et al.*, 1970) whereas the proportion was 21.5% in sheep (Rudolph and Heymann, 1970) and 23.2% in the baboon (Paton *et al.*, 1973). Another interspecies distinction is that preferential streaming of ductus venosus blood to the cerebral and coronary circulations occurs in the rhesus monkey but not in the fetal baboon and sheep. These individual physiological characteristics may significantly influence the distribution of drugs to the fetal nervous system in each species.

Angiograms performed in the human midgestational fetal liver reveal that a substantial portion of umbilical venous flow (estimated to be between one-third and two-thirds of the total) enters the ductus venosus. *In vitro* perfusion of livers obtained from stillborn infants has also demonstrated that 40 to 50% of the saline perfusate is diverted through the liver via the ductus venosus into the inferior vena cava (Meyer and Lind, 1966). Recently, the circulation of the previable human fetus has been studied with the radionuclide microsphere technique (Rudolph *et al.*, 1971). The proportion of total umbilical venous flow bypassing the liver via the ductus venosus varied from 8 to 92% in these subjects. However,

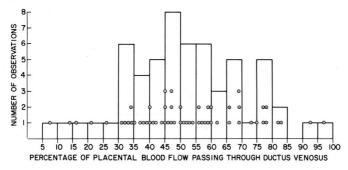

FIG. 2. Blood flow through the ductus venosus of the previable human infant. (Derived from Rudolph *et al.*, 1971.) See text for further discussion.

a more detailed analysis reveals that 30 of the 58 (52%) observations demonstrated ductus venosus flows exceeding 50% of umbilical venous flow and in 43 of the 58 (76%) it was greater than 40% (Fig. 2). These data are similar to the findings of Gurpide *et al.* (1972) who reported that 70% of the progesterone infused into an umbilical vein reached the fetal inferior vena cava and estimated that approximately 60% of the fetal placental flow was shunted through the ductus venosus. Collectively, therefore, the bulk of available quantitative data suggests that a variable but very significant portion of umbilical blood flow is diverted into the ductus venosus during *in utero* fetal existence.

The distribution of blood flow within the ovine liver has been determined by the indirect means of comparing oxygen saturation in blood samples obtained from the fetal pulmonary vein, umbilical vein, and inferior vena cava, both above and below the entry of the ductus venosus (Born *et al.*, 1954). The *left* lobe of the fetal liver appears to be perfused by oxygenated blood flowing directly from the umbilical vein (80% oxygen saturation). The *right* side of the fetal liver receives blood primarily from the portal venous system, which is mixed with umbilical venous blood, and the oxygen saturation of blood specimens taken from this confluence is only 27%. The mean oxygen saturation of blood specimens obtained from different regions of the fetal cardiovascular system has been used to predict drug concentrations which may occur in tissues perfused by these vascular segments. In a theoretical context, such data may have some relevance if blood flow alone were the primary determinant of drug distribution. At the present time, since many other factors affect this process, it appears hazardous to make predictions based upon the assumed, yet unproved, parallelism between oxygen saturation data and drug distribution in the fetus.

The concentration of a given drug in the blood perfusing the right side of the fetal liver is probably much lower than that flowing to the left or central lobular regions, due to the dilutional influence of the portal venous blood flow. The portal vein receives blood from the gastrointestinal tract, from which there is likely to have been considerable extraction of drug following perfusion of the visceral organs. The net result of these events is that prior to and probably after equilibrium is achieved, the fetal portal vein concentrations of maternally administered drugs are likely to be significantly below comparable fetal systemic blood levels. This concentration gradient would probably be reduced or perhaps reversed if drug were orally administered to the fetus or if absorption from the fetal gastrointestinal tract occurred over an extended period of time. While it is difficult to conceive of oral feedings to the fetus *in utero,* a situation closely simulating this may occur in the maternal–placental–fetal unit following chronic maternal drug tharapy or after the administration of drugs to the fetus via the transuterine intraperitoneal route. Drugs excreted into the amniotic fluid are very likely reingested by the fetus, establishing a renal–amniotic fluid–gastrointestinal pathway. This may represent an *in utero* mechanism enabling the fetus to mimic the postnatal oral route of drug administration.

There are, unfortunately, very few quantitative or qualitative data describing drug concentrations in regional vessels of the cardiovascular system or their segmental distribution to different areas of a common organ. Immunoassays for digoxin performed on extracts of specimens obtained from the right, left, and middle lobes of the fetal sheep liver did not reveal any significant differences in regional concentration 180 minutes after administering digoxin (i.v.) to the mother (Singh *et al.,* 1973). Radioautographic studies in pregnant mice have also not demonstrated any selective distribution patterns within the liver following injection of ^{14}C-diphenylhydantoin (Waddell and Mirkin, 1972) or ^{14}C-barbiturates (Waddell, 1971). Quantitative barbiturate analyses performed on specimens of fetal liver obtained after steady-state blood levels had been established in the pregnant ewe also failed to reveal any significant differences between the barbiturate concentrations of each hepatic lobe (Fehr and Mirkin, 1975). The hepatic distribution pattern of digoxin, diphenylhydantoin, and phenobarbital is relatively uniform, differing from that shown by thiopental *in situ* (Finster *et al.,* 1972).

While the factors which regulate the intrahepatic distribution of hepatic blood flow are not well understood, it does not appear to be influenced by total umbilical blood flow, fetal blood gas concentrations, or body weight (Rudolph *et al.,* 1971). Intrahepatic shunting of umbilical blood flow might result from an increase in hepatic portal vein resistance following the release of vasoactive substances in the fetus, possibly secondary to fetal distress; however, this is a completely speculative concept at the current time. Since the liver can effectively inactivate adrenergic neurotransmitters and vasoactive polypeptides, any chemical substance thus involved would probably have to be released in close proximity to the intralobular microvasculature. In this context, small amounts of norepinephrine have been identified in the fetal liver of the pregnant dog and rat (B. L. Mirkin, unpublished data, 1969; Mirkin, 1972a). Furthermore, it is highly probable that the intrahepatic vasculature would be reactive to such chemical stimuli during the last trimester of gestation. This area remains an important and highly significant one for further research, since it may help resolve the question of whether the fetal liver prevents excessively large concentrations of drugs from reaching vital fetal organs such as the heart and brain.

The pharmacokinetics of placental drug transfer are influenced not only by placental blood flow rates, but also by the integrity of the fetal circulation. Any impairment of the latter will exert significant effects upon the concentration of drug achieved in fetal tissues and the rate at which drugs enter and leave the fetal circulation. The interrelations between the fetal systemic circulation and placental drug transfer have been discussed by Heyman (1972).

Pharmacological agents can modify fetal hemodynamics directly by decreasing cardiac output and fetal heart rate. They may also exert a reflex or indirect effect on the fetal cardiovascular system which is generally mediated through depression of the fetal central nervous system. A change in the level of central nervous system activity can cause depression of the vasomotor center, with an associated decrease in the reflex tone of the adrenergic system, the fetal heart rate, and regional vascular resistance (Heyman, 1972).

B. Physicochemical Characteristics of Drugs

1. LIPID SOLUBILITY AND DEGREE OF IONIZATION (pK_a)

Most lipophilic compounds tend to diffuse quite readily across the placenta into the fetal circulation. Dancis and co-workers (1958) studied the relative rates at which estrogens and their glucuronides crossed the guinea pig placenta. Estriol and its lipid soluble metabolites rapidly traversed the placenta in either direction whereas the lipid-insoluble glucuronides did not.

Numerous studies have shown that drug molecules tend to penetrate biological membranes more quickly in an un-ionized state than in an ionized state (Mayer et al., 1959). Compounds such as antipyrine and thiopental, which are both poorly ionized at physiological pH, cross the placenta almost immediately with minimal resistance to their diffusion. In contrast, bases with high pK_a's and acids with low pK_a's diffuse across biological membranes poorly. The quarternary bases such as succinylcholine, d-tromethamine (THAM tris buffer) and the acidic sulfated mucopolysaccharides like heparin are highly ionized.* The placental passage of these compounds is so extremely slow, that under most therapeutic circumstances, very little passes into the fetal circulation. Only after administering doses 1000 times greater than the minimal maternal paralyzing dose has it been possible for sufficient succinylcholine to diffuse across the placenta and affect the newborn rabbit (Moya and Kvisselbaard, 1961). Despite the apparent impermeability of the rabbit placenta to succinylcholine, neonatal flaccidity and apnea have been observed in infants delivered from women receiving the muscle relaxant during parturition.

The impermeability of the placenta to polar compounds seems relative rather than absolute. If sufficiently high maternal-to-fetal concentration gradients are achieved, even polar compounds may cross the placenta and enter the fetal circulation. In this respect, it should be noted that some drugs, such as the salicylates, which are almost 100% ionized at pH 7.4, pass through the placental membranes quite rapidly. This probably occurs because even the very small amount of drug present in the un-ionized state readily moves across the placenta due to its high lipid solubility (Oh, 1973).

The placental transfer or drugs is also influenced by the respective pH of the maternal and fetal circulations, particularly when drugs possessing pK_a values close to that of blood are under consideration. The pH of umbilical vessel blood is normally 0.10 to 0.15 pH units lower than that of maternal blood. As a consequence, the concentration of undissociated basic drugs tends to be higher in the maternal circulation than in the fetal circulation. This partitioning leads to a net transfer of drug from the maternal organism to the fetus so that the final drug concentration in the fetus may exceed that of the mother at equilibrium (Asling and Way, 1971).

Previous studies on the passage of drugs across the blood–brain barrier and gastrointestinal tract have demonstrated that drug transfer is related not only to the degree of ionization of the compound but also to the lipid solubility of the un-ionized molecule (Hogben et al., 1959; Brodie et al., 1960). The rate of movement of drugs across biological membranes

---

* Succinylcholine and heparin also undergo enzymatic degradation by cholinesterase and heparinase, respectively, which are present in high concentrations in the placenta.

appears to be primarily governed by the lipid solubility of the nonionized drug molecule. Nonionized drugs with high lipid solubilities are transferred rapidly whereas, lipid-insoluble drugs penetrate poorly despite their low degree of ionization. The dissociation constant is primarily important because it determines the plasma concentration of the nonionized form of the drug.

2. MOLECULAR WEIGHT

Generally, compounds with low molecular weights tend to diffuse more rapidly across membranes than larger molecules, i.e., diffusion varies inversely with molecular weight. Most drugs possess molecular weights ranging from 250 to 500 and can cross the placenta quite easily, depending on their state of ionization, lipid solubility, and mechanism of transfer.

It has often been stated, despite the absence of substantive data, that compounds with molecular weights exceeding 1000 are severly retarded in their passage across the placenta. Recently, it has been shown that the cardiac glycoside, digoxin (molecular weight, 792), readily crosses the rodent (Mirkin and Singh, 1973) and human (Rogers et al., 1972) placentas; however, the ovine placenta is surprisingly impermeable to this drug (Singh et al., 1973).

3. PROTEIN BINDING

The binding of drugs to macromolecules inhibits their transfer across the placenta. If the association constant of the drug–macromolecular complex or the quantity of macromolecular binding sites in the maternal circulation is sufficiently large, the concentration of free drug in maternal plasma will be significantly reduced. Under these circumstances, the maternal-to-fetal diffusion gradient is diminshed as is the amount of drug entering the fetal circulation.

Protein binding does not appear to exert a significant effect on the placental passage of drugs which are highly lipophilic and nonpolar, since the transfer of these drugs seems to be proportional to placental blood flow. Compounds which move across the placenta more slowly, owing to higher degrees of ionization or lower lipid solubilities, may be drastically altered by protein binding in that diffusion is rate limiting for these agents (Goldstein et al., 1968).

Several studies have suggested that major distinctions in protein binding exist between fetal and maternal sera. Shoeman et al. (1972) found the total protein level of fetal goat serum (3.1 gm %) to be lower than that of maternal serum (6.4 gm %). This difference was attributable to a reduction in the albumin and gamma globulin content of the fetal serum. The maternal plasma proteins of the goat had a greater binding affinity for diphenylhydantoin than fetal plasma proteins. The much higher concentration of protein in maternal sera and the observed differences in diphenylhydantoin binding constants were considered to be responsible for the extremely low fetal serum levels observed after steady-state infusions of diphenylhydantoin to the mother.

Human fetal and maternal sera also exhibit differences in their capacity to bind local anesthetics (Mather et al., 1971). The binding of bupivicaine to maternal plasma proteins was twice that of fetal proteins when compared over the same range of drug concentrations. Ehrnebo et al. (1971) demonstrated that human fetal plasma had very little binding capacity for ampicillin, benzylpenicillin, phenobarbital, and diphenylhydantoin. Though the total concentration of plasma protein in the human fetus is significantly lower than that of the adult, this alone does not explain the decreased binding of drugs to fetal plasma proteins (Pruitt and Dayton, 1971).

Some compounds appear to bind equally well to maternal and fetal plasma proteins. Thus, Finster et al. (1966) was unable to observe any differences in the extent of protein binding of thiopental to either fetal or maternal plasma. A similar phenomenon was reported by Miller et al. (1972) with respect to iophenoxic acid, a radioopaque used for cholecystography. The recent data of Ganapathy and Cohen (1975) suggest that no qualitative distinctions in the physical or binding characteristics of albumin isolated from human cord and adult blood are discernible. This differs from other reports and the issue remains to be resolved.

4. PLACENTAL MATURATION

The rates of diffusion of specific drugs as well as the permeability of the placenta probably undergo continuous change during the lifespan of this organ. As the placenta matures, there is a decrease in the number of tissue layers interposed between the capillaries and the blood so that the thickness of the trophoblastic epithelium diminishes from 25 μm early in gestation to 2 μm at birth (Strauss et al., 1965). Most of the data obtained from studies in the pregnant rodent indicate that drug transfer is greatest in both the first and last trimesters with the least passage occurring at midgestation (Stevens and Harbison, 1974). The information available on this subject is rather inadequate and more data are necessary to adequately assess the influence of placental aging upon drug transfer.

5. PLACENTAL METABOLISM OF DRUGS

The therapeutic significance of drug biotransformation in the placenta remains to be clearly defined under *in vivo* conditions. It is known that the placenta can carry out numerous aromatic oxidase reactions (e.g., demethylation, hydroxylation, and N-dealkylation) when tissue extracts of this organ are incubated with an appropriate substrate *in vitro* (Juchau, 1972).

The drug-metabolizing activity of the human placenta on a weight basis is substantially less than that of either the maternal or fetal liver. Consequently, the role of the placenta as a major site of metabolism for xenobiotic substrates may be less important than it is for the biotransformation of endogenously synthesized substrates, such as steroidal hormones (see Chapter 2 for detailed discussion).

A summary of the factors which appear to influence the disposition of drugs in the maternal–placental–fetal unit is presented in Table V and Fig. 3.

TABLE V   Factors Modulating Drug Disposition in the Maternal–Fetal–Placental Unit

A. Placental transfer of drugs
    1. Physicochemical properties of drugs
        Lipid solubility (partition coefficient)
        Degree of ionization (pK_a)
        Molecular weight
        Protein binding
    2. Placental blood flow
        Maternal and fetal circulations
        Maternal–fetal blood pH gradient
    3. Stage of development of placenta
    4. Placental metabolism of drugs (?)
B. Drug disposition in the fetus
    1. Altered permeability of specific membrane-bound compartments
        Blood–brain barrier
        Total body water and lipid content
    2. Selective tissue uptake of drug
        Nonspecific lipid solubility
        Specific binding to cellular constituents
    3. Distribution of fetal circulation
    4. Metabolism of fetal liver
    5. Fetal swallowing of amniotic fluid
    6. Excretion by fetal kidney

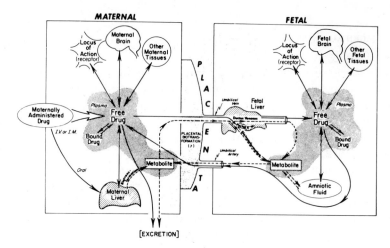

FIG. 3. Schematic illustration of drug disposition in the maternal–placental–fetal unit. (Adapted from Mirkin, 1973, with permission of Raven Press, New York.)

VI. Drug Disposition and Pharmacokinetics in the Maternal–Placental–Fetal Unit

A. Chemotherapeutic Agents

Antimicrobial compounds are commonly administered to pregnant women presenting with suspected amnionitis, prolonged rupture of placental membranes, and other causes of intrauterine infections. Precise and meaningful pharmacokinetic data describing the placental transfer of this class of compounds are unfortunately lacking. Most of the investigations have been carried out under poorly controlled conditions in conjunction with faulty experimental design. The studies generally consist of single pulse injections of drug to the mother followed by acquisition of maternal and cord blood specimens (occasionally amniotic fluid) at parturition. Despite the obvious limitations of such data, it is apparent that most antibiotics are transferred across the placenta to varying degrees and specific information pertaining to each agent has been summarized in this section.

1. PENICILLINS

a. *Ampicillin* (α-Aminobenzyl Penicillin). This antibiotic is rapidly transferred across the placenta into the fetal circulation and enters most fetal tissues (Bray *et al.*, 1966; MacAulay *et al.*, 1966). Some controversy exists regarding the maternal:fetal concentration ratios of ampicillin which are established after a maternal dose. Fetal and cord blood levels have been reported to be generally lower than maternal blood concentrations by Blecher et al. (1966) and William et al. (1966) whereas, Bray et al. (1966) and MacAulay et al. (1966) observed fetal levels to be higher than maternal. In each of these studies the fetal and maternal specimens were obtained at parturition. Since the maternal:fetal concentration gradient is directly proportional to the elapsed time between maternal drug administration and blood sampling, considerable attention must be given to this factor when attempting to compare and reconcile these apparently conflicting data.

The overall rate of clearance of ampicillin from the blood of pregnant women is slower than that occurring in nonpregnant females and detectable levels of ampicillin persist from 1 to 2 hours longer in pregnant subjects. Unfortunately, statistical analyses confirming the significance of these observations are lacking. This potentially important pharmacokinetic distinction has been attributed to the accumulation of drug in the amniotic fluid compartment which then functions as a slowly equilibrating reservoir and source of ampicillin. The concentration of ampicillin in amniotic fluid increases slowly and levels ranging from 0.25 to 6.00 μg/ml have been reported after administering either 250 or 500 mg ampicillin doses to pregnant women.

Ampicillin injected directly into the amniotic fluid is not rapidly cleared from the fetal environment. Maternal serum levels determined 90 minutes after an intra-amniotic instillation were very low, in contrast to fetal serum levels which were extremely high 6 hours later at parturition. It should be noted that equilibration of fetal and maternal serum concentrations of ampicillin has been reported to occur 1 hour after maternal administration (MacAulay et al., 1966).

b. *Penicillin G.* Doses of penicillin G administered parenterally to women at term, rapidly cross the placenta to establish therapeutic concentrations in fetal fluids (Woltz and Zintel, 1945; Charles, 1954). As mentioned previously, these early studies were generally based on single point determinations of cord and maternal blood specimens.

Recently, Kauffman et al. (1973) have observed that penicillin G traverses the goat placenta very slowly despite the maintenance of steady-state blood levels by constant infusion of the drug into the maternal circulation. At equilibrium, the ratio of fetal-to-maternal serum concentrations was 0.11. Injecting the drug directly into the fetal circulation caused a gradual increase in maternal serum levels; however, the maternal:fetal ratio ranged from 0.003 to 0.0006, at peak maternal and fetal concentrations. Infusions of penicillin into the fetus resulted in extremely high fetal blood levels and were associated with fetal death in nearly all experiments. These data illustrate that penicillin G diffuses through the goat placenta poorly in either direction in sharp contrast to the human. It is significant that penicillin G has been utilized extensively in pregnant women and no apparent adverse effects in the fetus have been reported (Adamsons and Joelsson, 1966).

c. Penicillinase-Resistant Penicillins. Methicillin crosses the placenta rapidly and equilibrium between the maternal and fetal circulations is established about 1 hour after administration. Clearance rates of this drug from both the maternal and fetal circulations appear to be similar (Depp *et al.*, 1970). Methicillin is initially detected in amniotic fluid 2 hours after a single maternal dose of 500 mg, reaching peak levels (5 μg/ml) about 6 hours later.

Dicloxacillin, which is highly protein bound (greater than 95%), appears to be limited primarily to the maternal circulation and only minute amounts are transferred to the fetus (MacAulay *et al.*, 1968). The amniotic fluid levels of this antibiotic are very low and the concentration gradient between maternal and fetal circulations extremely high. For all practical purposes therefore, equilibration between the fetus and mother does not occur under routine therapeutic conditions (Depp *et al.*, 1970). Thus, it would appear that methicillin constitutes a better choice of antibiotic than dicloxacillin when treatment for an intrauterine staphylococcal infection is indicated.

2. CEPHALOSPORINS

a. Cephalothin. This antibiotic can be assayed in amniotic fluid within 15 minutes of an intravenous injection to the mother. It is also transferred in the reverse direction (fetal to maternal) with the same apparent ease (Paterson *et al.*, 1970).

Despite the facility with which cephalothin moves across the placental membranes, umbilical cord blood concentrations of the antibiotic seem to be consistently lower than corresponding maternal blood levels and equilibrium occurs rather slowly (Morrow *et al.*, 1968). The rate constant for elimination (K_{el}) of cephalothin from the maternal–placental–fetal circulation has been estimated to be 0.0198 for the mother and 0.0111 for the fetus so that its clearance is substantially more rapid from the maternal circulation than the fetal. No adverse effects upon the fetus have been reported following the maternal administration of cephalothin (Youkilis, 1970).

Recent studies by Cooper *et al.* (1973) and Anders *et al.* (1974) suggest that the half-life of cephalothin is about 15 to 20 minutes in both children and adults. Approximately 20% of the antibiotic undergoes metabolism to form a more polar compound, deacetylcephalothin which is also an active antibiotic. Further investigation of this compound in the maternal-placental–fetal unit seems desirable to determine whether deacetylcephalothin enters the fetal circulation after maternal biotransformation of cephalothin and if the fetus has the capacity to metabolize cephalothin.

b. Cephaloridine. Therapeutic levels of cephaloridine are rapidly established in fetal sera due to the ease with which it crosses the placenta. The antibiotic is present in amniotic fluid 3 hours after a maternal dose and the concentration of drug in this compartment appears to increase over a period of several hours (Barr and Graham, 1967).

The rate of decline of serum cephaloridine levels in the fetus is less than that observed in the mother. The drug persists for almost 22 hours in fetal blood, whereas, maternal levels are very low 6 hours after a dose (Arthur and Burland, 1969). When cephaloridine was injected intramuscularly (1 gm every 12 hours), therapeutically effective, bactericidal concentrations were present in 76% of the cord sera tested; a twofold increment in the dose administered increased this to 90% of the cord sera studied (Barr and Graham, 1967).

3. ERYTHROMYCIN

This molecule is poorly transferred across the placenta. Erythromycin cannot be detected in fetal serum following the administration of single doses (200–800 mg) to the mother. Low levels of the antibiotic were detectable in 8 out of 12 fetal blood specimens obtained from subjects whose mothers had received repetitive doses of erythromycin (Kieffer *et al.*, 1955).

The placental transfer of erythromycin has been evaluated in humans prior to therapeutic abortion. The respective fetal and maternal blood concentrations of erythromycin were 0.02 (0–0.11) μg/ml and 2.55 (0.38–7.2) μg/ml after a single 500-mg oral dose. Antibacterial activity could not be demonstrated in any of the fetal tissues investigated. In subjects receiving multiple doses of the drug, fetal blood concentrations were still extremely low and averaged 0.06 (0–0.12) μg/ml in contrast to maternal concentrations of 4.94 (0.66–8.0) μg/ml. A major distinction between the single and multiple dosing regimens was the establishment of effective antibacterial drug levels in fetal tissues after the latter (Philipson *et al.*, 1973).

4. AMINOGLYCOSIDES

a. Kanamycin. The transplacental passage of kanamycin is quite rapid, and it has been assayed in umbilical cord sera 15 minutes after administration to pregnant women. Maternal blood levels (18.6 μg/ml) were highest 60 minutes following a maternal dose of kanamycin (500 mg intramuscularly) whereas peak umbilical cord levels (0 μg/ml) were established approximately 1 hour and 45 minutes thereafter (Good and Johnson, 1971).

b. Gentamicin. While this antibiotic traverses the placenta with no apparent difficulty, fetal serum concentrations lag behind maternal gentamicin serum levels by about 30 to 60 minutes. The ratio of peak umbilical to maternal serum levels of gentamicin is 0.34 after administering single parenteral doses. Equilibrium appears to be established some 3 to 6 hours later (Yoshioka *et al.*, 1972).

It is of interest that the placental transfer of gentamicin in pregnant goats is considerably slower than in pregnant women and that no drug can be demonstrated in fetal serum even after steady-state maternal blood levels have been established (Kauffman *et al.*, 1975).

c. Streptomycin. (See Antitubercular Drugs)

5. COLISTIMETHATE

This polypeptide antibiotic has a molecular weight of 1200 which might be expected to significantly retard its transfer across the placenta into the fetal circulation. Initial concentrations are low in fetal blood, and maternal–fetal equilibrium is established about 6 hours after maternal administration (MacAulay and Charles, 1967). The elimination of colistimethate from amniotic fluid is extremely slow and 20 to 30% of a dose injected into the amniotic sac can be detected in this compartment 18 to 20 hours later.

6. NITROFURANTOIN

Maternal infusions of nitrofurantoin (90 mg per 30-minute period) produced maternal serum levels ranging from 2.8 to 9.8 μg/ml in specimens obtained 1–5 minutes after completing the infusion. The drug concentration in cord serum did not exceed 2.5 μg/ml during this time period and was not detectable in specimens taken 1 hour after administration. The apparent half-life of disappearance in the mother was 32 ± 16 minutes but marked variations have been reported between subjects (Perry *et al.*, 1967; Perry and Le Blanc, 1967). Very little if any nitrofurantoin could be assayed in the amniotic fluid of these subjects, and these data parallel studies performed in the pregnant guinea pig (Buzard and Conklin, 1964).

7. Chloramphenicol

A single maternal dose (2 gm) of chloramphenicol produces bactericidal levels of antibiotic in cord blood in approximately 70 minutes (Scott and Warner, 1950). Fetal blood levels are approximately 25% of corresponding maternal concentrations but Charles (1954) was unable to find any drug in amniotic fluid after administering single doses of chloramphenicol (500 mg) to mothers.

Despite the well-described "gray syndrome" which may be produced by excessive amounts of chloramphenicol in young infants, virtually no untoward effects have been reported in the fetus following administration of this drug to the mother. This may be due to the fact that on a weight basis, the doses employed in treatment of the adult are rather small compared to those which have been utilized in the neonatal age group (Adamsons and Joelsson, 1966). In addition, the clearance of chloramphenicol from the fetus via the placenta may prevent excessive accumulation of the drug in fetal tissues.

8. Tetracyclines

The placental transfer of most tetracyclines and their derivatives (chlor-, oxy-, demethylchlor-) has been demonstrated in the human (Penman *et al.*, 1953; Monfort *et al.*, 1963; Gibbon and Reichelderfer, 1960). Tetracycline appears in cord blood about 10 minutes after its intravenous administration. Peak serum levels are attained by $1\frac{1}{2}$ hours with equilibrium between maternal and cord sera noted 4 to 8 hours thereafter. The antibiotic concentrations achieved in cord sera are only 60% of the maternal level. Tetracycline has been detected in amniotic fluid 18 minutes after maternal dosing and peak levels averaged about 20% of the maternal blood concentration (Le Blanc and Perry, 1967).

Every tetracycline antibiotic which has been investigated possesses an extremely high affinity for the skeletal structures of the developing fetus and neonate. These antibiotics, which fluoresce in ultraviolet light, are incorporated in a virtually irreversible manner into the matrix of osseous tissue to produce important cosmetic and developmental abnormalities. The major side effects of administering tetracyclines in the last trimester of pregnancy or during early childhood include tooth discoloration, enamel hypoplasia, and a tendency toward dental caries (Toaff and David, 1968).

In the pregnant rat, tetracycline (40 mg/kg/day) administered between the tenth and fifteenth days of gestation produced a 28% reduction in the anticipated size of each fetus. A similar phenomenon has been observed in a group of premature infants who manifest a 40% reduction in the length of their long bones after receiving this drug. The inhibition of skeletal growth appears to be reversible if the tetracycline has only been administered for a short term (Cohlan et al., 1963).

9. Sulfonamides

Most of the commonly used sulfonamides are readily transferred across the placenta. Equilibrium between maternal and fetal circulations has been reported to occur within 3 hours, with fetal levels remaining about 10 to 30% lower than corresponding maternal blood concentrations. Most of the studies in humans suggest that sulfadiazine develops the highest fetal blood concentration, though sulfanilamide appears in the umbilical circulation most rapidly (Pomerance and Yaffe, 1973).

The placental transfer rates and fetal distribution patterns of a large series of sulfonamides have been exhaustively studied in the pregnant rat (Oh, 1973; Mirkin, 1974b). A group of sulfonamide derivatives selected on the basis of differences in lipid solubility, pK_a, protein binding, and molecular weight have been shown to possess distinct pharmacokinetic and tissue distribution characteristics (Fig. 4). Some of these compounds, particularly the sulfanilylbenzamide derivatives, were barely detectable in fetal tissues after maternal administration and crossed the placenta very poorly whereas sulfapyridine and sulfanilamide achieved rather high concentrations in fetal tissues (Fig. 5).

There are virtually no documented reports which clearly describe, in a cause and effect manner, any adverse or deleterious actions of sulfonamides upon fetal development. Statistically, this seems rather unusual since there appear to be various biochemical and physiological processes in the fetus which are more vulnerable than in the adult. The fetal erythrocyte is deficient in glucose-6-dehydrogenase and glutathione so that hemolysis induced by sulfonamides might occur more readily in the fetal than adult red blood cell. Similarly, the well-known capacity of sulfonamides to produce hyperbilirubinemia in neonates receiving these drugs does not seem to be a major problem in the fetus. While sulfonamides

Name	Molecular structure	MW	pK_a	%un-ionized at pH 7.4	log P (Octanol)	Effective[*] log P
1. Sulfanilic acid	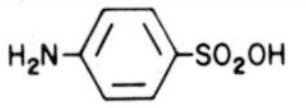	173.84	3.19	0.00616	2.384	0.0146
2. Sulfanilyl benzamide	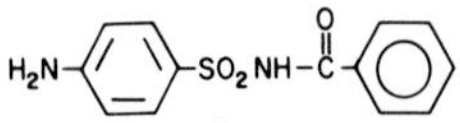	276.31	4.57	0.148	1.254	0.185
3. Sulfaethidole	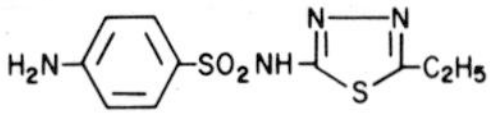	284.3	5.4	0.990	1.2273	1.215
4. Sulfisoxazole	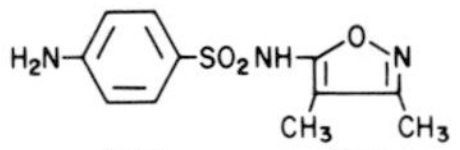	276.3	5.8	2.45	1.10	2.69
5. Sulfadiazine	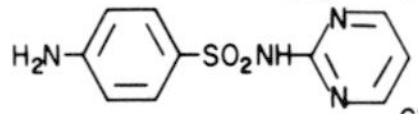	250.3	6.48	10.7	-0.08	-0.856
6. Sulfamerazine	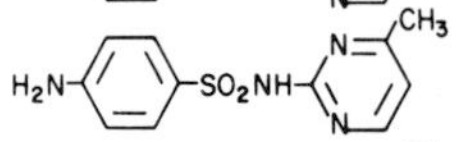	264.3	7.06	31.4	0.14	4.396
7. Sulfamethazine	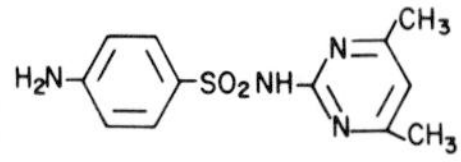	278.3	7.37	48.3	0.27	13.04
8. Sulfapyridine	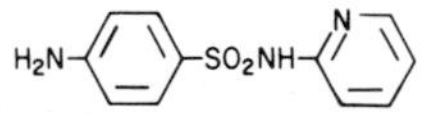	249.29	8.43	91.5	0.00	0.000
9. Sulfanilamide	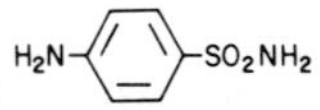	172.21	10.43	99.9	-0.72	-71.93

*Effective log P = (% un-ionized at pH 7.4) x log P (Oct/H₂O)

FIG. 4. Physicochemical properties of selected sulfonamide drugs. These compounds were used to investigate the relationship between pK_a, partition coefficient (log P or effective log P), and placental drug transfer. (Adapted from Oh, 1973.)

can compete with bilirubin for albumin-binding sites in the fetal circulation, increases in unconjugated bilirubin rarely reach hazardous levels, probably because this compound is cleared by the placenta into the maternal circulation.

10. ANTITUBERCULAR DRUGS

a. Streptomycin. The presence of streptomycin in amniotic fluid and umbilical cord blood has been demonstrated within 20 minutes of an intravenous administration (Woltz and Wiley, 1945). Streptomycin concentrations in these biological fluids are approximately 50% of comparable maternal levels (Heilman *et al.*, 1945; Charles, 1954).

Throughout the early stages of pregnancy, maternal and fetal cerebrospinal fluid concentrations of streptomycin are similar despite marked differences in their respective blood levels. However, during the last

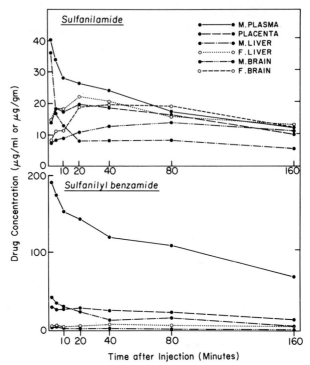

Fᴵɢ. 5. Pharmacokinetics and tissue distribution of sulfanilamide (top) and sulfanilylbenzamide (bottom) in the maternal–placental–fetal unit of the pregnant rat (21 days gestation). Each drug was administered to the maternal rat in a dose of 25 mg/kg i.v. (Adapted from Oh, 1973.)

month of gestation neither streptomycin nor dihydrostreptomycin enters the fetal cerebrospinal fluid to any appreciable extent. In view of the enhanced susceptibility of developing neural structures to streptomycin, maternal treatment with this antibiotic or other related aminoglycosides may result in vestibular or cochlear damage to the fetus. In this regard, it is worth noting that the incidence of deafness in the neonates of individuals so treated appears to be quite low (Adamsons and Joelsson, 1966; Vapela et al., 1969; Rasmussen, 1969). The abnormalities in hearing which have been described are usually minor with no noticeable influence upon those frequencies commonly associated with human speech (Conway and Birt, 1965).

b. Isoniazid. A single, 100-mg dose of isoniazid taken orally has been shown to produce umbilical vein concentrations ranging from 0 to 6.6 μg/ml and maternal blood levels of 0 to 10 μg/ml 4 hours after ingestion.

In 7 of 19 cases investigated by Bromberg *et al.* (1955) the concentration of isoniazid in cord blood was higher than in maternal blood samples obtained at the same time period. Encephalopathy occurring in some infants born to mothers who have received isoniazid has been attributed to this drug, though a direct cause and effect relationship has not yet been established (Pomerance and Yaffe, 1973).

c. Rifampin.   Therapeutic concentrations of rifampin are established in fetal blood and amniotic fluid following its oral administration to the mother. Initially, fetal blood levels are lower than corresponding maternal values but the rate of elimination of this drug from the fetus is slower than from the mother and accumulation may occur during chronic therapy. In some clinical situations a fetal-to-maternal blood concentration ratio of 3:1 has been reported following prolonged courses of therapy (Termine and Santuari, 1968).

B. Drugs Acting on the Central and Autonomic Nervous Systems

1. ANTICONVULSANT AGENTS

a. Diphenylhydantoin (DPH).   The rapid placental transfer of DPH has been demonstrated in the maternal–placental–fetal unit of the rodent (Mirkin, 1971; Harbison and Becker, 1971; Waddell and Mirkin, 1972), goat (Shoeman *et al.*, 1972), and human (Mirkin, 1971). Total body radioautography was utilized by Waddell and Mirkin (1972) to determine the distribution of ^{14}C-DPH in the maternal and fetal tissues of the mouse. Individual tissues were analyzed by thin-layer radiochromatographic techniques which provided semiquantitative data on ^{14}C-DPH and its metabolites in each specimen studied. ^{14}C-DPH was present in the fetal myocardium, liver, intestines, adrenal gland, and yolk sac 6-minutes after injecting the drug (i.v.) into the pregnant mouse. The highest concentrations of ^{14}C-DPH were found in maternal liver, heart, adrenal cortex, ovary (copora lutea), and kidneys in each of the time periods studies. The predominant isotope in these specimens was ^{14}C-DPH (95–99%) with minor quantities of ^{14}C-parahydroxydiphenyl-hydantoin (1–5%) also present.

Pharmacokinetic studies of DPH in the pregnant rat have suggested that body distribution patterns and kinetic parameters are similar in both the mother and fetus. The following tissue distribution pattern was observed 1 hour after administering DPH (25 mg/kg i.v.) to the mother (highest to lowest concentration): maternal liver, maternal and fetal heart, placenta, fetal liver, maternal and fetal brain, and maternal plasma (Fig. 6). The fetal clearance of DPH following a single maternal

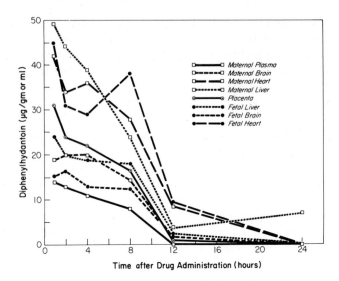

Fig. 6. Pharmacokinetics and tissue distribution of diphenylhydantoin in the maternal–placental–fetal unit of the pregnant rat (20 days gestation). The drug was administered to the maternal rat in a dose of 25 mg/kg i.p. (Adapted from Mirkin, 1974b, with permission of Yearbook Pub., Chicago.)

dose paralleled that of the mother with no evidence of any fetal accumulation or lag in elimination.

An extremely interesting effect of phenobarbital and SKF-525A, an inducer and inhibitor, respectively, of hepatic microsomal enzymes, on the disposition of DPH in pregnant mice has been reported by Harbison and Becker (1971). They demonstrated that pretreatment with phenobarbital enhanced, whereas SKF-525A retarded, the metabolism of DPH and its rate of disappearance from the plasma of both the mother and fetus. These data also indicated that DPH was present in the fetus primarily in its unmetabolized form, confirming the report of Waddell and Mirkin (1972).

The use of DPH for the control of convulsive disorders in pregnant women was initially described by Bergman (1942). Despite its widespread clinical use, identification of DPH (or metabolites) in the blood of infants delivered from women receiving the drug during gestation was not reported until quite recently (Baughman and Randinitis, 1970; Mirkin, 1971; Rane et al., 1973). These investigations clearly established that maternal plasma levels of DPH were equivalent to fetal umbilical cord levels when the drug had been chronically administered during gestation. The maternal venous plasma levels in a study involving eight subjects averaged 3.6 ± 0.7 μg/ml and the umbilical vein 3.4 ± 0.6 μg/ml when anticonvulsant therapy had been maintained throughout pregnancy. A marked maternal-to-fetal concentration gradient was observed in blood specimens obtained $\frac{1}{2}$ hour after administering the drug to the mother. The distribution of DPH in the aborted human fetus following a single maternal injection at hysterotomy was similar to the rat with the highest concentrations localized in the fetal liver, heart, and adrenal gland (Mirkin, 1971).

One of the major concerns regarding the use of anticonvulsant drugs in pregnant women is whether these agents increase the incidence of congenital anomalies in the offspring of such individuals. This possibility was suggested by Meadow (1968) who observed severe cleft lip and palate, congenital heart lesions, minor skeletal abnormalities, and unusual facies in the children of mothers who had received anticonvulsant agents such as DPH, phenobarbital, and primidone during pregnancy. In a follow-up study, Meadow (1970) summarized responses to a questionnaire sent to epileptic mothers in which he was able to identify 32 instances of cleft lip and/or palate in their offspring. Significantly, DPH had been taken by 29 of the subjects, either alone or in combination with other agents, during the initial trimester of pregnancy.

Hill et al. (1973, 1974) have proposed that infants born to mothers receiving anticonvulsant agents during pregnancy may exhibit a clustering of physical findings which makes them an identifiable population or syndrome among neonates. Their study contrasted 28 newly born infants, exposed to different anticonvulsant drugs in utero, with a cohort of 165 infants not exposed to these agents. The syndrome includes both major and minor anomalies such as cleft lip and/or palate (3.8%), malformations of the skeleton (1.9%), the heart (1.7%), and central nervous system (1.3%).

Retrospective epidemiologic investigations have been carried out by Monson et al. (1973) who analyzed a cohort of 50,000 pregnancies. The highest malformation rate (61 per 1000) was observed in 98 children exposed to DPH during the early months of pregnancy. The rate was lowest in children born to nonepileptic mothers who either did not receive any drug(s) during the early trimesters or were exposed to drug(s) in a somewhat sporadic manner. The incidence of malformations in children of drug-treated epileptic mothers when compared with those of epileptic mothers receiving no DPH during gestation was not significantly different. Consequently, it was concluded that the increased incidence of malformations in the children delivered from epilpeptic mothers receiving DPH during gestation reflected an impact of both the drug and possibly the disease itself.

The teratogenic action of DPH has been vividly demonstrated in mice where the drug must be administered on days 10–15 of gestation (equivalent to the first trimester) to produce a maximum effect (Harbison and Becker, 1969). The malformations observed were similar to those occurring in man consisting of cleft lip and palate, skeletal defects, long-bone shortening, and central nervous system lesions.

While it has not been possible at this time to establish a direct correlation between maternal anticonvulsant therapy and human teratogenesis, the Food and Drug Administration has recently concluded that a finite risk exists for children born to epileptic women receiving DPH. They suggest "that anticonvulsant medication should not be discontinued in pregnant epileptic women in whom the medication is necessary for the prevention of major seizures" but indicate that both the physician and patient should be fully informed regarding its potential hazards (Food and Drug Administration, 1974).

b. Diazepam. The transplacental passage of diazepam has been demonstrated in mice, hamsters, monkeys (*Cynomolgus iris*), and humans (Idänpään-Heikkilä *et al.*, 1971b). Diazepam levels (expressed as μCi ^{14}C-diazepam/100 ml) in paired maternal and fetal plasma specimens obtained from pregnant monkeys after the administration of ^{14}C-diazepam (i.v.) to the mother were as follows: $\frac{1}{2}$ hour postinjection (maternal 6.8; fetal 6.9); 2 hours postinjection (maternal 4.0; fetal 4.2) and 24 hours postinjection (maternal 1.2; fetal 1.5). Equilibrium between the fetal and maternal circulations was established 30 minutes after drug administration. The elimination rates of diazepam from both maternal and fetal plasma were similar; however, the compounds and its metabolite(s) were retained in the cerebellum, spinal cord, and spinal nerves of the fetal monkey for periods up to 24 hours later.

The placental transfer and fetal localization of diazepam in the human seem to differ in several respects from that observed in the subhuman primate. Maternal administration of ^{14}C-diazepam early in pregnancy (12–16 weeks gestation) produced higher drug concentrations in umbilical cord plasma than in maternal plasma after equilibrium had been attained. In these studies, postinjection levels of ^{14}C-diazepam in umbilical cord plasma (expressed as ng/ml) were 47.5, 49.0, and 19.0 at 1, 2, and 6 hours, respectively; maternal plasma concentrations were 25.6, 18.0, and 11.3 in corresponding samples (Cavanagh and Condo, 1964; DeSilva *et al.*, 1964; Shannon *et al.*, 1972; Cree *et al.*, 1973).

Fetal tissue levels peak 1 hour after a maternal dose of diazepam. The highest drug concentrations have been found in the fetal gastrointestinal tract, liver, and brain. Diazepam is cleared quite slowly from fetal brain in contrast to other fetal tissues which eliminate the drug more rapidly.

Diazepam localized in the fetal central nervous system does not rapidly equilibrate with other fetal compartments. Drug disposition studies in the maternal–placental–fetal unit based exclusively upon blood level data may not accurately reflect total body pharmacokinetics or drug distribution patterns in the fetus.

The human fetus cannot metabolize diazepam to any appreciable extent. Premature and term infants also exhibit a decreased capacity for biotransforming diazepam when compared with children and adults (Morselli et al., 1973). Despite the inability of the fetus to N-demethylate and conjugate diazepam, administration of this compound to pregnant ewes in doses of 0.1–0.5 mg/kg did not cause any significant alterations in either maternal or fetal hemodynamics; larger amounts produced a slight fall in blood pressure. Injection of diazepam directly into the umbilical vein of the pregnant ewe, in doses of 0.5–8.0 mg/kg, likewise exerted a negligible effect upon fetal cardiovascular function and tissue oxygenation (Mofid et al., 1973).

Diazepam has been used extensively in combination with meperidine and appears to reduce the quantity of the latter analgesic required for satisfactory obstetrical management (Flowers et al., 1969; Niswander, 1969). While few adverse effects of diazepam were reported during its early period of use, recent studies indicate that hypotonia, apneic spells, low Apgar scores, reluctance to feed, and impaired metabolic responses to cold can be observed in neonates born to mothers who have been given this drug (Shannon et al., 1972; Cree et al., 1973. A total maternal dose of diazepam which was 30 mg or less if administered within 15 hours of delivery exerted little or no influence upon the fetus. Doses exceeding this quantity were associated with some of the problems described above. Lethargy and impaired suckling have also been noted in the breast fed infants of mothers receiving diazepam (Patrick et al., 1972). Correlating with these clinical signs is the presence of diazepam and N-demethyldiazepam in maternal breast milk and the urine and blood of breast-feeding neonates (Erkolla and Kanto, 1972).

The hypotonia observed in some newborns exposed to diazepam during gestation may be related to the prolonged retention of this drug (and its metabolites) by the developing fetal nervous system. The persistence of active drug during extrauterine life is enhanced by the impaired metabolism of diazepam in the newborn infant. The half-life of diazepam is prolonged in the human neonate (Morselli et al., 1973) so that the parent compound and its active metabolites may persist for as long as 1 week after delivery (Cree et al., 1973). In the light of these observations it appears necessary to carefully observe all infants who have been exposed prenatally to high doses of diazepam and to exercise caution in the use of these drugs for obstetrical procedures.

2. BARBITURATES

All of the pharmacologically active derivatives of barbituric acid which have been investigated are able to cross the mammalian placenta with relative ease. As a consequence, equilibrium between the maternal and fetal circulations is often established within minutes (Crawford, 1956; Flowers, 1959; Root et al., 1961; Fehr and Mirkin, 1975).

The pharmacokinetics of barbiturates in the maternal–placental–fetal unit is significantly influenced by the specific physicochemical properties of each agent. This class of compounds generally have rather low molecular weights, are weak acids, and exist to a large extent in their un-ionized state at physiological pH, thereby enhancing their lipid solubility. Fehr and Mirkin (1975) demonstrated significant differences in the relative rates of diffusion of a homologous series of barbiturate acid derivatives. Pentobarbital (pK_a: 8.02) crossed the placenta more rapidly than amobarbital (pK_a: 7.78) even though they have similar partition coefficients. In contrast, amobarbital which is more lipid soluble than butethal diffuses across the placenta at a more rapid rate despite both compounds having similar pK_a values (Fig. 7; Table VI). Carrier et al. (1969) found a larger fraction of sodium barbital (partition coefficient: 0.072; log P^*: 0.65) in the amniotic fluid of pregnant dogs than of the more lipid-soluble pentobarbital (partition coefficient: 3.4; log P: 1.95). This difference was attributed to the smaller volume of distribution of sodium barbital in the fetus relative to pentobarbital. A larger fraction of the more water-soluble drug (sodium barbital) is thus available for rapid elimination via the fetal kidney into the amniotic fluid compartment.

* See footnote p. 11.

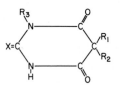

Compound	pK_a	log P	R_2 Side Chain	R_2 Side Chain Structure
Barbital	7.75	0.65	ethyl	CH_2-CH_3
Probarbital	7.90	0.95	isopropyl	$CH-CH_3$ / CH_3
Butabarbital	—	1.45	sec-butyl	$CH-CH_2-CH_3$ / CH_3
Pentobarbital	8.02	1.95	1-methyl-butyl	$CH-CH_2-CH_2-CH_3$ / CH_3
Amobarbital	7.78	1.95	isopentyl	$CH_2-CH_2-CH_2-CH_3$ / CH_3
Butethal	7.76	1.65	butyl	$CH_2-CH_2-CH_2-CH_3$

$R_1 = CH_2\,CH_3$
$R_3 = H$
$X = Oxygen$

FIG. 7. Physicochemical properties of selected barbituric acid derivatives. (Adapted from Fehr and Mirkin, 1975.)

TABLE VI   Placental Permeability Constants for Pentobarbital, Amobarbital, and Butethal in the Ovine Maternal–Placental–Fetal Unit[a]

	Mean		±SEM[b]	P[c]
Pentobarbital	0.01950	±	0.00119	0.05
Amobarbital	0.1522	±	0.00116	0.05
Butethal	0.01100	±	0.00115	0.05

[a] Adapted from Fehr and Mirkin, 1975.

[b] Data derived from steady-state infusion experiments carried out for each drug. The permeability constant represents the mean ± standard error of mean derived from 12 individual experimental observations.

[c] P represents placental permeability constant derived from the following equation:

$$P = \frac{1}{t} \ln \frac{C_m - C_f}{C_m}$$

where t = time of observation; $\ln$ = natural log; C_m = plasma concentration of drug in maternal femoral artery; C_f = plasma concentration of drug in umbilical vein. C_m and C_f corrected for protein binding.

a. *Thiobarbiturates.* While the thiobarbiturates are all highly lipid soluble and readily diffuse across the placenta, there is some delay in their passage from the maternal circulation to the fetal environment. Most of these compounds can be detected in the fetal circulation within a few minutes of their injection into the mother (McAllister and Flowers, 1956; Cassano *et al.*, 1967; Schechter and Roth, 1967). After administering a single pulse injection of any thiobarbiturate, the maternal blood level falls very rapidly as does the maternal–fetal concentration gradient. Equilibrium between the mother and fetus is established within minutes so that the total amount of drug transferred across the placenta is limited by these factors (Kosaka *et al.*, 1969). Barbituric acid derivatives such as phenobarbital which maintain elevated maternal blood levels over relatively prolonged periods generally achieve higher total concentrations in fetal tissues.

Studies in pregnant mice have shown that fetal tissue concentrations of thiopental peak 10 minutes after a maternal injection with most of the drug distributing to the fetal liver, brain, and lung. The levels in these tissues remain relatively constant over a 60-minute period with the exception of the brain, in which further accumulation appears to occur (Cassano *et al.*, 1967). Comparable observations have been made in the fetal liver of the pregnant guinea pig which accumulated two to four times more thiopental than did other fetal tissues (Finster et al., 1972).

In the human, the fetal liver also appears to take up a major proportion of any barbiturate entering the fetal circulation. The distribution pattern of thiopental in anencephalic fetuses following an intravenous dose to the mother is such that the highest concentrations are found in subcutaneous tissue, with intermediate amounts in the liver and lowest levels in the spinal cord. (See Section V, A, 2.)

b. *Oxybarbiturates.* Secobarbital moves across the human placenta very quickly, and an apparent equilibrium state between the maternal and fetal circulations is established within 4–5 minutes (Root et al., 1961). The ratio between mixed umbilical cord and maternal serum concentrations of secobarbital was less than 0.35 during the initial 2 minutes, increasing 3 minutes after maternal drug administration to 0.71. Significantly, the fetus rarely developed a blood level exceeding 20% of the initial maternal secobarbital concentration. There was virtually no correlation noted between the degree of neonatal depression, the time of drug administration and delivery, the extent of maternal sedation and the cord blood level of secobarbital.

The placental transmission of pentobarbital in pregnant women has been documented by Fealy (1958). The average fetal blood level was 74% of the maternal concentration and persisted in that range for at least 185 minutes after injection. Maternal:fetal plasma concentration ratios of pentobarbital in the pregnant dog reach equilibrium 15 minutes after intravenous administration. The rates of elimination of pentobarbital from the fetal and maternal circulations are similar and the compound can be detected in amniotic fluid as early as 10 minutes after injection (Carrier et al., 1969).

Dille (1956) initially demonstrated the presence of amobarbital in cord blood 15 minutes after injection into pregnant women. Umbilical cord and maternal plasma levels of amobarbital were subsequently shown to be similar in subjects delivered at varying times after maternal drug administration (Krauer et al., 1974). The average plasma half-life of this drug in the newborn infant was 38.9 ± 4.8 hours or two and one-half times greater than that of their mothers which was 15.8 ± 1.71 hours. Amobarbital is eliminated primarily by renal excretion after conversion to hydroxyamobarbital, and this metabolite can be found in the blood of mothers and infants. It is of interest that the plasma concentration of hydroxyamobarbital increases in neonates, 12 to 24 hours after delivery from mothers receiving amobarbital at parturition. This may be due to an impaired clearance of the hydroxy compound by the neonate.

Fehr and Mirkin (1975) have demonstrated that equilibrium between the maternal and fetal circulations of the pregnant sheep is established 20 minutes after giving an intravenous injection of amobarbital to the ewe. Fetal plasma concentrations were only 50 to 60% of corresponding maternal levels under experimental conditions in which steady-state maternal blood levels were maintained by constant infusions of drug.

c. Long-Acting Barbiturates. Infants delivered from epileptic mothers administered phenobarbital or primidone during pregnancy have umbilical cord blood levels of phenobarbital which are similar to maternal values (Melchior *et al.*, 1967). Studies in mice suggest that the transplacental passage of ^{14}C-phenobarbital is rather slow relative to other barbiturates. Utilizing radioautographic techniques, Cassano *et al.* (1967) have demonstrated an accumulation of ^{14}C-phenobarbital in the placenta and amnion following its administration to the pregnant dam. The concentration in fetal blood was very low 5 minutes after injection and remained significantly less than the maternal level during the course of the experiment. Fetal tissues reached their peak concentrations approximately 60 minutes later with the highest levels observed in the liver and brain. A similar distribution pattern has been noted in the human fetus (Ploman and Persson, 1957).

Sodium barbital moves across the placenta quickly so that maternal and fetal blood levels approximate one another within 2–5 minutes after injection (Flowers, 1957; Carrier *et al.*, 1969). When administered to mothers undergoing therapeutic abortion early in pregnancy, large amounts of the drug accumulated in the fetal brain. The highest concentrations were noted in the upper brain stem with lesser amounts in the cerebral cortex and the lowest levels observed in the fetal liver (Persson, 1961).

The effects of maternally administered barbiturates upon the neonate include hypotonia (Melchior *et al.*, 1967), diminished responsiveness (Brazelton, 1970), and a significantly lower rate and pressure of sucking (Kron *et al.*, 1966). A barbiturate withdrawal syndrome has been described in the neonate with signs closely resembling those observed during narcotic abstinence (Bleyer and Marshall, 1972; Desmond *et al.*, 1972). In one study of 15 infants who exhibited behavior patterns consistent with barbiturate withdrawal, a majority of the subjects had normal birth weights and satisfactory 1-minute Apgar scores. The most common acute clinical manifestation of the syndrome were hyperactivity, restlessness, disturbed sleep, excessive crying, tremors, hyperreflexia, and hypertonia. This phase may be followed by a subacute component lasting several months which is characterized by hyperphagia, periods of prolonged crying, episodic irritability, hyperacusis, and sweating. In general, the onset of these symptoms occurred later than those observed in a control group of infants delivered from mothers who were addicted to narcotics.

3. ETHANOL

The placental transfer of ethanol has been investigated in pregnant women receiving the drug prior to delivery (Idanpään-Heikkilä *et al.*, 1972). The mean concentration of ethanol in maternal and umbilical cord blood samples obtained 30 minutes after start of an infusion were 0.58 ± 0.08 and 0.36 ± 0.07 mg/ml, respectively. A gradient between maternal and fetal blood levels was not discernable 60 minutes after termination of the infusion and at parturition ethanol concentrations were identical in both circulations.

In contrast to the disposition of ethanol in the maternal–placental–fetal unit, the rate at which ethanol is removed from the neonate is substantially lower than that of the mother. The mean elimination rate of ethanol in newborns (up to 4 hours old) was 0.077 mg/ml/hour compared to 0.14 mg/ml/hour in the mother. The blood levels of ethanol in the neonate and the mother reflect this difference in clearance; 8 hours postpartum the maternal concentration was 0.06 ± 0.02 mg/ml and the fetal, 0.11 ± 0.03 mg/ml. A diminished rate of elimination of ethanol has also been observed in fetal monkeys and hamsters (Idanpään-Heikkilä *et al.*, 1971). The biochemical basis for this distinction between mature and immature organisms probably can be attributed to the reduced activity of alcohol dehydrogenase in fetal liver (Pikkarainen and Räihä, 1967).

It has been suggested that ethanol administration during gestation may cause a wide variety of adverse effects in both the mother and neonate. Since this agent has been widely used to inhibit uterine motility in human obstetrical practice, some of the more significant and potentially toxic actions of the compound are presented below:

(a) Severe central nervous system depression and transient muscular hypotonia has been observed in the neonates delivered from mothers receiving ethanol during the parapartum period (Pomerance and Yaffe, 1973). Blood glucose concentrations, insulin levels, or respiration are usually not affected.

(b) Ethanol is a potent inducer of specific hepatic microsomal enzymes. Chronic exposure to this compound could potentially create a degree of tolerance to therapeutic agents administered to the mother and fetus. Acute alcoholic intoxication, on the other hand, can significantly depress drug metabolism so that such individuals may experience a greater response to a given dose of drug than would normally be anticipated.

The reduction of serum bilirubin levels in neonates chronically exposed to alcohol is probably due to enzyme induction. The serum bilirubin concentrations on the third, fourth, and fifth days of life in this group of subjects were significantly lower than those of an untreated control group (Waltman et al., 1969).

(c) An association between maternal alcoholism, intrauterine growth retardation, and a syndrome of congenital malformations characterized by growth, mental retardation, and craniofacial, limb, and cardiac anomalies has been suggested by Jones et al. (1973).

4. ANALGESICS

a. Narcotic Agents. The placental transfer of narcotics from the mother to the fetus has been well described in the pediatric literature and is based primarily on detailed clinical observations (Shute and Davis, 1933; Eckenhoff et al., (1953). Changes in the rate and rhythm of the fetal heart, pinpoint pupils, addiction of the fetus in utero, withdrawal symptoms in infants born to addicted mothers, as well as respiratory depression at birth, have all been substantively documented (Goodfriend et al., 1956; Steg, 1957; Reddy et al., 1971; Zelson et al., 1973).

Despite the plethora of qualitative data describing the placental passage of narcotic agents, quantitative information in the human is remarkably scanty. Fetal distribution has been studied primarily in subhuman species, though the presence of narcotic drugs in biological fluids obtained from the human fetus has been reported (Way et al., 1949; Apgar et al., 1952; Crawford and Rudofsky, 1965; Jenkins et al., 1972; Moore et al., 1973).

i. Morphine. Sanner and Woods (1965) demonstrated that ^{3}H-dihydromorphine rapidly traverses the rat placenta when the drug is injected into the maternal circulation. Equilibrium between maternal and fetal plasma ^{3}H-dihydromorphine concentrations was established 2 hours after administration. At this time, maternal plasma levels were approximately two and one-half times greater than those of corresponding fetal plasma samples. Despite the much lower drug levels observed in fetal plasma, the ^{3}H-dihydromorphine content (μg/gm) of fetal brain was approximately three times that of maternal brain. Conjugated ^{3}H-dihydromorphine could not be detected in maternal brain during the entire 16-hour period of observation. However, low concentrations of the conjugate were present in fetal brain 2 hours after injection. These data strongly suggest that the fetal distribution of ³H-dihydromorphine and its major metabolite(s) differs significantly from that of the adult.

The partitioning of ³H-dihydromorphine between the mother and the fetus also seems to be influenced by prior exposure of the mother to the drug and whether or not tolerance has been established (Yeh and Wood, 1970). The tolerant animal differs from the nontolerant one in the following ways: the rate of removal of ³H-dihydromorphine from its site of injection is more rapid, the maternal plasma levels lower, the apparent rate of transfer of drug across the placenta faster and the fetal plasma and brain ³H-dihydromorphine levels higher than in the nontolerant animal.

Inturrusi *et al.* (1973) have shown that methadone crosses the human placenta and the compound has been identified in amniotic fluid as early as the sixteenth week of gestation. In a group of addicted women, maternal plasma concentrations of methadone ranged between 0.005 and 0.48 $\mu g/ml$, umbilical cord plasma from 0.03 to 0.25 $\mu g/ml$, and amniotic fluid levels from 0.07 to 0.39 $\mu g/ml$. The umbilical cord:maternal plasma ratio was 0.73. These data confirmed that maternal plasma levels were generally higher than those established in fetal plasma or amniotic fluid. Infants delivered from addicted mothers excreted methadone in their urine for at least 3 days following birth.

ii. Meperidine.   Pharmacokinetic studies carried out in the pregnant ewe have shown that fetal blood levels of meperidine peak less than 10 minutes after an intravenous infusion. Serum levels in the fetus were generally higher than those assayed in corresponding maternal plasma specimens. There appears to be no lag phase in removal of the drug from the fetal circulation since the elimination curves from both the maternal and fetal circulations were parallel exponential functions (Jenkins *et al.*, 1972).

Meperidine has been extracted and qualitatively assayed in urine (Way *et al.*, 1949) and blood obtained from neonates following maternal administration of the drug (Apgar *et al.*, 1952). The kinetics of placental transfer in the human have been described by Crawford and Rudofsky (1965) who found meperidine in fetal blood 2 minutes after its intravenous administration to the mother. In contrast to the data of Jenkins *et al.* (1972) and Apgar *et al.* (1952), none of the fetal meperidine plasma concentrations reported in this study exceeded the corresponding maternal levels. The ratio of maternal-to-fetal plasma concentrations in the initial minutes after injection was 3:1, and this value approached unity as a function of time.

The amount of drug excreted by the neonate differs depending upon whether the mother has received the compound intravenously or intramuscularly. Following a 50-mg maternal dose of meperidine, the total urinary excretion of meperidine in a group of neonates averaged 151 μg when the drug was given intramuscularly and 431 μg when administered by the intravenous route. If these elimination data are valid, less than 1% of the meperidine administered intramuscularly appears to reach the fetus. These observations provide substantive support for the frequently cited "clinical rule" that adverse effects in the neonate, such as diminished respiratory minute volume and decreased oxygen saturation (Roberts and Kane, 1957), are observed when meperidine is given 2–3 hours prior to delivery, but not when administered within 1 hour of parturition by the intramuscular route (Colburn and Saltzman, 1960; Shnider and Moya, 1964).

iii. Pentazocine. The analgesic properties of pentazocine are equivalent to meperidine, and it has been proposed as an alternative agent for use in obstetrical anesthesia (Duncan *et al.*, 1969; Mowat and Garrey, 1970; Moore and Hunter, 1970). This agent crosses the placenta to a lesser degree than meperidine and the ratio of fetal-to-maternal blood concentrations is 0.6 (Beckett and Taylor, 1967; Moore *et al.*, 1973). In general, an analysis of concurrently obtained blood samples has shown fetal levels of pentazocine to be lower than maternal concentrations in all of the studies published to date. It is important to note, however, that the adverse effects of pentazocine, particularly respiratory depression, do not differ significantly from meperidine when the former compound is administered in equipotent doses (Mowat and Garrey, 1970; Moore *et al.*, 1973).

iv. Narcotic addiction in the newborn. The etiology of the withdrawal syndrome observed in the narcotic addicted neonate appears to differ somewhat from that occurring in older individuals. In the newborn infant alterations in basic metabolic and physiological processes probably exert a predominant influence with minimal psychological overlay; in the more mature addict, psychological factors constitute a major component of the withdrawal phenomenon.

Symptoms of withdrawal are manifest in 50–90% of infants delivered from mothers addicted to narcotic agents. The onset of symptoms in such infants may occur any time after birth but generally is not observed beyond 4 days of age (Stevenson, 1973; Zelson *et al.*, 1973). Occasionally, the initial symptoms have been observed in infants 2–4 weeks after delivery (Kandall and Gartner, 1974). The elapsed time between birth and the onset of abstinence symptoms depends upon several factors: size of the maternal dose, duration of maternal addiction, time of the last maternal dose prior to parturition, and sensitivity of the fetus to these agents (Zelson *et al.*, 1971).

The neonate delivered from addicted mothers is frequently "small for dates" and exhibits tremors, hypertonicity, irritability, vomiting, respiratory distress, and a high pitched cry. Skin abrasions over points of contact with bedding may result from constant movement of the infant. Neonatal seizures occur more frequently in these subjects than in the general population. In contrast to the above, the incidence of hyperbilirubinemia is quite low and hyaline membrane disease has not been described in infants delivered to heroin addicted mothers (Glass *et al.*, 1971) but has been seen in the offspring of methadone addicted mothers (Zelson *et al.*, 1973).

Withdrawal symptoms occur with equal frequency in the infants of mothers on methadone maintenance regimens. The signs of withdrawal are much more severe in these individuals than in those delivered from heroin addicted subjects. The prognosis for any newborn experiencing symptoms of narcotic withdrawal varies and mortality rates up to 90% have been reported in untreated cases (Stevenson, 1973). Treatment of infants with barbiturates, chlorpromazine, or diazepam has been associated with a mortality in the range of 4 to 10%. However, it is not clear whether the reduction in mortality is directly related to this therapy or to an overall improvement in neonatal care and anticipation of these problems.

A long-term follow-up of infants exhibiting withdrawal signs after delivery from addicted mothers has not been completed and preliminary studies are somewhat controversial at this time. Hill and Desmond (1963) suggested that the development of such infants was not abnormal. However, Wilson *et al.* (1973) described a series of 34 infants with withdrawal symptoms who were tested at delivery and in whom age-appropriate levels of development were present. Reevaluation of 14 of these subjects at 1 year of age revealed 64% of them to be abnormal. The major symptoms being disturbances in behavior, such as hyperactivity and short attention span.

b. Nonnarcotic Analgesics. Salicylates.   In 1948, Jackson documented the passage of salicylate across the placentas of rats and rabbits receiving different dosages of sodium salicylate. A dose of 1.0 gm/kg subcutaneously produced a maternal serum concentration of 0.58 mg/ml and a fetal level of 0.37 mg/ml, 2 hours after injection; a larger dose (1.5 gm/kg subcutaneously) increased maternal and fetal serum levels, to 0.75 and 0.45 mg/ml, respectively. The fetus did not exhibit any selective toxicity or enhanced susceptibility to salicylate until doses lethal to the mother were utilized.

Palmisano and Cassidy (1969) assayed the salicylate content in umbilical cord sera obtained from 272 consecutive deliveries. Measurable drug levels were present in 26 samples (10%) and averaged 33 $\mu g/ml$ (range 12–109 $\mu g/ml$). While no adverse effects were noted in these infants, the mean albumin binding capacity of the salicylate exposed group differed significantly from the control group even though the total serum protein concentration of each group was similar.

Levy and Garrettson (1974) recently investigated the metabolic fate and elimination kinetics of salicylate in the infants of mothers who had ingested aspirin within 20 hours of delivery. The plasma salicylate concentration in four infants ranged from 8.3 to 30.8 $\mu g/ml$, whereas the maternal salicylate concentrations 8 to 30 minutes after delivery were between 2.0 and 26.0 $\mu g/ml$. The maternal:fetal plasma concentration ratio was equal to one in a single case and greater than unity in the other three subjects. The terminal exponential half-life of salicylate ranged from 4.5 to 11.5 hours in these infants, compared to an average value of 3 hours in the adult. Newborn infants were found to eliminate salicylate primarily by conjugation with glycine to form salicylphenolic glucuronide and approximately 2.3% of the salicylate dose administered to the mother could be recovered from neonatal urine. Salicylate was still detectable in the urine of these infants 3 days postpartum.

The effects of aspirin on hemostasis and platelet aggregation in the adult have been well defined. Similar changes in platelet function can occur in the fetus and neonate as a consequence of maternal aspirin administration. Bleyer and Breckenbridge (1970) demonstrated inhibition of collagen-induced platelet aggregation and diminished factor XII (Hageman factor) activity in infants born of mothers exposed to aspirin during the last week of pregnancy. Corby and Schulman (1971) confirmed the inhibition of collagen-induced platelet aggregation and also demonstrated that the platelets of such infants responded normally to exogenous ADP but exhibited an impaired reactivity to endogenously released ADP. The clinical significance of aspirin-induced abnormalities in platelet function and their role in bleeding disorders of the newborn remains to be clarified.

5. LOCAL ANESTHETICS

a. General Comments. Regional anesthesia employing local anesthetic agents is commonly used for the production of obstetrical analgesia. Since the initial report describing the placental transfer of lidocaine (Bromage and Robson, 1961), a massive literature on this subject has accumulated. These data indicate that local anesthetic agents injected into the maternal epidural or paracervical spaces are rapidly taken up by the maternal bloodstream and may traverse the placenta to enter the fetal circulation.

Several different types of local anesthetic agents have been used to induce paracervical and/or epidural nerve blockade. Currently, lidocaine, mepivacaine, and bupivacaine are the most extensively used in this regard (Thiery and Vroman, 1972). Unfortunately, a valid evaluation of the pharmacokinetic data currently available is complicated by the wide variety of procedures which have been used to assay these compounds. Methyl orange complexing or the cis-aconitic anhydride colorimetric technique are nonspecific and too insensitive for application to microsamples. Data based on these techniques often overestimate the true drug concentrations and recoveries frequently exceed 100%. Gas chromatographic assays are more reliable and specific.

Local anesthetics are basic drugs with pK_a's slightly higher than the physiological pH of blood. The pK_a of mepivacaine is 7.65, lidocaine 7.86, and bupivacaine 8.1. Consequently, a significantly large fraction of the drug may exist in its nonionized form in the maternal circulation. Since fetal blood is relatively more acidic than maternal blood, distribution of the un-ionized molecular species may be altered so that the concentration of local anesthetic in the fetus exceeds that of the mother at equilibrium.

Tucker et al. (1970) have reported that the binding of bupivacaine and lidocaine to fetal plasma proteins is significantly less than that occurring with maternal plasma proteins. The authors argued that differences in the placental transfer of bupivacaine, lidocaine, and mepivacaine were related to these distinctions in protein binding. Other investigators (Shnider and Way, 1968) were unable to detect any differences in the degree of binding of local anesthetics to either maternal or fetal plasma proteins.

Fetal bradycardia has been the most frequently reported and serious complication of regional obstetrical anesthesia. While the documented incidence of fetal bradycardia varies widely, it has been reported to occur in 2 to 70% of carefully observed cases (Thiery and Vroman, 1972). The bradycardia has its onset 10 to 15 minutes after induction of regional block and is generally shorter than 15 minutes in duration. A decrease in heart rate of 40–70 beats/minute may occur, and it is commonly associated with acidosis (Teramo, 1971). Morishima et al. (1972) infused lidocaine into fetal and newborn lambs and noted a brief bradycardia (16–30% decrease in heart rate lasting 10–17 minutes) followed by tachycardia. Fetal blood pressure was maintained until acute heart failure developed. Asphyxiated fetuses experienced cardiac failure and arrest at blood levels of lidocaine between 7.2 and 20 μg/ml, whereas normal fetuses tolerated blood concentrations of 36 to 42 μg/ml.

The bradycardia appears to result from a direct effect of these agents on the fetal myocardium (Asling *et al.*, 1970; Heymann, 1972). Others have suggested that the cardiovascular changes are secondary to stimulation of the central nervous system and convulsions induced by the local anesthetic (Teramo *et al.*, 1975). Mann *et al.* (1972) demonstrated that lidocaine toxicity in fetal sheep was manifest by a significant decrease in cerebral blood flow, though cerebral metabolism was unaffected. Since vagectomy did not prevent this bradycardia, they proposed that the observed effects were secondary to a direct action of the local anesthetic on both myocardial and neural elements.

b. Individual Agents. Local anesthetics can be broadly classified into two groups: (1) those possessing an amide linkage which confers relative resistance to enzymatic hydrolysis by plasma cholinesterase (lidocaine, mepivacaine, prilocaine, bupivacaine); and (2) those possessing an esteratic bond which is susceptible to enzymatic or nonenzymatic (alkaline) hydrolysis (procaine, tetracaine). Usubiaga *et al.* (1968) have reported that the apparent lack of transfer of procaine across the placenta is related to its rapid hydrolysis by maternal and fetal plasma cholinesterase. Thus, procaine could not be demonstrated in fetal blood when doses of less than 4 mg/kg of body weight were given to the mother. However, when doses up to 10 mg/kg were administered, the mean maternal procaine concentration was 6.2 ± 1.9 μg/ml and the corresponding cord blood procaine level was 3.0 ± 1.1 μg/ml.

i. Lidocaine. Injections of lidocaine administered for caudal, epidural, paracervical, or pudendal block procedures are promptly absorbed into the maternal circulation, reaching maximum maternal concentrations within 2–20 minutes (Thomas *et al.*, 1968; Lurie and Weiss, 1970; Petri *et al.*, 1974).

Shnider and Way (1968), in the course of a detailed pharmacokinetic study, administered lidocaine (2–3 mg/kg) intravenously to 16 women at the time of delivery. Maternal arterial lidocaine concentrations exhibited a biexponential decline with an α half-life of 30 seconds and a β half-life of 30 minutes. Lidocaine was detected in the umbilical vein within 2–3 minutes reaching peak values about 5–10 minutes thereafter. The drug was present in the fetal circulation for 30–45 minutes following its administration to the mother. Delivery of nine of these infants by Caesarean section occurred 7–39 minutes after administration of the drug and simultaneous blood samples were obtained from the mother and fetus. The mean maternal blood concentration of lidocaine was 2.8 ± 1.1 μg/ml, the mean umbilical vein concentration 1.6 ± 0.94 μg/ml, and the mean umbilical artery concentration 1.2 ± 0.85 μg/ml; these fetal values correspond to about 55% of the maternal levels. Lurie and Weiss (1970) found a mean maternal lidocaine concentration of 2.2 μg/ml with a corresponding neonatal concentration of 1.55 μg/ml. These authors estimated that the maternal:neonatal lidocaine concentration ratio was approximately 3:2. Petrie et al. (1974) reported an average maternal lidocaine level of 0.94 ± 0.11 μg/ml at delivery some 158 minutes (mean) after inducing paracervical blockade. The corresponding mean umbilical artery and vein concentrations were 0.54 ± 0.05 and 0.55 ± 0.05 μg/ml, respectively.

Some data suggest that lidocaine is not metabolized by placental homogenates and that the degree of plasma protein binding by maternal and fetal blood is identical. Other investigators attribute the persistent maternal-to-fetal gradient for lidocaine to the existence of a "placental barrier" (Shnider and Way, 1968). This conclusion has been questioned by Petrie et al. (1974) who have demonstrated monoethyl glycinexylidide, a metabolite of lidocaine, in approximately the same concentration in the maternal and fetal circulations. These observations imply that the increased ratio of lidocaine metabolites to lidocaine noted in the fetus is due to metabolism of the drug by the fetus or placenta.

ii. Mepivacaine.   This compound is rapidly absorbed into the maternal circulation from paracervical or epidural sites of administration. Peak maternal concentrations are generally reached within 5–30 minutes after the onset of nerve block and the drug can be identified in fetal blood at this time as well (Gordon, 1968; Lurie and Weiss, 1970; Asling et al., 1970).

Fetal blood concentrations of mepivacaine are approximately 50 to 70% of the corresponding maternal level (Tucker et al., 1970). Asling et al. (1970) studied the fetal and maternal mepivacaine concentrations in two groups of infants. They reported maternal arterial levels of 2.08 ± 0.55 μg/ml and fetal scalp blood levels of 1.16 ± 0.27 μg/ml in subjects without bradycardia and 4.11 ± 0.58 μg/ml in the group which developed bradycardia. The fetal levels were higher than corresponding maternal concentrations in two of the ten cases exhibiting no fetal bradycardia and in six of the seven cases with fetal bradycardia. In contrast to the elevated mepivacaine concentrations observed in scalp blood, cord blood samples were uniformly low, the levels frequently below 1.0 μg/ml. Lurie and Weiss (1970) and Teramo and Rajämaki (1971) have also reported that concentrations of mepivacaine in the umbilical vein and artery at birth were consistently lower than corresponding maternal levels.

iii. Bupivacaine. This agent is a long-acting local anesthetic and homologue of mepivacaine hydrochloride. Hyman and Shnider (1971) reported the mean bupivacaine concentration to be 0.14 ± 0.03 μg/ml in the maternal artery 127 ± 19 minutes after paracervical block. The umbilical venous blood level was 0.082 ± 0.02 μg/ml, the umbilical artery 0.048 ± 0.01 μg/ml, and the umbilical vein:maternal artery bupivacaine concentration ratio 0.60 ± 0.07. Comparable blood level data for epidural blockade follow: maternal arterial bupivacaine concentration at birth, 0.30 ± 0.08 μg/ml; umbilical venous level, 0.098 ± 0.02 μg/ml; and umbilical artery concentration, 0.072 ± 0.02 μg/ml. The umbilical vein: maternal artery concentration ratio 142 ± 42 minutes after injection was 0.26 ± 0.04 μg/ml.

The utilization of bupivacaine preparations containing epinephrine produced a significantly lower maternal blood concentration, however, the fetal levels were not significantly altered (Beazley *et al.*, 1972).

C. Drugs Acting on the Cardiovascular System

1. DIGITALIS GLYCOSIDES

Okita *et al.* (1952) have investigated the placental transfer of ^{14}C-digitoxin in guinea pigs and rats. One hour after administration to the mother $22.3 \pm 2.1\%$ of the total dose was present in the guinea pig fetus and $0.65 \pm 0.03\%$ in the rat fetus. The hearts of guinea pig fetuses contained six times as much digitoxin as the maternal heart when compared on a microgram/gram tissue basis.

The kinetics of digoxin transfer across the rodent placenta has been studied by injecting digoxin into pregnant rats and then sacrificing the animals at specific time intervals (Mirkin and Singh, 1973; Singh and Mirkin, 1975). This approach permits acquisition and analysis of comparable tissue specimens in both the mother and fetus. Fetal serum digoxin concentrations were approximately 50% of corresponding maternal serum levels after equilibration. The fetal tissue distribution pattern differed markedly from the mother. Maternal digoxin concentrations were greatest in the liver, followed (in descending order) by heart, kidney, and muscle. In contrast, fetal liver concentrations remained very low throughout the entire period of observation. Digoxin accumulated in the fetal myocardium and kidney, so that the fetal and maternal concentrations approximated one another 80 and 160 minutes after the maternal injection of digoxin.

Studies performed in the pregnant ewe have revealed major differences between the ovine and rodent maternal–placental–fetal unit. A large maternal-to-fetal gradient was observed in the sheep model. Following a single pulse injection, maternal serum concentrations of digoxin were 30 to 50 times greater than corresponding fetal samples and a large gradient was noted even after the initial distribution phase. There was a rapid falloff in both maternal and umbilical vein levels which resulted in extremely low fetal concentrations of digoxin at the 20- and 40-minute sampling period. The maternal:fetal tissue concentration gradient at the termination of these experiments (5 hours after drug administration) was as follows: kidney (67); heart (20); and liver (7) (Singh et al., 1973). Similar results were reported by Hernandez et al. (1973) who found only small quantities of ^{3}H-digoxin to be transferred across the placenta in both the exteriorized and in situ ovine fetus. The maternal serum half-life was estimated to be 3–5 minutes and the fetal 11–17 minutes. Marked differences were observed in the quantites of digoxin taken up by fetal and maternal tissues; the fetal:maternal ^{3}H-digoxin ratios for heart, kidney, and liver were 0.13.

Okita et al. (1956) studied the placental transfer of ^{14}C-digitoxin in 12-week-old human abortuses after its administration to the mother 3–5 hours prior to delivery. Less than 1% of the total maternal dose could be detected in the fetus as the parent compound, whereas 3.5% was present in the form of metabolite(s). All of the fetal tissues had higher levels of metabolite than the parent compound with the highest concentration noted in the fetal heart and kidney.

Administration of digitalis to pregnant women for a prolonged period results in a state of equilibration between the fetal and maternal circulations. Rogers et al. (1972) assayed the sera of subjects receiving chronic digoxin therapy throughout gestation. Maternal serum digoxin concentrations at delivery (5–7 hours after the last maintenance dose) averaged 0.6 ± 0.1 ng/ml and levels in umbilical cord sera were identical. Neonatal serum concentrations 12 hours after delivery were relatively unchanged $(0.5 \pm 0.1$ ng/ml) from those at parturition.

Digitalis glycosides have been used in pregnant women with myocardial decompensation for many years. The fetal consequences of such therapy has not been studied in detail despite report of a neonatal death allegedly due to digitalis intoxication in utero (Sherman and Locke, 1960). In general, there have not been any untoward effects noted in the fetus which can be attributed to the glycoside.

2. β-Receptor Blocking Agents

The placental transfer of several chemically different β-receptor blocking agents has been documented in the pregnant ewe (Truelove et al.,

1973). Maternal administration of propranolol, bunolol, butidrine, oxprenolol, and USVP 65–24 produced a measurable degree of β-blockade in both the fetus and the ewe. In contrast practolol, sotalol, and AH 3474 were effective in the ewe but not the fetus. It was assumed that these compounds crossed the placenta very slowly if at all. Since no analyses were performed on drugs other than propranolol this presumption remains to be validated. The duration of β-blockade produced by propranolol and oxprenolol was 3 hours in the pregnant ewe and 8–10 hours in the fetus.

A slow infusion of propranolol (1 mg/kg over 10 minutes) produced peak plasma concentrations of approximately 2.0 μg/ml in the ewe 8 minutes after terminating the infusion; maximum plasma levels in the fetus were established 14 minutes thereafter and averaged 0.8 μg/ml (Van Petten and Willes, 1970). The peak fetal plasma level was only 5% of the highest maternal plasma concentration and fetal plasma concentrations were equivalent to 10% of the corresponding maternal concentration at equilibrium (20 minutes after completing the infusion). The rates of elimination of propranolol from the maternal and fetal circulations appear to be similar in the postequilibrium period. Despite the extremely low fetal plasma levels of propranolol the persistence of β-blockade (determined by the chronotropic response to isoproterenol) was two to three times longer in the fetus than the ewe.

The transplacental passage of propranolol from the fetus to the mother has also been studied in the pregnant ewe (Van Petten and Willes, 1970). Propranolol (1 mg/kg estimated fetal body weight) injected via the umbilical vein caused bradycardia in the fetus and significantly inhibited the chronotropic response to isoproterenol. A decrease in maternal heart rate associated with this route of drug administration was attributed to the retrograde transfer of propranolol from the fetal to the maternal circulation. It is noteworthy that propranolol was not detectable in either the fetus or mother with the assay techniques employed.

In vitro experiments with isolated right ventricular tissue obtained from fetal sheep are more sensitive to the negative inotropic effects of propranolol than those prepared from adult myocardium (Friedman, 1972). Little or no difference was observed between fetal and adult myocardium with respect to the chronotropic effects of propranolol on sinoauricular node–right atrial tissue preparations. *In vivo* studies indicate that the reactivity and possibly the affinity of fetal β-receptors for isoproterenol and propranolol appears to be similar to that of adult animals. Van Petten and Willes (1970) demonstrated parallel shifts in the isoproterenol dose–response curve following propranolol infusions to both the dam and fetus.

The β-blockade induced in the fetus by maternal administration of propranolol in conventional doses appears to be minimal and of limited clinical consequence in the undisturbed fetus. However, such therapy may pose a distinct threat to the fetus under conditions of stress. In the presence of β-blockade, the asphyxiated fetus responds with a pronounced decrease in blood pressure, and the tachycardia usually seen following reversal of asphyxia is absent (Joelsson and Barton, 1969). The release of renin from the fetal sheep kidney is important in maintaining fetal cardiovascular homeostasis and inhibition of this process by β-adrenergic blockade may endanger the stressed fetus. Some infants born to mothers receiving propranolol during labor are depressed at birth, exhibit low Apgar scores, and may require resuscitation in the immediate postnatal period (Tunstall, 1969). Recent reports of bradycardia in neonates delivered from mothers receiving propranolol for thyrotoxicosis suggest a potential cause for concern.

3. Catecholamines

The adrenergic neuron undergoes profound changes in function and pharmacological reactivity during ontogenesis. Investigations in several different species (chicken, rat, rabbit, dog, lamb, and man) have demonstrated increases in the catecholamine content of the heart as it undergoes maturation (Mirkin, 1972a,b, 1974a).

Friedman et al. (1968) determined the concentration of norepinephrine in the developing rabbit heart and studied the anatomic distribution of the sympathetic neurons. The norepinephrine content of the fetal rabbit heart was extremely low (less than 0.2 μg/gm tissue) and reached adult levels by 3 weeks of age. The sympathetic innervation was immature and less dense in the fetal heart consisting of large, intensely fluorescent preterminal trunks. Partanen and Korkala (1974) were unable to demonstrate adrenergic terminal fibers in the atrial or ventricular wall of the human fetal heart. However, the nerve trunk contained small intensely fluorescent cells similar to those seen in the sympathetic ganglia. The absence of morphologically demonstrable adrenergic nerve synapses in the myocardium has suggested that the human fetal heart is influenced more by humoral than neural factors, at least during the first half of gestation. Similar observations have been made in other mammalian species during ontogenesis.

The activities of specific catecholamine synthesizing and metabolizing enzymes differ in the fetus, neonate, and adult. Fetal sheep heart contains less than one-seventh the tyrosine hydroxylase activity of the adult myocardium (Friedman, 1972). The catechol-O-methyltransferase activity of the fetal ovine myocardium is significantly higher than that of the adult myocardium, whereas, monoamine oxidase activity in the fetus is lower. There appears to be an orderly and sequential development of catecholamine synthesizing enzymes in the chick embryo; tyrosine hydroxylase, dopa decarboxylase, dopamine β-oxidase, and phenylethanolamine-N-methyltransferase activity can be assayed on the first, second, fourth, and sixth day of incubation, respectively (Ignarro and Shideman, 1968).

Many metabolic processes which are dependent upon the integrity of the adenylcyclase-phosphodiesterase system, undergo significant changes during maturation. Phosphodiesterase activity increases in the human fetus from the eighth to the seventeenth weeks of gestation and is inhibited by aminophylline from the tenth through the fifteenth week. The highest basal activities of adenylcyclase are found during the sixth week of fetal life and glucagon stimulation of this enzyme has been demonstrated at the seventeenth week of gestation (Dail and Palmer, 1973).

Mirkin (1972a) administered ^{3}H-norepinephrine (100 μCi) intravenously to pregnant rats at various gestational ages. The animals were sacrificed 1 hour later and the hearts fractionated by density gradient procedures. Uptake of ^{3}H-norepinephrine was not observed in the 16-day-old fetal heart and was barely detectable in hearts obtained on the eighteenth or twenty-first gestational day. It was possible to detect uptake when fetal hearts were incubated in vitro with ^{3}H-norepinephrine. Since endogenous norepinephrine had been demonstrated in the whole rat fetus as early as the thirteenth day of gestation, the poor in vivo uptake of catecholamine by the 18- and 21-day-old fetal heart was attributed to the impaired placental transfer of ^{3}H-norepinephrine. Further study demonstrated a marked accumulation of ^{3}H-norepinephrine and metabolites in the rat placenta.

The active metabolism of ^{3}H-norepinephrine to a variety of methylated and deaminated metabolites has been reported after incubation with extracts of human placental tissue (Castren and Saarikoski, 1968). In humans, administration of ^{14}C-dl-norepinephrine to pregnant women resulted in cord sera levels which ranged between 2 and 18% of the maternal concentration (Sandler et al., 1963).

REFERENCES

Abdul-Karim, R. W., and Bruce, N. (1973). *Fert. Steril.* **24**, 44.
Adams, F. H., Assali, N., Cushman, M., and Westersten, A. (1961). *Pediatrics* **27**, 627.
Adamsons, K., and Joelsson, I. (1966). *Amer. J. Obstet Gynecol.* **96**, 437.
Adamsons, K., Mueller-Heubach, E., and Meyers, R. E. (1971). *Amer. J. Obstet. Gynecol.* **109**, 248.
Aherne, W., and Dunhill, M. (1966). *Brit. Med. Bull.* **22**, 5.

Amoroso, E. C. (1952). *In* "Marshall's Physiology of Reproduction" (A. S. Parkes, ed.), 2nd ed., Vol. 2, p. 127. Longmans, Green, New York.

Anders, M. W., Cooper, M. J., Rolewicz, T., and Mirkin, B. L. (1974). *Proc. Int. Symp. Pediat. Pharm., 1st, 1974* (in press).

Apgar, V., Burns, J. J., Brodie, B. B., and Paper, E. M. (1952). *Amer. J. Obstet. Gynecol.* **64**, 1368.

Arthur, L. J., and Burland, W. L. (1969). *Arch. Dis. Childhood* **44**, 82.

Asling, J. H., and Way, E. L. (1971). *In* "Fundamentals of Drug Metabolism and Drug Disposition" (LaDu, B. N., Mandel, H. G., and Way, E. L., eds.), p. 88. Williams & Wilkins, Baltimore, Maryland.

Asling, J. H., Shnider, S. M., Margolis, A. J., Wilkinson, G. L., and Way, E. L. (1970). *Amer. J. Obstet. Gynecol.* **107**, 626.

Assali, N. S., Douglass, R. A., Baird, W. W., Nicholson, D. B., and Suyemoto, R. (1953). *Amer. J. Obstet. Gynecol.* **66**, 248.

Assali, N. S., Rauramo, L., and Peltonen, T. (1960). *Amer. J. Obstet. Gynecol.* **79**, 86.

Barclay, A., Franklin, K., and Prinhard, M. (1944). *In* "The Foetal Circulation and Cardiovascular System, and the Changes that They Undergo at Birth," 1st ed., pp. 207–251. Blackwell, Oxford.

Barr, W., and Graham, R. M. (1967). *J. Obstet. Gynaecol. Brit. Common.* **74**, 739.

Baughman, F. A., and Randinitis, E. J. (1970). *J. Amer. Med. Ass.* **213**, 466.

Beazley, J. M., Taylor, G., and Reynolds, F. (1972). *Obstet. Gynecol.* **39**, 2.

Beckett, A. H., and Taylor, J. F. (1967). *J. Pharm. Pharmacol.* **19**, Suppl., 505.

Behrman, R. E., and Kittinger, G. W. (1968). *Proc. Soc. Exp. Biol. Med.* **129**, 305.

Behrman, R. E., Lees, M. H., Peterson, E. N., De Lannoy, C. W., and Seeds, A. E. (1970). *Amer. J. Obstet. Gynecol.* **108**, 956.

Bergman, H. (1942). *Med. Rec.* **155**, 105.

Blecher, T. E., Edgar, W. M., Melville, H. A. H., and Peel, K. R. (1966). *Brit. Med. J.* **1**, 137.

Bleyer, W. A., and Breckenbridge, R. T. (1970). *J. Amer. Med. Ass.* **213**, 2049.

Bleyer, W. A, and Marshall, R. E. (1972). *J. Amer. Med. Ass.* **221**, 185.

Bonica, J. J. (1969). *In* "Principles and Practice of Obstetric Analgesia," p. 147. Davis, Philadelphia, Pennsylvania.

Born, G. V., Dawes, G. S., Mott, J. C., and Widdecomb, J. G. (1954). *Cold Spring Harbor Symp. Quant. Biol.* **19**, 102.

Borrell, V., Fernstrom, I., Ohlson, L., and Wiqvist, N. (1965). *Amer. J. Obstet. Gynecol.* **93**, 44.

Bray, R. E., Roe, R. W., and Johnson, W. L. (1966). *Amer. J. Obstet. Gynecol.* **96**, 938.

Brazelton, T. B. (1970). *Amer. J. Psychiat.* **126**, 9.

Brodie, B. B. (1964). *In* "Animal and Clinical Pharmacological Techniques in Drug Evaluation" (Nodine, J. H., and Siegler, P. E., eds.), p. 69. Yearbook Publ., Chicago, Illinois.

Brodie, B. B., Kurz, H., and Schanker, L. S. (1960). *J. Pharmacol. Exp. Ther.* **130**, 20.

Bromage, P. R., and Robson, J. G. (1961). *Anaesthesia* **16**, 461.

Bromberg, Y. M., Salzberger, M., and Bruderman, I. (1955). *Gynaecologia* **140**, 141.

Brunton, W. J., and Brinster, R. L. (1971). *Amer. J. Physiol.* **221**, 658.

Buzard, J. A., and Conklin, J. D. (1964). *Amer. J. Physiol.* **206**, 189.

Campbell, A. G., Dawes, G. S., Fishman, A. P., *et al.* (1966). *J. Physiol.* (*London*) **182**, 439.

Carrier, G., Hume, A. S., Douglas, B. H., Hyman, A. I., James, G. B., and Wiser, W. L. (1969). *Amer. J. Obstet. Gynecol.* **105**, 1069.

Cassano, G. B., Ghetti, B., Gliozzi, E., *et al.* (1967). *Brit. J. Anaesth.* **39**, 11.

Castren, O., and Saarikoski, S. (1968). *Acta Obstet. Gynecol.* **47**, 151.

Cavanagh, D., and Condo, C. S. (1964). *Curr. Ther. Res.* **6**, 122.

Charles, D. (1954). *J. Obstet. Gynaecol. Brit. Emp.* **61**, 750.

Cohlan, S. Q., Bevelander, G., and Tiamsic, T. (1963). *Amer. J. Dis. Child.* **105**, 65.

Colburn, D. W., and Saltzman, M. (1960). *N.Y. State J. Med.* **60**, 246.

Conner, E., and Miller, J. (1973). *J. Pharmacol. Exp. Ther.* **184**, 291.

Conway, N., and Birt, B. D. (1965). *Brit. Med. J.* **2**, 260.

Cooper, M. J., Anders, M. W., and Mirkin, B. L. (1973). *Drug Metabl. Disposition* **1**, 659.

Corby, D. G., and Schulman, I. (1971). *J. Pediat.* **79**, 307.

Corney, G., and Aherne, W. (1965). *Arch. Dis. Childhood* **40**, 264.

Crawford, J. D., and McCance, R. A. (1960). *J. Physiol.* (*London*) **151**, 458.

Crawford, J. S. (1956). *Brit. J. Anaesth.* **28**, 146.

Crawford, J. S., and Rudofsky, S. (1965). *Brit. J. Anaesth.* **37**, 929.

Cree, J. E., Meyer, J., and Hailey, D. M. (1973). *Brit. Med. J.* **4**, 251.

Dail, W. G., and Palmer, G. C. (1973). *Anat. Rec.* **177**, 265.

Dancis, J., Money, W. L., Condon, G. P., and Levitz, M. (1958). *J. Clin. Invest.* **37**, 1373.

Danielli, J. F. (1970). *In* "The Permeability of Natural Membranes" (Davson, H., and Danielli, J. F., eds.). Hafner, New York.

Davis, R. P. (1969). *In* "Biological Membranes" (Dowben, R. N., ed.), p. 109. Little, Brown, Boston, Massachusetts.

Davson, H. (1970). *In* "The Permeability of Natural Membranes" (Davson, H., and Danielli, J. F., eds.). Hafner, New York.

Dawes, G. S. (1968). *In* "Foetal and Neonatal Physiology," p. 27. Yearbook Publ., Chicago, Illinois.

Depp, R., Kind, A. C., Kirby, W. M. M., and Johnson, W. L. (1970). *Amer. J. Obstet. Gynecol.* **107**, 1054.

DeSilva, J. A., D'Areonte, L., and Kaplan, J. (1964). *Curr. Ther. Res.* **6**, 115.

Desmond, M. M., Schwanecke, R. P., Wilson, G. S., Yasunaga, S., and Burgdorff, I. (1972). *J. Pediat.* **80**, 190.

Dille, J. M. (1956). *J. Pharmacol. Exp. Ther.* **52**, 129.

Dilts, P. V. (1970). *Amer. J. Obstet. Gynecol.* **108**, 221.

Dowben, R. M. (1969). *In* "Biological Membranes," (Dowben, R. M., ed.), p. 1. Little, Brown, Boston, Massachusetts.

Duncan, S. B. (1969). *J. Physiol.* (*London*) **204**, 421.

Duncan, S. B., Ginsburg, J., and Morris, N. F. (1969). *Amer. J. Obstet. Gynecol.* **105**, 197.

Eckenhoff, J. E., Hoffman, G. L., and Funderburg, L. W. (1953). *Amer. J. Obstet. Gynecol.* **65**, 1269.

Ehrnebo, M., Agurdl, S., and Jalling, B. (1971). *Eur. J. Clin. Pharmacol.* **3**, 189.

Ely, P. A. (1966). *J. Physiol.* (*London*) **184**, 225.

Enders, A. C. (1967). *Amer. J. Anat.* **116**, 29.

Erkolla, R., and Kanto, J. (1972). *Lancet* **1**, 1235.
Fabro, S., and Sieber, S. M. (1969). *In* "The Foeto-Placental Unit" (A. Pecile and C. Finzi, eds.), Int. Congr. Ser. No. 183, p. 313. Exerpta Med. Found., Amsterdam.
Fealy, J. (1958). *Obstet. Gynecol.* **11**, 342.
Fehr, P., and Mirkin, B. L. (1975). Unpublished observations.
Finster, M., and Mark, L. C. (1971). *In* "Handbuch der experimentellen Pharmakologie" (Brodie, B. B., Gillette, J. R., and Ackerman, H. S., eds.), Vol. 28, Part 1, p. 276. Springer-Verlag, Berlin and New York.
Finster, M., Mark, L. C., Morishima, H. O., Moya, F., Perel, M. J., James, L. S., and Dayton, P. G. (1966). *Amer. J. Obstet. Gynecol.* **95**, 621.
Finster, M., Morishima, H. O., Mark, L. C., Perel, J. M., Dayton, P. G., and James, L. S. (1972). *Anesthesiology* **36**, 155.
Flexner, L. B., and Gellhorn, A. (1942). *Amer. J. Obstet. Gynecol.* **43**, 965.
Flowers, C. E. (1957). *Obstet. Gynecol.* **9**, 332.
Flowers, C. E. (1959). *Amer. J. Obstet. Gynecol.* **78**, 730.
Flowers, C. E., Rudolph, A. J., and Desmond, M. M. (1969). *Obstet. Gynecol.* **34**, 62.
Food and Drug Administration (1974). *FDA (Food Drug. Admin.) Drug Bull.*, July.
Fouts, J. R., and Adamson, R. H. (1959). *Science* **129**, 897.
Franklin, K., Barclay, A., and Prichard, M. (1940). *J. Anat.* **75**, 75.
Friedman, W. F. (1972). *Progr. Cardiov. Dis.* **15**, 97.
Friedman, W. F., Pool, P. E., Jacobowitz, D., Seagren, S. C., and Braunwald, E. (1968). *Circ. Res.* **23**, 25.
Ganapathy, S. K., and Cohen (1975). *Pediat. Res.* **9**, 283.
Gibbon, R. J., and Reichelderfer, R. (1960). *Antibiot. Med.* **7**, 618.
Glass, L., Rajegowda, B. K., and Evans, H. E. (1971). *Lancet* **2**, 685.
Goldstein, A., Aronow, L., and Kalman, S. M. (1968). *In* "Principles of Drug Action," p. 189. Harper, New York.
Good, R. G., and Johnson, G. H. (1971). *Obstet. Gynecol.* **38**, 60.
Goodfriend, M. J., Shey, I. A., and Klein, M. D. (1956). *Amer. J. Obstet. Gynecol.* **71**, 29.
Gordon, H. R. (1968). *N. Engl. J. Med.* **279**, 910.
Greiss, F. C. (1965). *Amer. J. Obstet. Gynecol.* **93**, 917.
Gurpide, E, Tseng, J., Escarcena, L., Fahning, M., Gibson, C., and Fehr, P. (1972). *Amer. J. Obstet. Gynecol.* **113**, 21.
Hagerman, D. (1970). *Environ. Res.* **3**, 145.
Hamner, C. E., and Fix, S. B. (1969). *In* "The Mammalian Oviduct" (Hafez, E. S., and Blendau, R. J., eds.), p. 333. Univ. of Chicago Press, Chicago, Illinois.
Hansch, C. (1968). *Farmaco, Ed. Sci.* **23**, 293.
Hansch, C. (1971). *In* "Drug Design" (E. J. Ariens, ed.), Vol. 1, p. 271. Academic Press, New York.
Harbison, R. D., and Becker, B. A. (1969). *Teratology* **2**, 305.
Harbison, R. A., and Becker, B. A. (1971). *Toxicol. Appl. Pharmacol.* **20**, 573.
Hart, L. G., Adamson, R. H., Dixon, R. L., and Fouts, J. R. (1962). *J. Pharmacol. Exp. Ther.* **137**, 103.
Heilman, D. H., Heilman, F. R., Hinshaw, H. R., Nichols, D. R., and Herrell, W. E. (1945). *Amer. J. Med. Sci.* **210**, 576.
Hernandez, A., Burton, R. M., Goldring, D., and Klint, R. (1973). *Amer. Heart J.* **85**, 511.

Heymann, M. A. (1972). *Fed. Proc., Fed. Amer. Soc. Exp. Biol.* **31,** 44.

Hill, R. M., and Desmond, M. M. (1963). *Pediat. Clin. N. Amer.* **10,** 67.

Hill, R. M., Horning, M. G., and Horning, E. C. (1973). *In* "Fetal Pharmacology" (Boreus, L. O., ed.), p. 375. Raven, New York.

Hill, R. M., Verniaud, W. M., Horning, M. G., *et al.* (1974). *Amer. J. Dis. Child.* **127,** 645.

Hogben, C., and Adrian, M. (1971). *In* "Handbuch der experimentellen Pharmakologie" (Brodie, B. B., Gillette, J. R., and Ackerman, H. S., eds.), Vol. 28, p. 1. Springer-Verlag, Berlin and New York.

Hogben, C. A., Tocco, D. J., Brodie, B. B., and Shanker, L. S. (1959). *J. Pharmacol. Exp. Ther.* **125,** 275.

Huckabee, W. E., Metcalfe, J., Prystowsky, H., and Barron, D. H. (1961). *Amer. J. Physiol.* **200,** 274.

Hyman, M. D., and Shnider, S. M. (1971). *Anesthesiology* **34,** 81.

Idanpään-Heikkilä, J., Fritchie, G. E., Ho, B. T., and McIssac, W. M. (1971a). *Amer. J. Obstet. Gynecol.* **110,** 426.

Idanpään-Heikkilä, Taska, R. J., Allen, H. A., and Schoolar, J. C. (1971b). *J. Pharmacol. Exp. Ther.* **176,** 752.

Idanpään-Heikkilä, J., Joupilla, P., Akerblom, H. K., Isoahor, R., Kauppila, E., and Koivisto, M. (1972). *Amer. J. Obstet. Gynecol.* **112,** 1.

Ignarro, L. J., and Shideman, F. E. (1968). *J. Pharmacol. Exp. Ther.* **159,** 38.

Inturrusi, C. E., Blinick, G., and Lipsitz, P. J. (1973). *Pharmacologist* **15,** 71.

Jackson, A. V. (1948). *J. Pathol. Bacteriol.* **60,** 587.

Jaszczak, S., Choroszewska, A., and Bentyn, K. (1970). *Pol. Med. J.* **9,** 1308.

Jenkins, V. R., Talbert, W. M., and Dilts, P. V. (1972). *Obstet. Gynecol.* **39,** 254.

Joelsson, I., and Barton, M. D. (1969). *Acta Obstet. Gynecol. Scand.* **48,** 75.

Jones, K. L., Smith, D. W., and Ulleland, C. N. (1973). *Lancet* **1,** 1267.

Juchau, M. (1972). *Fed. Proc., Fed. Amer. Soc. Exp. Biol.* **31,** 48.

Kandall, S. R., and Gartner, L. M. (1974). *Amer. J. Dis. Child.* **127,** 58.

Kauffman, R. E., Boulos, B. M., and Aazarnoff, D. L. (1973). *Amer. J. Obstet. Gynecol.* **117,** 64.

Kauffman, R. E., Boulos, B. M., and Azarnoff, D. L. (1975). *Pediat. Res.* **9,** 104.

Kavanau, J. L. (1963). *Nature (London)* **198,** 525.

Kennedy, J. S., and Waddell, W. (1972). *Toxicol. Appl. Pharamcol.* **22,** 252.

Kieffer, L., Rubin, A., McCoy, J. B., and Foltz, E. L. (1955). *Amer. J. Obstet. Gynecol.* **69,** 174.

Klebe, J., and Ingomar, C. (1972). *Pediatrics* **49,** 112.

Kosaka, Y., Takahashi, T., and Mark, L. C. (1969). *Anesthesiology* **31,** 489.

Krauer, B., Draffan, G. H., Williams, F. H., *et al.* (1974). *Clin. Pharmacol. Ther.* **14,** 442.

Kron, R. E., Stein, M., and Goddard, K. E. (1966). *Pediatrics* **37,** 102.

Larkin, E. C., Weintraub, L. R., and Crosby, W. H. (1970). *Amer. J. Physiol.* **218,** 7.

Le Blanc, A. L., and Perry, J. E. (1967). *Tex. Rep. Biol. Med.* **25,** 541.

Leduc, B. (1972). *J. Physiol. (London)* **225,** 339.

Lees, M. H., Hill, J. D., Ochsner, A. J., III, Thomas, C. L., and Novy, M. J. (1971). *Amer. J. Obstet Gynecol.* **110,** 68.

Levy, G., and Garrettson, L. K. (1974). *Pediatrics* **53,** 201.

Lien, E. J. (1970). *Drug. Intel. & Clin. Pharm.* **4,** 7.

Ling, G. M. (1965). *Fed. Proc., Fed. Amer. Soc. Exp. Biol.* **24,** Suppl. 15, 103.

Lurie, A. O., and Weiss, J. B. (1970). *Amer. J. Obstet. Gynecol.* **106**, 850.
Lust, J. E., Hagerman, D. D., and Villee, C. A. (1953). *J. Clin. Invest.* **33**, 38.
Lutwak-Mann, C., and Hay, M. F. (1962). *Brit. Med. J.* **2**, 944.
McAllister, H. A., and Flowers, C. E. (1956). *S. Med. J.* **49**, 1028.
MacAulay, M. A., and Charles, D. (1967). *Clin. Pharmacol. Ther.* **8**, 578.
MacAulay, M. A., Abou-Sabe, M., and Charles, D. (1966). *Amer. J. Obstet. Gynecol.* **96**, 943.
MacAulay, M. A., Berg, S. R., and Charles, D. (1968). *Amer. J. Obstet. Gynecol.* **102**, 1162.
McClure-Browne, J. C. (1959). *In* "Oxygen Supply to the Human Foetus" (Walker, J., Turnbull, A. C., Smith, C. A., and Baron, D. H., eds.), p. 113. Blackwell, Oxford.
McLachlan, J. A., Sieber, S. M., and Fabro, S. (1970). *Fed. Proc., Fed. Amer. Soc. Exp. Biol.* **28**, 744.
McNay, J. L. and Dayton, P. G. (1970). *Science* **167**, 988.
Mann, L. I., Bailey, C., Carmichael, A., and Duchin, S. (1972). *Amer. J. Obstet. Gynecol.* **112**, 789.
Martin, C. B. (1968). *In* "Intra-Uterine Development" (Barnes, A. C., ed.), p. 35. Lea & Febiger, Philadelphia, Pennsylvania.
Martin, C. B., McGaughey, H. S., Kaiser, I. H., Donner, M. W., and Ramsey, E. M. (1964). *Amer. J. Obstet. Gynecol.* **90**, 819.
Mastroianni, L., Beer, F., Shah, U., and Clewe, T. (1961). *Endocrinology* **68**, 92.
Mather, L. E., Long, G. J., and Thomas, J. (1971). *J. Pharm. Pharmacol.* **23**, 359.
Mayer, S., Maikel, R., and Brodie, B. B. (1959). *J. Pharmacol. Exp. Ther.* **127**, 205.
Meadow, S. R. (1968). *Lancet* **2**, 1296.
Meadow, S. R. (1970). *Proc. Roy. Soc. Med.* **63**, 48.
Melchior, J. C., Svensmark, O., and Trolle, D. (1967). *Lancet* **2**, 860.
Mellor, D. J. (1969). *J. Physiol. (London)* **204**, 395.
Meschia, G., Battaglia, F., and Bruns, P. (1967). *J. Appl. Physiol.* **22**, 1171.
Metcalfe, J., Romney, S. L., Ramsey, L. H., Reid, D. E., and Burwell, C. S. (1955). *J. Clin. Invest.* **34**, 1632.
Metcalfe, J., Bartels, H., and Moll, W. (1967). *Physiol. Rev.* **47**, 782.
Meyer, W. W., and Lind, J. (1966). *Arch. Dis. Childhood* **41**, 606.
Miller, R. K., Ferm, V. H., and Mudge, G. H. (1972). *Amer. J. Obstet. Gynecol.* **114**, 259.
Mirkin, B. L. (1971). *J. Pediat.* **78**, 329.
Mirkin, B. L. (1972a). *Fed. Proc., Fed. Amer. Soc. Exp. Biol.* **31**, 65.
Mirkin, B. L. (1972b). *In* "Immunosympathectomy" (Steiner, G., and Schönbaum, E., eds.), p. 79. Elsevier, Amsterdam.
Mirkin, B. L. (1973). *In* "Fetal Pharmacology" (Boreus, L., ed.), p. 1. Raven, New York.
Mirkin, B. L. (1974a). *In* "Drugs and the Developing Brain," p. 199. Plenum, New York.
Mirkin, B. L. (1974b). *In* "Modern Perinatal Medicine" (Gluck, L., ed.), p. 307. Yearbook Publ., Chicago, Illinois.
Mirkin, B. L., and Oh, Y. (1974). *Pharmacologist* **16**, 305.
Mirkin, B. L., and Singh, S. (1973). *Proc. Int. Congr. Pharmacol., 5th, 1972* p. 215.
Mofid, M., Brinkmann, C. R., and Assali, N. S. (1973). *Obstet. Gynecol.* **41**, 364.
Monfort, J. A., Diamond, I., MacGregory, A., and Peluso, J. (1963). *N.Y. State J. Med.* **26**, 263.

Monson, R. R., Rosenberg, L., Hartz, S. C., Shapiro, S., Heineman, O. P., and Slone, D. (1973). *N. Engl. J. Med.* **289**, 1049.
Moore, J., and Hunter, R. J. (1970). *J. Obstet. Gynaecol. Brit. Commonw.* **77**, 830.
Moore, J., McNabb, G., and Glynn, J. P. (1973). *Brit. J. Anaesth.* **45**, Suppl., 798.
Morishima, H. O., Heymann, H. A., Rudolph, A. M., and Barrett, C. T. (1972). *Amer. J. Obstet. Gynecol.* **112**, 72.
Morrow, S., Palmisano, P., and Cassady, G. (1968). *Tex. Rep. Biol. Med.* **26**, 567.
Morselli, P. L., Principi, N., Tognoni, G., Real, E., Belvedere, G., Standen, S. M., and Serini, F. (1973). *J. Perinatal Med.* **1**, 133.
Mowat, J., and Garrey, M. M. (1970). *Brit. Med. J.* **2**, 757.
Moya, F., and Kvisselbaard, N. (1961). *Anesthesiology* **22**, 1.
Naeye, R. (1963). *N. Engl. J. Med.* **268**, 804.
Niswander, K. R. (1969). *Obstet. Gynecol.* **34**, 62.
Ogawa, J. (1966). *Acta Paediat. Jap.* **71**, 997.
Oh, Y. (1973). Doctoral Dissertation, University of Minnesota, Minneapolis.
Oh, Y., and Mirkin, B. L. (1971). *Fed. Proc., Fed. Amer. Soc. Exp. Biol.* **30**, 2034.
Okita, G. T., Gordon, R. B., and Geiling, E. M. (1952). *Proc. Soc., Exp. Biol. Med.* **80**, 536.
Okita, G. T., Plotz, E. J., and Davis, M. E. (1956). *Circ. Res.* **4**, 376.
Palmisano, P. A., and Cassidy, G. (1969). *J. Amer. Med. Ass.* **209**, 556.
Partanen, S., and Korkala, O. (1974). *Experientia* **30**, 798.
Paterson, L., Henderson, A., Lunan, C. B., and McGurk, S. (1970). *J. Obstet. Gynaecol., Brit. Commonw.* **77**, 565.
Paton, J., Fisher, D., Peterson, E., De Lannoy, C. W., and Behrman, R. E. (1973). *Biol. Neonate* **22**, 50.
Patrick, M. J., Tilstone, W. J., and Reavey, P. (1972). *Lancet* **1**, 542.
Pelkonen, O., Arvela, P., and Karki, N. T. (1971). *Acta Pharmacol. Toxicol.* **30**, 385.
Peltonen, T., and Hirronen, L. (1965). *Acta Paediat. Scand., Supp.* **161**, 5–55.
Penman, W. R., Wilson, T. M., Gaby, W. I., and Heller, E. M. (1953). *J. Obstet. Gynaecol. Brit. Emp.* **61**, 750.
Penniston, J. T., Beckett, L., Bentley, D. L., and Hansch, C. (1969). *Mol. Pharmacol.* **5**, 333.
Perry, J. E., and Le Blanc, A. L. (1967). *Tex. Rep. Biol. Med.* **25**, 265.
Perry, J. E., Toney, J. B., and Le Blanc, A. L. (1967). *Tex. Rep. Biol. Med.* **25**, 270.
Persson, B. H. (1961). *Acta Gynecol.* **39**, 88.
Peterson, E. N., and Behrman, R. E. (1969). *Amer. J. Obstet. Gynecol.* **104**, 988.
Petri, R. H., Paul, W. L., Miller, F. C., Arce, J. J., Paul, R. H., Nakamura, R. M., and Hon, E. H. (1974). *Amer. J. Obstet. Gynecol.* **120**, 791.
Philipson, A., Sabath, L. D., and Charles, D. (1973). *N. Engl. J. Med.* **288**, 1219.
Pikkarainen, P. H., and Räihä, N. C. (1967). *Pediat. Res.* **1**, 165.
Ploman, L., and Persson, B. H. (1957). *J. Obstet. Gynaecol. Brit. Emp.* **64**, 706.
Pomerance, J. J., and Yaffe, S. J. (1973). *Curr. Probl. Pediat.* **4**, 2.
Prakash, A., Chalmers, J. A., Onojobi, O. I., Henderson, R. J., and Cummings, P. (1970). *J. Obstet. Gynecol.* (Brit. Commonwlth) **77**, 247.
Pruitt, A. W., and Dayton, P. G. (1971). *Eur. J. Clin. Pharmacol.* **4**, 59.
Räihä, N. C. (1958). *Acta Physiol. Scand.* **45**, Suppl. 155, 1.
Rane, A., and Ackermann, E. (1972). *Clin. Pharmacol. Ther.* **13**, 663.
Rane, A., Garle, M., Borgå, O., and Sjoquist, F. (1973). *Clin. Pharmacol. Ther.* **15**, 39

Rankin, J., Meschia, G., Makowski, E. L., and Battaglia, F. F. (1970). *Amer. J. Physiol.* **219**, 9.

Rasmussen, F. (1969). *Scand. J. Resp. Dis.* **50**, 61.

Reddy, A. M., Harper, R. G., and Stern, G. (1971). *Pediatrics* **45**, 353.

Roberts, H., and Kane, K. M. (1957). *Lancet* **1**, 128.

Rogers, M. C., Willerson, J. T., Goldblatt, A., and Smith, T. W. (1972). *N. Engl. J. Med.* **287**, 1010.

Romney, S. L., Gabel, P. V., and Takeda, Y. (1963). *Amer. J. Obstet. Gynecol.* **87**, 636.

Root, B., Eichner, E., and Sunshine, I. (1961). *Amer. J. Obstet. Gynecol.* **81**, 948.

Rudolph, A. M., and Heymann, M. A. (1967). *Circ. Res.* **21**, 163.

Rudolph, A. M., and Heymann, M. A. (1970). *Circ. Res.* **26**, 289.

Rudolph, A. M., Heymann, M. A., Teramo, K. A., Barrett, C. T., and Räihä, N. C. (1971). *Pediat. Res.* **5**, 452.

Sandler, M., Ruthren, C. R., Contractor, S. F., Wood, C., Booth, R. T., and Pinkerton, J. H. (1963). *Nature (London)* **197**, 598.

Sanner, J. H., and Woods, L. A. (1965). *J. Pharmacol. Exp. Ther.* **148**, 176.

Schechter, P. J., and Roth, L. J. (1967). *J. Pharmacol. Exp. Ther.* **158**, 164.

Scott, W. C., and Warner, R. F. (1950). *J. Amer. Med. Ass.* **142**, 1331.

Seydel, J. K. (1971). *In* "Drug Design" (E. J. Ariens, ed.), Vol. 1, p. 343. Academic Press, New York.

Shannon, R. W., Fraser, G. P., Aitken, R. G., and Harper, J. R. (1972). *Brit. J Clin. Pract.* **26**, 271.

Sherman, J. L., and Locke, R. V. (1960). *Amer. J. Cardiol.* **6**, 834.

Shibata, T., Koike, K., and Ogawa, J. (1969). *Ann. Paediat. Jap.* **15**, 33.

Shnider, S. M., and Moya, F. (1964). *Amer. J. Obstet. Gynecol.* **89**, 1009.

Shnider, S. M., and Way, E. L. (1968). *Anesthesiology* **29**, 944.

Shoeman, D. W., Kaufmann, R. E., Azarnoff, D. L., and Boulos, B. M. (1972). *Biochem. Pharmacol.* **21**, 1237.

Shute, E., and Davis, M. E. (1933). *Surg., Obstet. Gynecol.* **57**, 727.

Sieber, S. M., and Fabro, S. (1971). *J. Pharmacol. Exp. Ther.* **176**, 65.

Singh, S., and Mirkin, B. L. (1975). *Biochem. Pharmacol.* (submitted for publication).

Singh, S., Fehr, P., and Mirkin, B. L. (1973). *Pediat. Res.* **7**, 318.

Sjöstrand, F. S. (1963). *Proc. Int. Pharmacol. Meet., 1st, 1961* p. 1.

Steg, N. (1957). *Amer. J. Dis. Child.* **94**, 286.

Stevens, M. W., and Harbison, R. D. (1974). *Teratology* **9**, 317.

Stevenson, R. E. (1973). *In* "The Fetus and Newly Born Infant. Influences of the Prenatal Environment" (Stevenson, R. E., ed.), p. 96. Mosby, St. Louis, Missouri.

Strauss, L., Goldenberg, N., Hirota, K., and Okudaira, Y. (1965). *Birth Defects, Orig. Art. Ser.* **1**, 13–26.

Teramo, K. (1971). *Acta Obstet. Gynecol. Scand., Suppl.* **16**, 7.

Teramo, K., and Rajämaki, A. (1971). *Brit. J. Anaesth.* **43**, 300.

Teramo, K., Benowitz, N., Heymann, M. A., Kahampää, K., Sumes, A., and Rudolph, A. M. (1975). *Amer. J. Obstet. Gynecol.* (in press).

Termine, A., and Santuari, E. (1968). *Ann. Ist. "Carlo Forlanini"* **28**, 431.

Thiery, M., and Vroman, S. (1972). *Amer. J. Obstet. Gynecol.* **113**, 988.

Thomas, J., Climie, C. R., and Mather, L. E. (1968). *Brit. J. Anaesth.* **40**, 965.

Tien, H. T., and James, L. K. (1971). *In* "Chemistry of the Cell Interface," Part

A, p. 205. Academic Press, New York.
Toaff, R., and David, R. (1968). *In* "Drug Induced Diseases" (Meyler, L., and Peck, H. M., ed.), Vol. 3, p. 117. Excerpta Med. Found., Amsterdam.
Truelove, J. F., Van Petten, G. R., and Willes, R. F. (1973). *Brit. J. Pharmacol.* **47**, 161.
Tucker, G. T., Boyes, R. N., Bridenbaugh, P. O., and Moore, D. C. (1970). *Anesthesiology* **33**, 304.
Tunstall, M. E. (1969). *Brit. J. Anaesth.* **41**, 792.
Ussing, H. H. (1949). *Acta Physiol. Scand.* **19**, 43.
Ussing, H. H. (1963). *Proc. Int. Pharmacol. Meet., 1st, 1961* Vol. 4, p. 15.
Usubiaga, J. E., Iuppa, M. L., Moya, F., Wikinski, J. A., and Velazco, R. (1968). *Amer. J. Obstet. Gynecol.* **100**, 918.
Van Bruggen, J. T. (1971). *In* "Chemistry of the Cell Interface," p. 1. Academic Press, New York.
Van Petten, G. R., and Willes, R. F. (1970). *Brit. J. Pharmacol.* **38**, 572.
Varpela, E., Hietalahti, J., and Aro, M. J. T. (1969). *Scand. J. Resp. Dis.* **50**, 101.
Vishwakarma, P. (1962). *Fert. Steril.* **13**, 481.
Waddell, W. (1971). *In* "Fundamentals of Drug Metabolism and Drug Disposition" (La Du, B. N., Mandel, H. G., and Way, E. L., eds.), p. 505. Williams & Wilkins, Baltimore, Maryland.
Waddell, W., and Mirkin, B. L. (1972). *Biochem. Pharmacol.* **21**, 547.
Waltman, R., Nigrin, G., Bonura, F., and Pipat, C. (1969). *Lancet* **2**, 1265.
Way, L. E., Gimble, A. I., McKelway, W. P., Ross, H, Sung, C., and Ellsworth, H. (1949). *J. Pharmacol. Exp. Ther.* **96**, 477.
William, J. D., and Felton, D. J. C. (1966). *J. Obstet. Gynaecol. Brit. Commonw.* **73**, 654.
Wilson, G. S., Desmond, M. M., and Verniaud, W. M. (1973). *J. Amer. Med. Ass.* **126**, 457.
Wilson, J. G. (1973). *In* "Pathobiology of Development" (Perrin, E. V., Finegold, M. J., and Brunson, J. G., eds.), Chapter 2, p. 11. William & Wilkins, Baltimore, Maryland.
Wimsatt, W. A. (1962). *Amer. J. Obstet. Gynecol.* **84**, 1568.
Woltz, J. H. E., and Wiley, M. M. (1945). *Proc. Soc. Exp. Biol. Med.* **60**, 106.
Woltz, J. H., and Zintel, H. A. (1945). *Amer. J. Obstet. Gynecol.* **49**, 663.
World Health Organization. (1974). *World Health Organ., Tech. Rep. Ser.* **540**.
Yaffe, S. J., Rane, A., Sojqvist, F., Boreus, L., and Orrenius, S. (1970). *Life Sci.* **9**, 1189.
Yeh, S. Y., and Woods, L. A. (1970). *J. Pharmacol. Exp. Ther.* **174**, 9.
Yoshioka, H., Monna, T., and Matsuda, S. (1972). *J. Pediat.* **80**, 121.
Youkilis, M. H. (1970). *Ohio State Med. J.* **66**, 50.
Zelson, C., Rubio, E., and Wasserman, E. (1971). *Pediatrics* **48**, 178.
Zelson, C., Lee, S. J., and Casalino, M. (1973). *N. Engl. J. Med.* **289**, 1216.

2

Drug Biotransformation Reactions in the Placenta

Mont R. Juchau, Ph.D.

I. Introduction

Drug biotransformation refers to those reactions in which drug molecules are converted from one chemical species to another as a result of the sojourn of the drug molecule in a biological system. Such reactions commonly are referred to in terms of catalysis by enzymes present within that biological system. It is clear, however, that biotransformations may occur entirely unaided by catalysts, or they also may be hastened toward equilibrium by nonprotein catalysts (nonenzymatic). Most frequently they are catalyzed by enzymes existing within the biological entity. Recognition of changes in chemical species of drug molecules is of utmost interest and importance pharmacologically since each chemical species will influence the organism in a qualitatively or quantitatively different manner, thus resulting in a different type of pharmacological response. Research in recent years has demonstrated amply that drug biotransformation is not equivalent to drug inactivation or detoxication. The study

71

of drug metabolism has, in fact, been of great value in elucidating mechanisms by which drugs are able to interact with endogenous chemical species to produce specific pharmacological or toxicological effects, including carcinogenesis, mutagenesis, drug allergies, antitumor activity, tolerance, and a host of other effects for individual drugs. In many instances the observed pharmacological effect occurs as a *result* of the biotransformation of the drug molecule.

Axiomatic in pharmacology and therapeutics is the principle that a drug should not be administered unless the potential benefits derived clearly outweigh the potential harmful effects. A completely rational approach, therefore, presupposes that whosoever administers the drug has a perfect knowledge of all of the beneficial and harmful effects which will accrue following introduction of that chemical into the biological system. It is probably safe to say that no drug has ever been administered with the utilization of a completely rational approach. Rationality, of course, increases toward this goal with increases in the knowledge of chemical–biological interactions and factors which affect such interactions. Acquisition of such knowledge must be approached from at least two directions: first, a determination of those biological processes which lead to the optimal functioning of the individual (as well as his descendants) in his environment; second, a delimitation of the ways in which drugs (chemicals) introduced into the biological system will affect those same processes. The second aspect appears, at the outset, to be a particularly formidable problem because of the many thousands of possible chemicals which could affect a large number of biological processes in a variety of ways. The problem is compounded when it is considered that any given chemical species introduced into the system frequently is converted to a large number of other chemical species, each capable of exerting a different spectrum of pharmacological effects. In addition, the practical situation demands knowledge of the interactions of various drugs within the biological system since it is often the case that two or more drugs and chemicals will have been administered concurrently. Upon consideration of the many permutations and combinations, the varieties of possible pharmacological effects are truly astronomical in number. By comparison, only a very few have been described.

The situation is far worse for the developing infant since the developmental processes themselves are poorly understood and studies of the effects of drugs on the control of development (particularly with respect to humans) have only just begun. Research which is meaningful to the clinical situation is particularly difficult because of the prevalence of marked species differences in drug response to agents which influence developmental processes. These differences prevent the direct application of knowledge derived from work with experimental animal models. The differences have been particularly noticeable in teratological studies and reasons for such species specificity remain unclear. It has been suggested (Tuchmann-Duplessis, 1969) that various animal species react differently to teratogenic drugs because they handle the drugs through different metabolic pathways at different rates. This, of course, is only one of a number of possibilities, but in view of the insights into carcinogenesis and mutagenesis that studies of drug metabolism have provided, this clearly is an area which should be explored with great vigor.

This chapter deals with the role of the placenta as a determinant of the actions of drugs and foreign chemicals on the fetus, neonate, and pregnant female. During the past, most treatises on pharmacology have tended to regard the placenta as a somewhat inert distribution barrier to the transfer of drugs between the maternal and fetal bloodstreams. Research was confined largely to studies on the passage of drugs across the so-called "placental barrier" but very few detailed or systematic investigations were carried out even in this limited area. From such studies it has been learned that highly lipid-soluble drugs and anesthetic gases pass rapidly across the membranes of the placenta to enter the fetal circulation, whereas drugs which are highly water soluble (succinylcholine, d-tubocurarine, etc.) tend to pass across such membranes at slower rates. Such phenomena are comparable to those observed in the passage of chemicals across other lipid membranes which are ubiquitous in biological systems. The passage of drugs across the "placental barrier" has frequently been compared with distribution across other biological membrane "barriers," i.e., the "blood–brain barrier," membranes of the gastrointestinal tract, and renal tubules, all of which are of considerable significance with respect to the control of drug distribution within the organism. A more detailed discussion of these aspects of placental pharmacology have been dealt with in Chapter 1.

It now is becoming increasingly evident that the critical role of the placenta in the regulation of optimal development of the individual demands that pharmacological studies assume a variety of fresh approaches. The placenta performs an astounding number of complex functions, each of which is essential to optimal development of the evolving infant. This bewilderingly complex organ has been referred to as a combination gastrointestinal tract, kidney, lung, liver, spleen, thymus, and multifunctional endocrine organ with functions analgous to the anterior pituitary, ovarian follicle, and corpus luteum (Szabo and Grimaldi, 1970). The placenta transports several nutrient chemicals (i.e., amino acids, vitamins, carbohydrates, minerals, and lipids) from the maternal to fetal blood via energy-requiring transport systems. It synthesizes and catabolizes proteins, carbohydrates, lipids, nucleic acids, and steroid hormones. It possesses immunologically competent cells and hemopoietic cells. It performs many other functions, the significances of which are unknown in many cases. Yet, the manner in which drugs and foreign compounds affect these functions remains largely unexplored.

From the discussion above, it would appear that approaches to placental pharmacology should consist of at least three aspects: (a) the disposition (transport, binding, degradation, and bioactivation) of pharmacological and toxicological agents that come in contact with placental tissues; (b) the capacity of the placenta to synthesize substances capable of modifying the pharmacological–toxicological effects of biologically active chemicals; and (c) the effects of drugs and other chemicals upon the multiple functions of the placenta. Some of these aspects have been the subject of recent critical reviews (Juchau, 1973; Yaffe and Juchau, 1974). Knowledge of each aspect seems essential to a rational approach to therapeutic drug usage during pregnancy and also should better equip the physician in advising the expectant mother with regard to environmental chemicals which should be avoided as potential hazards to herself or to the developing conceptus.

II. Drug Metabolism in the Human Placenta

A. General Principles of Xenobiotic Biotransformation

The distinction which normally is made in order to distinguish drug-metabolic processes from other forms of metabolism is based on the foreign or nonendogenous nature of the substrate under investigation. Foreign, nonendogenous compounds also are referred to as xenobiotics and, since most drugs are xenobiotics, it is convenient to refer to the metabolism of foreign substances as drug metabolism or, less commonly, xenobiotic metabolism. Owing to the ambiguous nature of the word "drug," however, many scientific writers do not confine their discussions of drug metabolism to analyses of xenobiotic biotransformation. Frequently included are certain considerations of the metabolism of important biogenic amines which are of considerable interest to pharmacologists. In this chapter an attempt is made to distinguish between processes involved in the metabolism of foreign versus endogenous substrates in placental tissues. While such a distinction might seem completely arbitrary it appears to be necessary at the present time. Although the emphasis will be directed toward xenobiotic biotransformation mechanisms, other aspects of placental metabolism which are of interest pharmacologically will be discussed.

CLASSIFICATION OF DRUG-METABOLIC PROCESSES

A large number of the enzymes involved in the catalysis of xenobiotic biotransformation reactions are concentrated in the liver. Most of the studies of drug metabolism have described reactions occurring in hepatic tissues, tissue slices, homogenates, or homogenate subfractions. The rat has been employed extensively as a model in which to study such metabolic processes. Therefore, most of the classificatory nomenclature and descriptions of drug-metabolic reactions are based upon observations of these phenomena in rat liver preparations.

Lyases, isomerases, and ligases traditionally are not considered to participate in drug-metabolic reactions, and the usual statement is that drug biotransformations occur via four principal processes: oxidation, reduction, hydrolysis, and conjugation mechanisms. These four reaction types would involve oxidoreductases, transferases, and hydrolases insofar as enzymatic participation is concerned. Oxidoreductases and hydrolases catalyze nonsynthetic reactions which also frequently are referred to as "phase I" reactions because they sometimes precede reactions catalyzed by transferase enzymes. Transferases catalyze synthetic reactions (conjugations) which may be referred to as "phase II" reactions although they do not always succeed nonsynthetic reactions. Since a large number of drug-metabolizing enzymes are concentrated in the endoplasmic reticulum, such biotransformation reactions also have been classified on a morphological basis. Homogenized isolated fragments of the endoplasmic reticulum are referred to as microsomes and drug-metabolic reactions have been categorized as microsomal versus nonmicrosomal. Therefore, drug-metabolic reactions may be classified according to Table I.

It should be emphasized that the classification in Table I is by no means complete, and in addition, it is still unclear as to whether certain of these reactions occur microsomally, extramicrosomally, or perhaps both. For additional details of classification of drug biotransformation reactions, one should refer to the *Handbook of Experimental Pharmacology*, Volume 28, Part 2 (1971).

Because of the extreme importance of mixed-function oxidation reactions and glucuronidation, it is not surprising that these have received the greatest attention. Fortuitously, both of these reaction types are "microsomal," thus providing an explanation for the large numbers of studies performed on microsomal drug-metabolizing enzymes and the corresponding relative neglect of drug biotransformations occurring outside the endoplasmic reticulum.

TABLE I   Classification of Drug-Metabolic Reactions

Microsomal	Nonmicrosomal
1. *Oxidation*	1. *Oxidation*
Hydroxylation	Dehydrogenation
Epoxide formation	Deamination
N-Oxidation	Aldehyde oxidation
Dealkylation	Alcohol oxidation
Deamination	Amine oxidation
Desulfuration	Aromatization (alicyclic)
Sulfoxide formation	Oxidative ring scission
Dehalogenation	Dehydration
2. *Reduction*	2. *Reduction*
Aromatic nitro group reduction	Hydrogenation of double bonds
Azo linkage reduction	Aldehyde reduction
Dehalogenation	Dehydroxylation
	N-Oxide reduction
	Sulfoxide reduction
	Dehalogenation
3. *Hydrolysis*	3. *Hydrolysis*
Carboxylic acid ester hydrolysis	Carboxylic acid ester hydrolysis
Amide hydrolysis	Amide hydrolysis
Sulfate ester hydrolysis (type I)	Ring scission
	Hydroxamic acid hydrolysis
	Hydrazide hydrolysis
	Carbamate hydrolysis
	Nitrile hydrolysis
	Dehalogenation
	Glucuronide hydrolysis
	Sulfate ester hydrolysis (type II)
	Phosphate ester hydrolysis
4. *Conjugation*	4. *Conjugation*
Glucuronidation	Sulfation
	Acetylation
	Amino acid conjugation
	Riboside formation
	Methylation
	Mercapturic acid formation
	Thiocyanate formation
	Phosphorylation

B. Oxidative Reactions

Of the microsomal mixed-function oxidative reactions, hydroxylations
and dealkylations have been the most intensively investigated. On the
basis of sex differences in the rates of biotransformation (in rats), of
the types of spectral changes produced when added to suspensions of rat

liver microsomes, and on differences in the rates of metabolism following pretreatment of rats with various chemicals which produce induction of drug-metabolic pathways, substrates for hydroxylation and dealkylation reactions may be placed arbitrarily into three categories. Substrate prototypes of the first category (Group I) include hexobarbital, pentobarbital, ethylmorphine, aminopyrine, and benzphetamine. Hexobarbital and pentobarbital undergo extensive hydroxylation whereas the latter three compounds undergo biotransformation via oxidative N-demethylation reactions. Substrates and primary reaction products are illustrated in reactions (1)–(5).

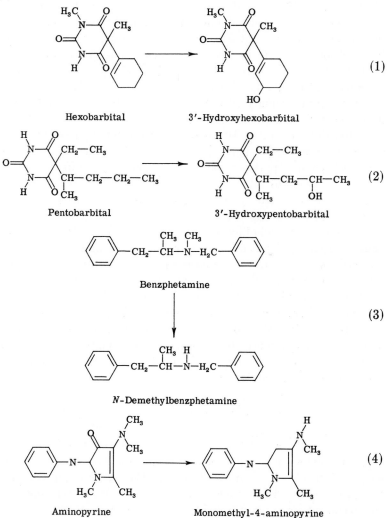

Hexobarbital   3′-Hydroxyhexobarbital   (1)

Pentobarbital   3′-Hydroxypentobarbital   (2)

Benzphetamine   (3)

N-Demethylbenzphetamine

Aminopyrine   Monomethyl-4-aminopyrine   (4)

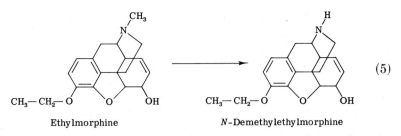

Ethylmorphine   N-Demethylethylmorphine

(5)

When added to suspensions of rat liver microsomes these substrates produce a characteristic "type I" difference spectrum with maxima at approximately 385 nm and minima at approximately 420 nm. These same substrates are metabolized much more rapidly by male rats than by females both *in vivo* and *in vitro*. (Such sex differences in drug metabolism do not appear to be marked in most other species of experimental animals or in humans. In certain strains of mice, the females metabolize substrates of Group I more rapidly than do the males.) Pretreatment of experimental animals with phenobarbital, a powerful inducer of certain drug-metabolic reactions, markedly increases the rates of oxidation of this group of substrates. However, pretreatment with certain polycyclic aromatic hydrocarbon-inducing agents (e.g., 3-methylcholanthrene or benzo[a]pyrene) appears to produce a slight decrease in rates of metabolism of this group of substrates.

The substrate prototype of the second category (Group II) is aniline. Members of this group usually are considered to include basic nitrogeneous compounds including primary amines, whereas typical amine compounds of Group I are most frequently tertiary amines. When added to suspensions of rat liver microsomes, Group II compounds produce a difference spectrum with a maximum in the area of 430 nm and a minimum at approximately 390 nm. Pretreatment of experimental animals with either phenobarbital or 3-methylcholanthrene can markedly increase the rate of aniline hydroxylation and the magnitude of the difference spectrum. Sex differences in the rate of hydroxylation of Group II compounds do not appear to exist. The predominant reaction in liver microsomes is shown in reaction (6).

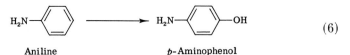

Aniline   p-Aminophenol

(6)

A third category of substrates for hepatic microsomal mixed-function oxidases can also be envisioned (Group III). This group would include benzo[a]pyrene, 3-methylcholanthrene, and 3'-methyl-4-monomethyl-aminoazobenzene (3-methyl-MAB) as prototype substrates. Although such compounds may yield the typical type I difference spectra when added to suspensions of rat liver microsomes, they display characteristics which differ markedly from substrates of Group I. Pretreatment of experimental animals with phenobarbital produces low to moderate induction of the enzymes which catalyze hepatic metabolism of these substrates, but pretreatment with 3-methylcholanthrene or benzo[a]pyrene results in very rapid reaction rates. In addition, it has been demonstrated recently that compounds in Group I exhibit a preference for one microsomal cytochrome (P-450) as the terminal oxidase in the system whereas benzo[a]pyrene apparently prefers a different cytochrome (P-448) as the terminal oxidizing enzyme (Lu et al., 1971). Reactions for substrates of the third category are illustrated in reactions (7)–(9). It should be borne

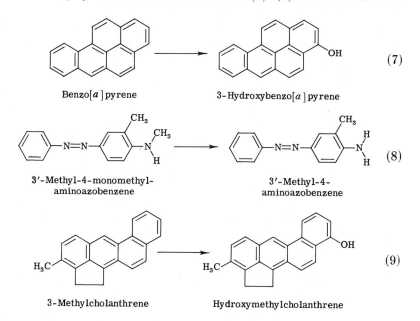

Benzo[a]pyrene → 3-Hydroxybenzo[a]pyrene (7)

3′-Methyl-4-monomethyl-aminoazobenzene → 3′-Methyl-4-aminoazobenzene (8)

3-Methylcholanthrene → Hydroxymethylcholanthrene (9)

in mind that a very large number of oxidized metabolites can be produced and that the reactions illustrated provide only examples of possible reactions.

Oxidation of substrates of each of the three categories requires molecular oxygen and a reduced pyridine nucleotide (NADPH is the preferred electron donor). One atom of the oxygen molecule is incorporated into the drug substrate, and the other atom is reduced to water. A unique electron transport system, present predominantly in the smooth-surfaced endoplasmic reticulum of hepatic cells functions in the catalysis of these mixed-function oxidase systems. A highly simplified version of the sequence is illustrated in reaction (10). Reducing equivalents (NADPH)

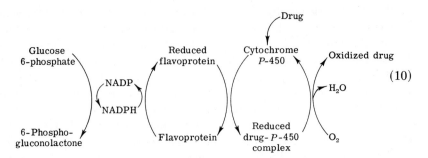

$$(10)$$

appear to be generated principally via the hexosemonophosphate shunt pathway. Electrons are transferred then to a membrane-bound, NADPH-specific flavoprotein (microsomal NADPH cytochrome c reductase) which in turn reduces microsomal cytochrome P-450 (or P-448) that previously, in the oxidized form, had combined with the drug substrate. Molecular oxygen reacts with the reduced drug–cytochrome complex to eventually result in the formation of water and the oxidized drug substrate which dissociates from the cytochrome. The oxidized form of the cytochrome also is regenerated. A research question which has aroused considerable interest in recent years asks whether cytochrome P-450 and cytochrome P-448 (also called cytochrome P-466 and cytochrome P_1-450) are two separate cytochromes or two interconvertible forms of the same cytochrome. At present the question remains unresolved. The components of the electron transport complex, however, have been isolated and a functional system (which apparently requires the addition of phosphatidylcholine) has been reconstituted *in vitro* (Autor *et al.*, 1971). The same complex appears to catalyze the ω-oxidation of fatty acids, and certain steroid hydroxylations, which occur in hepatic microsomes, also will proceed in the presence of the reconstituted system.

Of the extramicrosomal xenobiotic oxidative biotransformation enzyme catalysts, alcohol dehydrogenase (EC 1.1.1.1) has been studied extensively. Other extramicrosomal oxidations which have received attention, however, are frequently considered in discussions of drug metabolism. Most prominent among these are the amine oxidases, certain dehalogenations, and deaminations.

Interest in the capacity of the placenta to oxidize foreign compounds first became apparent in 1965 when Creaven and Parke (1965) reported negative results with respect to the biotransformation of some typical drug substrates. This report, however, was in abstract form; thus details of these early attempts were not universally available. Shortly thereafter, however, several reports—many negative—concerning placental drug-metabolic reactions began to appear in the permanent literature. Some of the major factors which appear to have encouraged investigators to search for drug-oxidizing capacity in the placenta include:

1. The fact that the placenta is an organ of major metabolic capacities with respect to catalysis of the biotransformation of a multitude of endogenous substrates tends to indicate that it also should contain enzyme systems for catalysis of drug biotransformation reactions as well.

2. The presence of significant quantities of smooth endoplasmic reticulum in trophoblastic cells, while not evidence for, is consistent with the concept of placental drug-hydroxylating systems. (Mixed-function oxidases for drug substrates are highly concentrated in the smooth endoplasmic reticulum of hepatic cells.)

3. A concept has emerged which suggests that steroids and fatty acids are "natural" substrates for the enzymes which catalyze drug hydroxylation reactions. The concept developed in tandem to a growing awareness that some of the most important functions of the placenta were connected with steroid hydroxylation reactions, particularly on the 19, 20, and 22 carbon atoms of the steroid molecule.

4. The fact of a growing concern for the effects of drugs on the fetus, neonate, and pregnant female. Each of these organisms has been referred to as a "therapeutic orphan" due to lack of knowledge concerning mechanisms of drug effects within those species. The presence of drug biotransformation systems in the placenta could help to explain such effects.

5. The easy availability of large quantities of human tissues at several stages of development rendered the placenta an attractive organ for study, particularly in view of the difficulties involved in obtaining suitable quantities of fresh human liver tissue for drug-metabolism research.

Almost simultaneously, reports on placental drug metabolism from eight widely scattered laboratories appeared in the literature in 1968 and 1969. As might be expected, many of these reports were of a preliminary nature and contained much descriptive rather than rigorously quantitative information. Some of the most interesting data originated from the laboratories of Welch and his co-workers. In preliminary experiments with rats, Welch and Harrison (1967) were able to detect placental hydroxylation of benzo[a]pyrene between 14 and 21 days gestation. The ability of placental homogenates to metabolize benzo[a]pyrene was increased approximately 15 times at 24 hours after oral administration of 3-methylcholanthrene or benzo[a]pyrene. Twofold increases were observed following administration of chlorpromazine, but pretreatment of pregnant rats with phenobarbital, chlorcyclizine, acetanilide, acetophene-tidin, or zoxazolamine did not appear to affect rat placental benzpyrene hydroxylase activity. (Benzpyrene hydroxylase is also referred to as aryl hydrocarbon hydroxylase.) On the basis of these studies, interest was generated in determining whether the human placenta contained a similar enzyme system. Subsequently, Welch *et al.* (1968a,b, 1969) reported that hydroxylation of benzo[a]pyrene could be detected in homogenates of placentas from women who smoked cigarettes, whereas activity was not detectable in placentas of nonsmokers. However, there appeared to be no relationship between the number of cigarettes smoked and the specific activity of the human hydroxylase system, even though a good dose–response relationship between the dose of polycyclic hydrocarbon inducer and specific enzymatic activity could be shown in the case of rat placentas (Welch *et al.*, 1968a). It was also shown that the rate of N-demethyl-ation of 3′-methyl-4-monomethylaminoazobenzene was closely correlated with the rate of benzpyrene hydroxylation in human placental homoge-nates at term (Welch *et al.*, 1969). Thus it was demonstrated that two substrates of the third category (Group III) could be oxidized by virtue of mixed-function oxidases present in human placental tissues. The same workers, however, were unable to detect any significant hydroxylation of [2-^{14}C]pentobarbital (a Group I substrate) following incubation of homogenates equivalent to 400 mg of human placental tissue for 30 min-utes. Negative results were obtained in placentas of four nonsmokers as well as in the corresponding preparations of smokers. They also tested several polycyclic hydrocarbons known to be present in cigarette smoke for their ability to induce benzpyrene hydroxylase in rat placentas. 1,2-Benzanthracene, 1,2,5,6-dibenzanthracene, benzo[a]pyrene, and chrysene were approximately equipotent in stimulating the hydroxylase system. 3,4-Benzofluorene, anthracene, pyrene, fluoranthrene, perylene, and phen-anthrene also induced the enzyme in decreasing order of potency.

In a separate study, Nebert *et al.* (1969) found less correlation between smoking habits and human placental benzpyrene hydroxylase activity. In determining activity from 97 placentas they observed significantly higher activity in homogenates of smokers but they also observed com-paratively high activity in placentas of some nonsmokers and no measur-able activity in placentas of a few smokers. This contrasts with the stud-ies of Welch *et al.* (1969) who found no activity in the placentas of nonsmokers and activity in all of the placentas from smokers. In studies with hamster placentas, Nebert and his co-workers were unable to induce benzpyrene hydroxylase activity by pretreatment with phenobarbital, although activity of the same enzyme system was elevated in maternal liver and lung as well as in the fetal liver. Also, two nonsmoking women to whom phenobarbital was administered throughout pregnancy did not show elevated hydroxylating capacity.

Juchau et al. (1968a) had previously reported absence of detectable levels of benzpyrene hydroxylase in placentas obtained from therapeutic abortions at 9–12 weeks gestation. In that study the women had not been screened with regard to smoking habits. In a later study (Juchau, 1971b) it was found that placentas of 8–12 weeks gestation displayed only negligible levels of activity regardless of the smoking habits of the mother. The activity in smokers appeared to increase with gestational age, and these studies have been confirmed by other workers in more recent experiments (Pelkonen et al., 1972). Lack of placental enzymes which catalyze xenobiotic biotransformations during the first trimester of pregnancy, however, could have important implications with respect to the effects of foreign compounds on the fetus, particularly since the majority of known teratogens appears to be most deleterious when administered during this period. A teratogen could be more inaccessible to the fetus because of its conversion to polar or nontoxic derivatives by placental catalytic systems. On the other hand, the placenta conceivably could convert an inactive chemical to an active teratogen, mutagen, or carcinogen.

In studies of some of the characteristics of rat and human placental benzpyrene hydroxylase, it was found that, although some differences between these systems were observed, the similarities appeared to be more striking (Bogdan and Juchau, 1970; Juchau, 1971b). The systems were similar with respect to kinetic parameters (although V_{max} values for the human system appeared somewhat higher), the effects of various inhibitors, subcellular localization, pH optima, and apparent inducibility. The more important question that arises regards the comparison of capacities of maternal liver, fetus, and placenta to metabolize this important environmental carcinogen. A direct comparison of rat maternal liver, fetal liver, placenta, and hepatectomized fetus has been made (Bogdan and Juchau, 1970). The placenta also has been compared with several human fetal tissues (Juchau et al., 1972; Juchau and Pederson, 1973). Rat and human placentas have been compared but no direct comparisons have been made between human hepatic versus human placental enzymatic activity. Such comparisons would be extremely important but should be made with caution since profound differences between rat maternal hepatic and placental benzpyrene hydroxylase activities have been observed, the maternal liver preparations catalyzing the reaction at rates which were one to two orders of magnitude higher than placental preparations. Early studies (Welch and Harrison, 1967; Bogdan et al., 1969) indicated a difference in the subcellular distribution of the placental versus hepatic enzyme systems; however, later studies (Juchau and

Smuckler, 1973; Gough *et al.*, 1975) have revealed that the placental
hydroxylase system is localized primarily in the endoplasmic reticulum
of the syncitium. One of the principle differences between maternal hepatic and placental benzpyrene hydroxylating systems is with respect
to the apparent affinity of NADPH for the two systems (Bogdan and
Juchau, 1970; Juchau, 1971b). Plots of reciprocal activity versus reciprocal NADPH concentrations revealed that K_m values for maternal liver
preparations were at least one order of magnitude lower than values derived from studies on placental tissues. Both human and rodent placental
systems were much more difficult to saturate with NADPH than the
corresponding hepatic system. The difficulty is not due to a rapid degradation of the nucleotide (Juchau and Zachariah, 1975). The maternal
system also appeared to be more sensitive to induction by 3-methyl-
cholanthrene and more sensitive to inhibition by flavins. All systems exhibited approximately equal sensitivity to carbon monoxide inhibition.

It thus appears to be well established that placentas of experimental
animals and humans possess an enzyme system capable of catalyzing
mixed-function oxidase reactions involving xenobiotic substrates from
Group III. An important question which arises asks whether this enzyme
system also catalyzes the hydroxylation of steroids or is important to
other placental functions. Evidence has been obtained which indicated
that the benzo[*a*]pyrene hydroxylating system differs from either the cholesterol side-chain oxidizing system, which is rate limiting for placental
progesterone production, or the aromatase system, which is rate limiting
for estrogen biosynthesis in human placentas. Substrates for the side-
chain oxidizing system (cholesterol) or aromatase complex (dehydroepiandrosterone, androstenedione, testosterone) were not particularly potent
inhibitors of the human placental benzpyrene hydroxylase (Juchau,
1971b), which might be expected if the same system catalyzed hydroxylation of both drug and steroid molecules. Estrogens and progesterone, on
the other hand, were relatively potent inhibitors of benzpyrene hydroxylation even though they are products rather than substrates of these
two important placental steroid-synthesizing systems. Even so, substrates
for aromatase and side-chain oxidation of cholesterol appeared to exert
slightly more pronounced effects in human placental preparations than
in the corresponding rat placental or rat liver preparations (Bogdan and
Juchau, 1970; Juchau, 1971b). Such an observation might be expected
in view of the fact that rodent placentas or livers do not appear to synthesize progesterone or estrogens (Ryan, 1969). Carbon monoxide was
found to have little or no effect on the aromatization reaction (Meigs
and Ryan, 1968, 1971), whereas cyanide inhibits this system. The converse is true for placental benzpyrene hydroxylase since 10^{-3} *M* KCN

had no effect on the system, and carbon monoxide inhibited the placental system as effectively as it inhibited the hepatic system. Recently, Meigs and Ryan (1971) have reported that carbon monoxide would inhibit the conversion of 19-norsteroids to estrogens in tissues of the human placenta. Yet if carbon monoxide did not inhibit the overall reaction, this would seem to indicate either that a carbon monoxide sensitive component of the reaction was not rate limiting or that the cytochrome exhibited a low affinity for carbon monoxide as compared to its affinity for oxygen. Thompson and Siiteri (1974) have speculated that lack of inhibition by CO may be due to a limited rate of entry of the first electron into the oxidized P-450 substrate complex. Zachariah and Juchau (1975) however, have shown that endogenous substrates may prevent CO from binding to the cytochrome.

Side-chain oxidation of cholesterol occurs in mitochondrial fractions and is sensitive to carbon monoxide inhibition (Mason and Boyd, 1971). Significant quantities of cytochrome P-450 have been detected within this fraction, and P-450 is assumed to act as a terminal oxidase for the rate-limiting step in progesterone biosynthesis. However, cytochrome P-450 is present in abundance in adrenal mitochondria and microsomes, yet these homogenate fractions do not catalyze most of the classic drug hydroxylations. Therefore, the common requirements for NADPH, molecular oxygen, NADPH-specific flavoprotein, and cytochrome P-450 do not necessarily indicate common metabolic pathways, and it now appears that enzyme systems which catalyze placental oxidation of steroid carbons 19, 20, or 22 are not the same systems which catalyze hydroxylation of benzo[a]pyrene and that they exhibit a high specificity for their steroid substrates. It may be more logical to expect that placental systems that catalyze 6-hydroxylation of a number of steroid molecules or 2-hydroxylation of estrogens could be the same as those which catalyze benzpyrene hydroxylation since, of the steroids tested, estrone and β-estradiol were the most potent inhibitors of placental benzpyrene hydroxylase. This possibility has not yet been investigated.

Still another important question pertaining to placental benzpyrene hydroxylase concerns the significance of the hydroxylating system to the fetus, newborn infant, or pregnant mother. Benzo[a]pyrene is a potent carcinogen, but the hydroxylated product is noncarcinogenic. This consideration could lead one to believe that the placental hydroxylase is acting as an additional protective mechanism for the fetus and/or mother. It should be noted, however, that studies with cultured cells have shown that those cells which hydroxylate polycyclic hydrocarbons at significant rates are more susceptible to toxicity (cell death) than cells which lack this capacity (Nebert and Gelboin, 1968). Also it has been shown (Gel-

boin, 1969) that the rat hepatic enzyme system which catalyzes
benzo[a]pyrene hydroxylation also catalyzes the formation of hydrocarbon–DNA complexes indicating that the enzyme may be important in
the binding of the hydrocarbon to DNA *in vivo*. It is considered possible
that intermediate epoxides may be carcinogenic and mutagenic and,
therefore, possibly also teratogenic. Therefore, it is of interest that the
epoxide hydrase activity observed in human placentas is very low, does
not increase with cigarette smoking, and is not correlated with benzo-
[a]pyrene hydroxylase activities (Juchau and Namkung, 1974).

The principal observed effect of cigarette smoking during pregnancy
concerns a significantly decreased birth weight (approximately 13 ounces
lighter on the average) and a possibly higher infant mortality. At present,
it is not known whether the marked increases in drug hydroxylation observed in placentas of cigarette smokers are causally related to decreases
in birth weight of the offspring. This remains an extremely interesting
question for future investigations. The question of transplacental carcinogenesis via cigarette smoking is possibly even more important.

Although by far the most extensively investigated, benzo[a]pyrene is
not the only substrate which has been reported to be metabolized via
monooxygenase enzymes in placental tissues. Compounds of Group I have
been the substrates most frequently investigated. A critical review of
studies in this area has recently appeared (Juchau, 1973). Only a very
few studies have been carried out, however, and much of the data appears
to be conflicting. In one early study (Van Petten *et al.*, 1968), it was
reported that 9000 *g* supernatant fractions of homogenates of human
placentas obtained at term would catalyze the oxidation of pentobarbital
at rates which approached those observed in corresponding preparations
of rat liver. The women in the study had received only meperidine as
medication immediately prior to delivery. The results obtained in these
investigations, however, have not been substantiated by the results obtained in other laboratories. As previously mentioned, Welch *et al.* (1969)
were unable to detect any significant hydroxylation of pentobarbital in
their experiments with human placentas at term. Juchau and Yaffe
(1969) were unable to demonstrate hexobarbital oxidation at several gestational stages and also reported that metabolisms of other Group I substrates (aminopyrine, codeine) were undetectable during early gestation
or at term. Creaven and Parke (1965) also were unable to detect typical
oxidations of foreign compounds in the placenta. More recent investigations (Symms and Juchau, 1973; Bergheim *et al.*, 1973; Juchau *et al.*,
1974; Juchau and Zachariah, 1975; Zachariah and Juchau, 1975) have
shown that type I substrates do not bind to human placental cytochrome

P-450 and that lack of measurable drug hydroxylation is most probably
due to a high substrate specificity of the placental microsomal mixed-
function oxidase system. The problem is deserving of further attention,
particularly in view of the reports of hydroxylation of Group I substrates
by preparations of placentas from experimental animals and of the hydroxylation of various substrates in the presence of cultures of human
trophoblasts. Dixon and Willson (1968) reported that homogenate fractions of rabbit placentas would not metabolize hexobarbital at 2, 3, or
4 weeks gestation but that pretreatment of the pregnant animals with
chlordane caused significant placental hexobarbital oxidation at 2 weeks,
Pretreatment with phenobarbital, however, did not produce an observable
effect on hexobarbital metabolism. This is a somewhat surprising observation in view of the very similar nature of the enzyme-inducing properties
of chlordane and phenobarbital. This apparent discrepancy may be explicable in terms of a differential capacity of chlordane and phenobarbital
to gain access to trophoblastic cell components. Also, it should be regarded with rather strong reservations due to difficulties in the assay of
hexobarbital oxidation. A disappearance assay was employed with all
the attendant difficulties in the interpretation of results, but in addition,
these investigators admitted to the extraction of substances from their
incubation flasks which absorbed ultraviolet light at the same wave-
lengths in which hexobarbital was being determined. In addition, Pecile
et al. (1969) have examined rat and rabbit placentas for capacity to
oxidize strychnine, a compound which displays characteristics of those
in Group I. Reaction (11) is believed to occur. They were unable to dem-

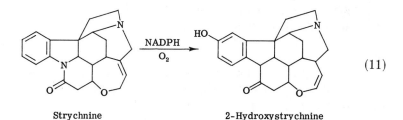

$$\text{Strychnine} \qquad\qquad \text{2-Hydroxystrychnine} \tag{11}$$

onstrate significant metabolism of this substrate in either species near
the end of gestation but reported that pretreatment of the pregnant animals with phenobarbital resulted in measurable rates of placental hydroxylation in both species. Partial maternal hepatectomy did not appear
to enhance phenobarbital induction. Again, disappearance assays were
utilized and recovery data were not reported, rendering the results subject
to uncertainty.

Uher (1969) has reported hydroxylation of drugs in the presence of cultures of human trophoblasts. The substrates examined were keto-phenylbutazone, benzopyrazone, and mebrophenhydramine, which, though not determined, probably fit best into the category of Group I substrates. The structures of these compounds are given below; however, no details of the hydroxylations have been reported as yet.

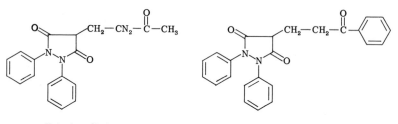

Ketophenylbutazone   Benzopyrazone

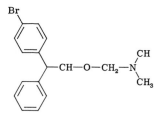

Mebrophenhydramine

In an earlier report, Uher et al. (1966) had found that the chorion and fetus from a pregnant woman which had been given benzopyrazone contained a metabolite more polar than benzopyrazone. This metabolite did not appear in the serum or urine of the mother indicating a possible role of the placenta in the metabolism of the anti-inflammatory drug.

The metabolism of three compounds which might be placed in the Group II category have been investigated with respect to placental hydroxylation catalysis. These are aniline (the prototype of this group), amphetamine, and zoxazolamine. Amphetamine can produce a "type II" difference spectrum when added to suspensions of rat liver microsomes but has not been investigated with respect to sex differences in rates of metabolism in rats. No sex differences appear to occur in the case of zoxazolamine metabolism; phenobarbital and polycyclic hydrocarbons both markedly increase metabolic rates, but addition of zoxazolamine to rat liver microsomal suspensions yields "type I" difference spectra. Typical reactions for zoxazolamine and amphetamine are given in (12) and (13). Steps 1 and 2 are catalyzed by the typical hepatic microsomal

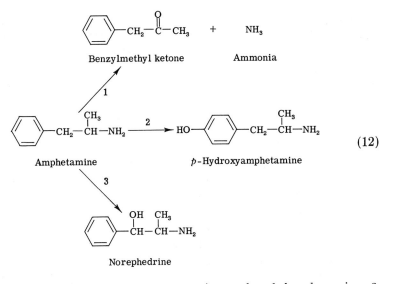

(12)

mixed-function oxidase system; step 3 is catalyzed by dopamine β-hydroxylase (EC 1.14.1.7.1).

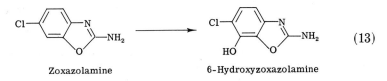

(13)

Van Petten *et al.* (1968) reported that human placental 9000 *g* supernatant fractions would catalyze NADPH-dependent oxidation of amphetamine at rates which were approximately equivalent to those observed in corresponding rat liver preparations (on the basis of micromoles metabolized per gram protein per hour). Substrate disappearance was measured in these experiments but recovery from reaction flasks reportedly was 98 ± 5%. Juchau *et al.* (1968a) were unable to detect significant rates of amphetamine metabolism in placentas from 9 to 12 weeks gestation or at term (Juchau and Yaffe, 1969). The woman involved in the latter study, however, had received several drugs prior to operations or delivery, whereas those in the former study had received only meperidine. The discrepancy may be explicable upon that basis but more studies clearly are required to answer the question.

Dixon and Willson (1968) reported that 9000 *g* supernatant fractions of rabbit placental homogenates would catalyze hydroxylation of zoxazolamine at 1, 2, and 3 weeks gestation. Pretreatment of the pregnant animals with phenobarbital did not appear to affect the rate of placental metabolism but chlordane pretreatment appeared to accelerate the reactions somewhat. These observations may indicate a species difference since Juchau and Yaffe (1969) were unable to detect significant hydroxylation of zoxazolamine in human placentas at 9–12 weeks or at term. What initially appeared to be zoxazolamine metabolism in human placental homogenates from early gestation was found to be incomplete extraction of zoxazolamine from reaction vessels. (Substrate disappearance is measured in these assays.) Since Dixon and Willson did not report recovery data, it is feasible that incomplete extraction of zoxazolamine in their experiments may have been interpreted as hydroxylation.

Symms and Juchau (1971) have reported the presence of an unusual aniline-hydroxylating system in placental homogenates of humans and rodents. Surprisingly, the placental aniline-hydroxylating system was localized in 104,000 g supernatant (soluble) fractions and was not detectably present in particulate subfractions; even in those subfractions with extremely high benzpyrene hydroxylase activity (Juchau, 1971a). Kinetic analyses indicated a very low affinity of the substrate (aniline HCl) for the placental enzyme system which could account for the very low specific activities observed. Pretreatment of experimental animals with phenobarbital or 3-methylcholanthrene did not affect the placental catalysis of aniline hydroxylation but markedly accelerated the reaction in maternal livers. Later studies with human placentas at term (Juchau and Symms, 1972) with ammonium sulfate fractionation and column chromatography have indicated that placental aniline-hydroxylating activity was associated almost exclusively with hemoglobin-rich fractions. (Placental soluble fractions contain varying quantities of hemoglobin owing to the difficulty of clearing placental tissues of blood prior to homogenizing.) Substitution of highly purified crystalline hemoglobin (recrystallized three times) for placental soluble fractions in reaction vessels resulted in an easily measurable reaction. Cytochrome c also could substitute for hemoglobin but was a much less efficient catalyst. Addition of xanthine oxidase to flasks containing cytochrome c, however, markedly accelerated the reaction rate. A flavin was not required as a component of the tissue-free reaction system but markedly accelerated the rate of the ferrihemoglobin-catalyzed reactions. The para-hydroxylated derivative appeared to be the major metabolite, in consonance with the reaction catalyzed in hepatic microsomes. These results indicated that the presence of heme compounds (primarily hemoglobin) in soluble fractions of human placental homogenates is responsible for catalysis of p-hydroxylation of aniline and that human placental cells possess very little hydroxylating capacity with respect to aniline hydrocholoride as substrate (Juchau and Symms, 1972; Symms and Juchau, 1974; Juchau and Zachariah, 1975). These observations also may relate to the capacity of both polycyclic hydrocarbon inducers and phenobarbital to accelerate hepatic microsomal aniline hydroxylation. Polycyclic hydrocarbons increase predominantly the microsomal content of cytochrome P-448, whereas pentobarbital pretreatment results in a greater increase of cytochrome P-450 than P-448. Since it seems apparent that a variety of heme compounds will catalyze the reaction (particularly in the presence of flavins), increases in any microsomal cytochrome (P-450, P-448, b_5, etc.) could increase the reaction rate. Also, since microsomal fractions of placental homogenates did not measurably catalyze aniline hydroxylation, this would tend to indicate that such fractions possessed low levels of all hemoproteins. Recent measurements of concentrations of various hemoproteins in washed placental microsomes (Juchau and Zachariah, 1975) indicated that as compared to rat hepatic microsomes, these subfractions contained less than one-sixth the concentration of total heme (per gram of protein). In addition, only slightly more than one-half of the heme could be accounted for in terms of cytochrome P-450, cytochrome b_5, and hemoglobin.

Various investigators have reported mixed-function oxidation of several other xenobiotics in placental tissues *in vitro* including biphenyl (Lake et al., 1973), N-methyl aniline (Pelkonen et al., 1972), methylaminobenzoic acid (Juchau and Zachariah, 1975), 3-methylcholanthrene (Guibbert et al., 1972), aminopyrine, codeine, and phenazone (Traeger et al., 1972), hexobarbital (Keyegombe et al., 1973), coumarin (Feuer, 1973), and aminopyrine (Rane et al., 1973). These reports remain to be confirmed.

Of xenobiotic oxidations which proceed other than via mixed-function oxidative mechanisms, alcohol dehydrogenase has been reported to occur in placental tissues (Hagerman, 1969). The enzyme reportedly is linked to NAD and is present in the soluble fraction of human placental homogenates but has not been purified or studied in detail. Monoamine and diamine oxidase are present in relatively high concentrations in human placental tissues and may play an important role in placental drug-metabolic processes (Bardsley et al., 1974).

C. Reduction Reactions

Although normally considered to be of lesser significance than oxidation reactions in drug metabolism, reductions of xenobiotic substrates have commanded attention for a number of compelling reasons. Reduction reactions are frequently simpler, both from a mechanistic viewpoint as well as in terms of analysis facility. Several compounds to which the human population is frequently exposed, medicinally or otherwise, are metabolized via reduction processes.

The principal xenobiotic reduction reactions which have been studied in mammalian systems include the reductions of azo linkages, aromatic nitro groups, double bonds, disulfides, sulfoxides, N-oxides, and aldehydes. In particular, azo linkage and nitro group reduction have been studied rather intensively because of rapid catalysis of these reactions by hepatic microsomal components. However, by definition, the acceptance of one or more electrons by any xenobiotic compound within a biological system constitutes a drug biotransformation reaction. Thus, indicator dyes reduced in tissues in histochemical studies provide examples of xenobiotic reduction reactions. These reactions occur ubiquitously and normally are given little consideration. Thus, it was not extremely surprising when Juchau and Yaffe (1967) demonstrated that placental homogenates would catalyze the transfer of electrons from NADPH or NADH to single electron acceptors such as potassium ferricyanide (KCN) or cytochrome *c* and two electron acceptors such as 2,6-dichlorophenolindophenol (DCPIP) even though these experiments were some of the first to focus attention on placental drug metabolism. NADPH and NADH appeared to serve equally well as electron donors in reactions involving potassium ferricyanide, but NADH was more efficient in the reduction of cytochrome *c* and DCPIP. Reduction of menadione and biliverdin which are two-electron acceptor molecules, could not be demonstrated although the former substrate was not studied intensively. Lack of a biliverdin reducing system in placental tissues may provide a partial explanation for the occurrence of biliverdin in amniotic fluid during early stages of gestation (Krasner *et al.*, 1971).

Of considerably greater interest was the demonstration that reduction of the azo linkage of neoprontosil was markedly accelerated in the presence of several human placental homogenate subfractions [reaction (14)].

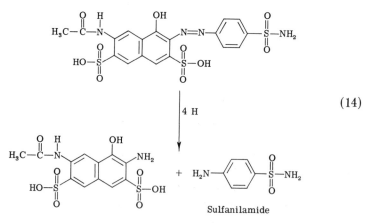

$$(14)$$

Sulfanilamide

The reaction proceeds via a hydrazo intermediate (—NH—NH—) and requires the transfer of four electrons to form the final reaction products. Initial studies of the reaction in homogenates of placental tissue provided some surprising results (Juchau et al., 1968b) that indicated striking differences in comparison to the azo reductase system(s) present in hepatic tissues. Although NADPH appeared to be the preferred electron donor, the placental reaction system was not inhibited significantly by carbon monoxide or oxygen and was inhibited rather than activated by flavins. Also in contrast to the hepatic system, placental azo reductase appeared to be localized in the soluble fraction rather than the microsomal fraction of tissue homogenates. In marked contrast to the hepatic azo reductase, the placental system was not influenced by pretreatment of experimental animals with phenobarbital or 3-methylcholanthrene. Recognition of the previously unreported fact that NADPH could reduce neoprontosil at significant rates without the aid of catalysts provided the clue needed to solve the apparent enigma. It was discovered that considerable quantities of substrates (or substrate precursors) for dehydrogenase enzymes (EC 1.1.1.44 and 1.1.1.49) of the placental hexosemonophosphate shunt pathway were present in the placental incubation mixtures. The presence of comparatively high quantities of the dehydrogenase enzymes in soluble fractions of placental homogenates ensured the maintenance of high levels of NADPH in incubation flasks. NADPH oxidized in the process of spontaneous reduction of neoprontosil could be re-reduced by virtue of the dehydrogenases. It was shown in these studies that the entire increase in rate of azo-linkage reduction observed in placental soluble fractions was attributable to the above described enzymatic–nonenzymatic coupled mechanism.

In view of the relatively high cytochrome c reductase activities observed in placental microsomes, it was somewhat surprising that significant enzymic catalysis of the reduction of the azo linkage of neoprontosil could not be detected in incubation flasks containing these same microsomal preparations. A rapid nonenzymatic reduction of neoprontosil by NADPH could be observed in the presence of placental microsomes, indicating that degradation of NADPH was not a significant factor in the observance of negative results with respect to placental microsomal drug-metabolic activities. A comparison of rates of neoprontosil reduction by NADPH in the presence of human placental versus rat hepatic preparations from which NADPH-regenerating systems were omitted from both preparations revealed that the rate of reduction was considerably more rapid in preparations containing placental microsomes than in those containing hepatic microsomes. Additions of FMN or FAD to the incubation flasks containing placental microsomes also did not result in the detection of observable enzymatic reduction. For these experiments, it should be emphasized that incubation mixtures containing placental microsomes exhibited no capacity to reduce NADP.

Studies of azo-linkage reduction in placental tissues utilizing other azo compounds have not been carried out but preliminary studies (M. R. Juchau, unpublished results) indicate that cleavage of the azo linkages of 3′-methyl-4-monomethylaminoazobenzene or of 4-dimethylaminoazobenzene will not occur in fortified placental homogenate subfractions. These observations are consistent with the concept that azo linkages of certain compounds are more resistant to reduction than others (Walker, 1970).

The reduction of the aromatic nitro group of p-nitrobenzoic acid (PNBA) in the presence of human placental tissues has been reported from four laboratories (Juchau, 1969; Symms and Juchau, 1972; Van Petten et al., 1968; Keyegombe et al., 1973; Lake et al., 1973). In each of these laboratories p-nitrobenzoic acid was utilized as substrate. [See reaction (15).] Presumably because of the rapid reoxidation of the hy-

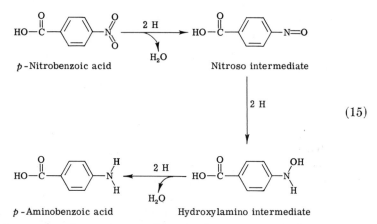

p-Nitrobenzoic acid   Nitroso intermediate

(15)

p-Aminobenzoic acid   Hydroxylamino intermediate

droxylamino to the nitroso intermediate in the presence of air or oxygen, the reaction proceeds best under anaerobic conditions. The reaction is catalyzed by preparations of hepatic microsomes, and this aspect has received considerable attention from a number of investigators. It is well known that the reaction proceeds well in the presence of either hepatic microsomes or the soluble fraction of the same tissue (as well as certain other tissues, notably the kidney). However, uncertainty exists as to which cells or cell components are most important in vivo. Pretreatment of experimental animals with phenobarbital, chlordane, or 3-methylcholanthrene markedly increases the rate of the reaction in hepatic microsomes in vitro but has little or no effect upon the reaction catalyzed in the presence of hepatic soluble fractions. Pretreatment of experimental animals with phenobarbital surprisingly does not produce increases in the quantities of p-aminobenzoic acid (PABA) excreted in the urine. On the other hand urinary excretion of PABA is decreased in animals placed on molybdenum deficient diets. These observations may be related to the fact that intestinal microflora very effectively convert PNBA to PABA (Zachariah and Juchau, 1974).

In very early studies on aromatic nitro group reduction in placental homogenates, it was reported that the reaction could not be detected in human placentas but was readily measurable in homogenates of rodent placentas (Juchau and Yaffe, 1967). Later it was discovered that additions of FAD, FMN, or riboflavin to reaction flasks containing human placental homogenates resulted in the observation of readily measurable reactions (Juchau, 1969). Dialysis of rodent homogenates resulted in profound losses in activity which could be restored by the addition of flavin to reaction vessels. Also measurements of the flavin content of rat versus human placental homogenates indicated a much higher flavin content in the rodent preparation. Thus it seemed that the apparent biochemical difference between human and rodent placentas with respect to aromatic nitro group reduction was explicable in terms of differences in tissue concentration of flavin compounds. However, when sufficient flavin was added to human placental homogenates to render the concentration equal to that found in the rodent placentas, a measurable reaction still could not be observed. This indicated that differences in flavin content could at best provide only a partial explanation for the observed species difference.

More recent studies (Symms and Juchau, 1974) provide evidence that flavoproteins play an extremely important role in the control of reaction rates; i.e., hepatic microsomal flavoproteins effect a much more rapid reduction reaction than free flavins.

The results obtained in the aforementioned experiments appeared to conflict with those observed in the laboratory of Van Petten et al. (1968). The latter investigators reported that aromatic nitro group reduction of PNBA proceeded in 9000 g supernatant fractions of human placental homogenates at easily measurable rates (approximately 6% that observed in rat liver 9000 g supernatant fractions). However, no flavins were added to their preparations. They were unable to detect significant activity when 100,000 g hepatic supernatant fractions were employed. Reasons for these discrepant observations have been discussed in a recent review (Juchau, 1973).

The human placental nitroreductase reaction appeared to prefer NADPH as the initial electron donor, but when NADPH generation or regeneration were eliminated as factors in the reaction system, it became apparent that NADH was at least as efficient as NADPH. Attempts to accelerate the reaction in rodent placentas by pretreatment with phenobarbital or 3-methylcholanthrene were not successful even though the hepatic reaction was markedly accelerated in the same animals. In human placental subfractions the reaction proceeded at approximately equal rates in soluble, "mitochondrial" and "microsomal" fractions if the regeneration of NADPH were eliminated as a factor. Heat inactivation of enzymes by boiling reduced the activity observed in the particulate fractions but had no apparent effect on the rate of the reaction in the soluble fraction. Very surprisingly it was found that carbon monoxide markedly inhibited the reaction which proceeded in the presence of a dialyzed, boiled human placental soluble fraction. Since the reaction was not detectable in the absence of tissue, it was assumed that a heat-stable, nondialyzable, carbon monoxide sensitive factor which catalyzed aromatic nitro group reduction was present in soluble fractions of human placental homogenates. This factor was sought by a variety of techniques. Ammonium sulfate fractionation, diaflo ultrafiltration, differential solvent extraction, and ion-exchange chromatography were utilized (Symms and Juchau, 1971) but the activity could not be separated from hemoglobin-rich fractions. Catalytic activity of purified (twice recrystallized) bovine methemoglobin, substituted for tissue-homogenate subfraction, displayed biphasic effects with variation in concentration. This explained earlier negative results when an attempt was made to demonstrate reduction in the presence of whole blood homogenates. In tissue-free systems (Juchau et al., 1970) it could be shown that compounds containing sulfhydryl groups (reduced glutathione, cysteine, mercaptoethanol) could substitute for placental soluble fractions in reaction flasks but, regardless of incubation conditions or substrate and cofactor concentrations, these compounds would catalyze the reaction at only about one-tenth the rate observed in the presence of placental soluble fractions. Substitution of several heme-containing compounds, including hematin, in concentrations approximately equal to the hemoglobin concentration in placental soluble fractions would catalyze nitro group reduction at rates approaching those of the tissue-catalyzed reactions. Purified milk xanthine oxidase also catalyzed the reduction of PNBA to the primary amine (Symms and Juchau, 1972). NADPH and NADH appeared to be equally efficient as electron donors in these tissue-free, heme-catalyzed systems, but NADPH was only approximately one-tenth as efficient in the xanthine oxidase-catalyzed reactions. Riboflavin 5-phosphate (FMN), at concentrations which were optimal for increasing rates of the heme-catalyzed reactions, exhibited inhibition in xanthine oxidase systems. Concentrations of xanthine oxidase exhibiting only very low activity markedly stimulated

the catalytic efficiency of the heme model systems, particularly cytochrome c. Carbon monoxide inhibited almost completely the reactions
catalyzed by xanthine oxidase, cytochrome c, hematin, and methemoglobin. Carbon monoxide had been assumed to inhibit the microsomal
reaction by binding with cytochrome P-450, but since cytochrome c had
been reported not to bind carbon monoxide at the pH of the reaction
medium, the mechanism by which this gas is inhibitory to the reaction
was unclear. It is possible that a large percentage of the commercially
available form (Sigma) occurs as the tetramer which does bind carbon
monoxide (Dupré et al., 1974).

Hemoglobin, methemoglobin, hematin, cytochrome c, and xanthine oxidase were all capable of catalyzing the reaction. Myoglobin and catalase
appeared to be very efficient catalysts, but the reaction could not be
demonstrated when cyanocobalamin, chlorophyllin, copper phthalocya-
nine, or ferrous salts (with or without EDTA) were utilized as potential
catalysts for the aromatic nitro group reduction system.

In terms of placental xenobiotic metabolism, these results indicated
that a wide variety of heme compounds as well as a variety of compounds
bearing sulfhydryl groups present in placental tissues would catalyze the
reaction. In soluble fractions, hemoglobin appears to play a dominant
role, but the mechanisms by which particulate fractions of placental
homogenates catalyze this reaction remain to be elucidated. If placental
particulate heme compounds are catalyzing aromatic nitro group reduction, they do not appear to be capable of catalyzing measurable aniline
hydroxylation even though hemoglobin catalyzed both reactions.

Results obtained in the above described experiments indicated that a
most important factor, both for catalysis of placental xenobiotic reduction as well as oxidation, is the quantity of available NADPH or NADH
as reducing equivalents in the tissues. Thus the activity of the placental
hexose monophosphate shunt enzymes may play a critical role in regulation of rates of oxidation and reduction of drug substrates *in vivo*. The
fact that the activity of these enzymes can vary considerably with
changes in a number of physiological or pathological conditions (notably
nutritional status) may have an important bearing on the capacity of
foreign compounds to produce mutagenic, carcinogenic, teratogenic, or
other effects in the developing organism.

D. Hydrolytic Reactions

Hydrolysis of drug substrates represents the third and last of the so-
called "Phase I" reaction types. Oxidation, reduction, and hydrolysis
reactions all result in the formation of compounds with polar reactive

moieties such as carboxyl, hydroxyl, amino, keto, sulfhydryl, and many other groups. Thus, even though they are excreted more rapidly by virtue of the increased water solubility, they are sometimes even more (or differently) biologically active than the parent compounds. Conjugation of such groups with glucuronic acid, sulfate, or other endogenous compounds in "Phase II" reactions fortunately normally masks the activity of the reactive moieties formed in "Phase I" and frequently renders the conjugated derivative even more highly water soluble and excretable.

Hydrolysis reactions are extremely ubiquitous in biological systems which is not surprising since the only coreactant required for such systems is water. As might be expected, then, enzymes which catalyze such reactions (hydrolases) also are biologically omnipresent and often exhibit less substrate specificity than other enzyme classes. However, certain hydrolases exhibit considerable specificity and may be discretely localized both on a gross anatomic basis as well as subcellularly. As indicated earlier in this chapter, the placenta represents an organ in which hydrolases may play a unique role in the regulation of the endocrinology of pregnancy. Thus the role of placental hydrolases in the metabolism of foreign compounds is of considerable interest.

Hydrolyses of drug (xenobiotic) substrates in placental tissues have not been investigated systematically. Nevertheless, judging from the comparatively large number of reports concerning hydrolysis of endogenous substrates, it would appear probable that many drugs bearing hydrolyzable moieties would undergo hydrolytic biotransformation during their sojourn in placental tissues. There are also reports in the literature which tend to confirm such an expectation. In fact, most of the observations on placental xenobiotic hydrolyses have been made by investigators who were interested primarily in studying the enzymatic hydrolysis of endogenous substrates, such as steroids.

Meperidine hydrolysis in human placental 9000 g supernatant fractions at term has been reported by Van Petten et al. (1968) [reaction (16)].

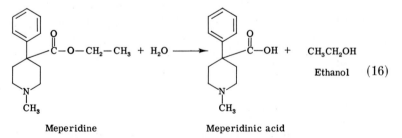

Meperidine   Meperidinic acid

Although a disappearance assay was employed for analysis of the reaction, their results indicated that no formaldehyde was formed in these preparations (formaldehyde is formed as a product of the oxidative N-demethylation of meperidine) and control experiments indicated that no nonenzymatic breakdown of meperidine was occurring. These observations are interesting because plasma esterases do not catalyze this reaction whereas hepatic microsomal esterases will attack meperidine (Parke, 1968).

Juchau and Yaffe (1969) reported enzymatic hydrolysis of acetylsalicylic acid (aspirin) and procaine in soluble fractions of human placentas but the enzymes responsible for these reactions appeared to be contaminating plasma esterases for the most part [reactions (17) and (18)].

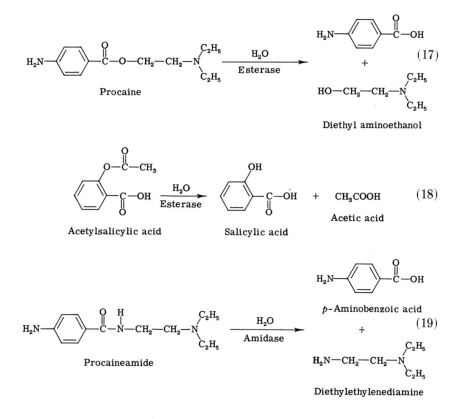

Nevertheless, procaine hydrolysis in thoroughly washed human placental "microsomes" was observed (M. R. Juchau, unpublished results). Procainamide hydrolysis [reaction (19)] in the same homogenate subfraction or other subfractions could not be detected even though naphthylamidases with a low degree of substrate specificity are known to be present in the placenta (Beckman *et al.*, 1969). Bastide *et al.* (1963) were able to detect only low levels of carboxylesterase activity in blood-free homogenates of human placentas at term using benzoylarginine ethyl ester as substrate. Hydrolyses of several acetate esters of nonendogenous substrates by placental tissues have been reported by several investigators (Christie, 1968; Hagerman, 1969). These include naphthyl acetate, norethindrone acetate, and 5-bromoindoxyl acetate, and it appears that at least three nonspecific carboxylic acid esterases (designated A, B, and C by Christie) are present in human placental cells. The synctiotrophoblast appears to possess the highest concentration of these enzymes with activity decreasing slightly toward term. These enzymes do not appear to be the same as those which catalyze the placental hydrolysis of acetylcholine. The presence of β-glucuronidase in the placenta is particularly interesting from the viewpoint of pharmacology, and certain species appear to exhibit high activity. The human placenta, however, appeared to contain only traces of activity when naphthol-AS-B1-β-D-glucuronide was utilized as substrate (Christie, 1968).

From these scattered observations it would *appear* that while placental cells may contain enzymes for catalyzing hydrolysis of xenobiotic compounds with carboxylic acid ester moieties, the relative contribution of such enzymatic activity might be low when compared to the ester-hydrolyzing capacity of the blood. Nevertheless, any categorical statements in this regard are premature since studies on substrate specificity, quantitative rate comparisons with other tissues, etc., are lacking. Likewise, generalizations concerning placental hydrolysis of amide linkages of foreign compounds cannot be made at this time even though a large number of amidases and peptidases are known to be present in placental tissues (Christie, 1968).

In view of the extensive hydrolysis of endogenous phosphates and sulfates, foreign compounds with sulfate or phosphate ester groups might be expected to undergo rapid hydrolysis during their presence in placental tissues. Indeed this has been demonstrated for naphthyl and phenyl phosphates and phenolic and catechol sulfates (Hagerman, 1969). A large number of highly active phosphatase enzymes are present in microsomal, lysosomal, and soluble fractions of placental homogenates and appear to be important for hydrolysis of such important endogenous compounds as ATP and FAD. These will also hydrolyze glucose 6-phosphate even though specific glucose-6-phosphatase reportedly is absent from the placenta. Lust *et al.* (1954) hypothesized that the conversion of FAD to FMN (catalyzed by nucleotide pyrophosphatase) in the placenta was involved in the transport of the vitamin from maternal to fetal blood.

Whether foreign phosphorylated compounds can compete for hydrolysis of endogenous phosphates, however, remains to be determined.

Placental sulfatase enzymes are considered to be extremely important in the overall scheme of the physiology of pregnancy. The fetal liver and adrenal gland contain large quantities of sulfokinase enzymes which catalyze sulfation at several positions on steroid molecules. Once sulfated, these molecules become considerably less lipid soluble and, hence, pass from fetal to maternal tissues much less readily than do the unconjugated stroid forms. The placental enzymes, however, catalyze hydrolytic cleavage of the sulfate ester bonds facilitating transfer from fetal to maternal blood and thus appear to prevent the accumulation of such steroids in fetal tissues. Although experimental evidence for such a phenomenon is lacking, it seems probable that this also may be a mechanism for regulation of feto–maternal xenobiotic distribution. Drugs such as phenols, naphthols, and catechols are sulfate acceptors and are conjugated as such by fetal tissues enzymes (Percy and Yaffe, 1964) which catalyze extensive sulfation of such compounds. An interesting and perhaps important question to ask is whether sulfated drug molecules would compete with sulfated steroids or other endogenous entities for placental sulfatase enzymes. Such competitive inhibition feasibly could disturb hormonal balance and disrupt certain developmental processes.

Two general classes of sulfatase enzymes occur in the placenta; the aryl sulfatases, of which there are at least three present in "microsomal" fractions (French and Warren, 1967; Pasqualini et al., 1967), and sterol sulfatases which attack nonphenolic sulfate esters. Sterol sulfatases also occur predominantly in "microsomal" fractions of placental homogenates but appear to exhibit considerable substrate specificity. It would appear that estrogens sulfated in either the 3 or 2 positions would be the most likely endogenous compounds to compete for placental enzymes which catalyze hydrolysis of sulfated xenobiotics. At present, however, these concepts are largely in the realm of speculation.

E. Conjugation Reactions

In hepatic tissues the enzymes which catalyze conjugation of xenobiotic substrates are localized in extramicrosomal fractions of homogenates. Amino acid conjugations (glycine, glutamine, etc.) occur predominantly in the mitochondria whereas sulfation, acetylation, methylation, and other reactions catalyzed by transferase enzymes, occur largely in the soluble fraction. An important exception to this rule, however, is glucuronide formation. Transfer of the glucuronic acid moiety from uridine diphosphoglucuronic acid (UDPGA) to xenobiotic acceptor molecules is one of the most important drug metabolic reactions as judged from the quantities of glucuronidated drugs excreted in the human urine. Glucuronidation also is extremely important from the viewpoint of termination of drug effects. Acquisition of the glucuronic acid moiety almost invariably results in rapid inactivation of the drug by virtue of any one or a combination of three possible effects:

1. A marked increase in water solubility which greatly impedes reabsorption from kidney tubules and thus facilitates a rapid excretion into the urine.
2. Active transport of the conjugated derivative into the urine or bile. The glucuronic acid moiety is a strong anion which is actively transported via anion transport systems.
3. Masking of reactive groups to which transfers occur.

UDP-glucuronosyltransferase (EC 2.4.1.17) is capable of catalyzing transfer of the glucuronic acid moiety from UDPGA to an amazingly wide variety of acceptor groups on drug molecules. Some of the more common acceptor groups include carboxyl, aromatic and aliphatic hydroxyl, amino, hydroxylamine, and sulfhydryl groups but there also are many others (Smith and Williams, 1966). This contrasts with the extramicrosomal transfer reactions in which the endogenous moieties frequently are transferred predominantly to a limited number of acceptor groups. Some of the most important endogenous acceptors are steroids and bilirubin, and it is noteworthy that attempts to demonstrate glucuronidation of these substrates in placental tissues have indicated either extremely low or negligible activity (Troen et al., 1966; Levvy and Storey, 1959).

Utilizing a highly sensitive fluorometric method and digitonin-activated human placental microsomes, Aito (1974) was able to detect only extremely low rates of glucuronidation of 4-methylumbelliferone. Idäpään-Heikkilä et al. (1971) could find no evidence for metabolism of diazepam in human placentas during early gestation or at term. Likewise, Juchau and Yaffe (1969) were unable to demonstrate glucuronidation of p-aminophenol in placental homogenates from early gestation or at term. Glucuronide conjugation of o-aminophenol, bilirubin, estrogens, or p-nitrophenol could not be demonstrated in placentas of humans and experimental animals (Dutton, 1966), and it is commonly felt that glucuronidation reactions are not catalyzed extensively in placental tissues. Using a 9000 g supernatant fractions of rabbit placental homogenates, however, Berté et al. (1969) reported glucuronide conjugation of oxazepam [reaction (20)].

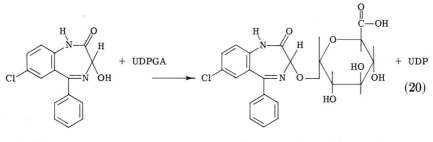

Oxazepam   Oxazepam glucuronide

These investigators reported that placental glucuronidating activity was approximately five times higher at day 14 than at day 30 of gestation. They also reported that pretreatment of the pregnant rabbits with phenobarbital produced a twofold increase in activity at day 14 and a four- to fivefold increase at day 30. These somewhat surprising results could indicate a species difference with respect to placental glucuronidating enzymes or perhaps an unusual facility of glucuronidation for this particular substrate.

Placental catalysis of sulfate transfer via aryl sulfotransferase (sulfokinase) from 3'-phosphoadenosine-5'-phosphosulfate (PAPS) to a variety of steroid acceptors has been reported by several authors (Hagerman, 1969). The bovine placenta is much more active than the human placenta to catalyze such reactions. However, the hepatic enzyme which catalyzes transfer from PAPS to xenobiotic phenols has been distinguished from estrone sulfokinase (Parke, 1968). Current consensus appears to favor the view that the human placenta contains little if any sulfokinase activity and that highly active placental sulfatases would tend to overwhelm any sulfate transfer activity (Diczfalusy, 1969). Juchau et al. (1968a) were unable to demonstrate transfer of sulfate groups of m-aminophenol utilizing tissue from 9 to 12 weeks gestation.

Acetylation of xenobiotic molecules possessing primary amino groups has been reported by several laboratories to occur in placental tissues (Juchau et al., 1968a; Van Petten et al., 1968; Berté et al., 1969; Uher, 1969). Sulfamethyoxypyrimidine, 4-aminoantipyrine (4-AAP), and p-aminobenzoic acid (PABA) were utilized as acceptors in these experiments [reactions (21)–(23)].

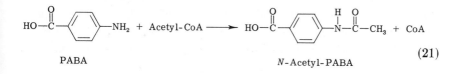

PABA N-Acetyl-PABA

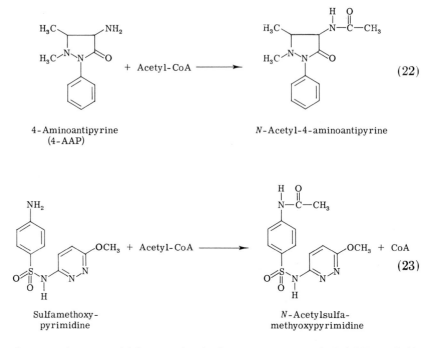

In experiments which examined the appearance of 4-AAP and its acetylated derivative in various tissues following perfusion of the utero-placental–fetal circulation of dogs *in situ* with aminopyrine, Benzi *et al.* (1968) reported that significant quantities of these two metabolites were formed within the complex at 8–9 weeks gestation. Tissues responsible for the biotransformations were not investigated at that time but in a later study (Berté *et al.*, 1969) it was reported that 9000 *g* supernatant fractions of rabbit placental homogenates catalyzed a fairly rapid acetyl-ation of 4-AAP. They also reported that this reaction proceeded seven times as rapidly at 14 days of gestation than at 30 days and that pre-treatment of the pregnant rabbits with phenobarbital increased placental acetylating activity by 44% at day 14 and 53% at day 30. The results were somewhat surprising since phenobarbital theretofore had not been known to induce xenobiotic acetylation reactions. Acetylation of 4-AAP also was observed in 9000 *g* supernatant fractions of human placental homogenates at term (Van Petten *et al.*, 1968). According to the results reported, activity in the human placenta was two- to fourfold higher than that observed in a corresponding preparation of rat liver. These experi-ments will require confirmation since disappearance of 4-AAP from incu-bation flasks was assayed. Nevertheless, other investigators have reported a high acetylating capacity of human placental tissues. Examination of the acetylation of sulfamethoxypyrimidine in cultures of human tropho-blasts (Uher, 1969) indicated that these cells were capable of catalyzing the reaction at a rapid rate. It was found that the proportion of the acety-lated derivative to unmetabolized drug was higher in the trophoblast tissue culture than in the blood of adults. Juchau and Yaffe (1969) also reported acetylation of p-aminobenzoic acid in some human placental soluble (104,000 g supernatant) fractions during early gestation but for unex-plained reasons, reported inability to detect the reaction in certain other placentas. They also reported negative results with respect to the acetyla-tion of sulfanilamide, isoniazid and p-aminosalicylic acid at 9–12 weeks gestation in humans. It should be noted that in those cases where signifi-cant acetylating activity was observed in placental homogenate fractions, the possible contribution of contaminating blood was not evaluated. It is well known that red blood cells and reticuloendothelial cells contain enzymes which catalyze the transfer of acetate to foreign molecules (Govier, 1965) and in each of the experiments either 9000 g or 104,000 g supernatant fractions were utilized. These fractions could be expected to contain varying quantities of contaminating blood. Nevertheless, the demonstration of the reaction in trophoblast tissue cultures tends to indi-cate that placental cells also contain enzymes which catalyze acetate transfer. Since many drug substrates are acetylated in a genetically poly-morphic pattern in humans, it would appear that studies in human placental tissues could provide much needed information in this area. Also it would be interesting to determine whether any of the drug acetyla-tion reactions reported to occur in placental tissues were catalyzed by the same or a similar enzyme system which catalyzes the acetylation of choline in this organ. Choline acetyltransferase appears to be present in placentas of primates but not of other species (Hebb and Ratkovic, 1962).

Only one other reaction (24) involving the conjugation of drug sub-strates in placental tissues has been reported in the literature. Conjuga-

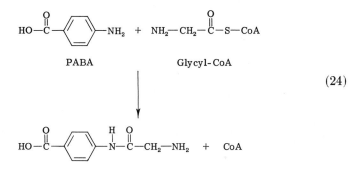

(24)

tion of glycine with PABA was observed in "mitochondrial" fractions of human placental homogenates during early gestation (Juchau and Yaffe, 1969).

The reaction occurred only about 10% as rapidly as in a corresponding preparation of rat liver mitochondria, but only preliminary studies were accomplished. It might be expected that other mitochondrial amino acid conjugation reactions would occur in placental tissues but attempts to demonstrate conjugation of glycine with salicylic acid at 9–12 weeks gestation yielded negative results (Juchau and Yaffe, 1969). The same investigators also were unable to detect significant conjugation of glutathione with bromsulphthalein (BSP) either during early gestation or at term. The reaction was examined in the soluble fraction since it is known to occur in that fraction in hepatic tissues.

Methylation of xenobiotic substrates has not been investigated systematically in placental tissues although this appears a likely mechanism of drug biotransformation since N-methylation of the imidazole ring of histamine and O-methylation of the 2-hydroxyl group of estrogens are known to proceed within the placenta. Also, the enzyme which catalyzes the synthesis of S-adenosylmethionine (SAM) from ATP and methionine was reported to occur in the human placenta at term (Hagerman, 1969). Recently, human placental catechol-O-methyltransferase (EC 2.1.1.6) has been isolated and partially characterized in a purified form (Gugler et al., 1970). The enzyme was localized in the soluble fraction and had a molecular weight of 52,000. The purified enzyme catalyzed the methylation of epinephrine, norepinephrine, and 2-hydroxyestradiol-17β in both the 2 and 3 positions. It was also reported that the 2-hydroxylated estrogen competitively inhibited the methylation of epinephrine to metanephrine. Since DL-3,4-dihydroxybenzaldehyde and DL-3,4-dihydroxymandelic acid also were methylated under the influence of the partially purified enzyme, it is to be expected that other xenobiotic compounds could act as methyl acceptors in their system.

Important drug conjugation reactions which remain to be investigated in placental tissues include glutamine conjugation (known to occur only in primates), glucoside formation, riboside formation, mercapturic acid formation, and thiocyanate formation. It is to be expected that at least some of these reactions would be detected.

F. Miscellaneous Drug-Metabolic Reactions

In previous sections the placental biotransformation of foreign, nonendogenous (xenobiotic) substrates has been emphasized. To many pharmacologists, however, the concept of drug metabolism extends to a consideration of certain chemicals normally present in the biological system but which are frequently used as medicines and hence also referred to as "drugs." The best examples of such chemicals include certain steroids, epinephrine, norepinephrine, oxytocin, insulin, acetylcholine, and many others. Thus, biotransformation of such highly active (particularly vaso-active) substances in placental tissues and the enzymes which catalyze such reactions should be of significant pharmacological interest, particularly in those instances in which xenobiotics and endogenous compounds may compete for the same enzyme system.

Enzymes involved in one of the most intriguing aspects of placental functions are choline acetyltransferase (EC 2.3.1.6) and acetylcholinesterase (EC 3.1.1.7), enzymes involved in the biosynthesis and degradation of acetylcholine. Normal human placentas have relatively high concentrations of acetylcholine (Goodlin, 1970), and it has been suggested that a correlation exists between placental acetylcholine levels and induction of labor. Acetylcholine apparently is capable of effecting increased myometrial contractions although atropine and neostigmine appear to exert no significant effects on myometrial contractility. (Interestingly, estrogens appear to increase placental acetylcholine content.) Both cholinesterase (EC 3.1.1.6) and acetylcholinesterase have been detected in human placental tissues (Zacks and Wislocki, 1953). The acetylcholinesterase activity appears to be low but the cholinesterase, which attacks a number of important xenobiotic esters of choline such as succinylcholine, exhibits about one-half the activity observed in human blood. Placental acetylcholinesterase is inhibited by diisopropylfluorophosphate, and the inhibition constants and kinetic parameters appear similar to those of the brain enzyme (Hagerman, 1969).

Choline acetyltransferase appears to be more active in the human placenta (at 24 weeks gestation) than any other vertebrate tissue (Bull et al., 1961). Activity of the enzyme at term, however, is only about one-third that observed at 24 weeks. The enzyme is present in placentas of humans and monkeys but appears to be absent from placentas of a variety of other mammalian and rodent species (Hebb and Ratkovic, 1962).

Monoamine oxidase (MAO, EC 1.4.3.4) normally is considered to be localized in the outer mitochondrial membrane of mammalian cells. This enzyme catalyzes the oxidative deamination of a number of pharmacologically important compounds including tyramine, dopamine, epinephrine, norepinephrine, tryptamine, and serotonin. Amphetamine and various other amines also are deaminated via MAO catalysis but some are poor substrates. Phenethylamines with a methyl group on the α carbon, for example, are not metabolized well. Using histochemical methodology, human placental MAO activity was found to be localized primarily in the syncytiotrophoblast (De Maria, 1963). Since the placental content of serotonin increases throughout gestation in rats (Fahim *et al.*, 1966) and falls sharply prior to parturition, interest in placental MAO is expectedly high, but little can be said at present concerning the overall significance of the placental enzyme during human pregnancy. This appears to be an extremely important area for future investigations.

Diamine oxidase (DAO, EC 1.4.3.6) occurs in the soluble fraction of cell homogenates and with respect to the placenta, appears to be concentrated in decidual tissues. This enzyme also catalyzes oxidative deamination of pharmacologically important compounds, the most notable of which is histamine. Thus, the enzyme also is referred to as histaminase. Other compounds which are good substrates for DAO include putrescine and cadaverine, but its substrate specificity overlaps that of MAO. Because of the known effects of histamine on vascular systems and the presence of relatively high quantities of histamine in placental tissues (Wicksell, 1949) considerable interest in placental DAO exists. Also, correlations have been made in which low levels of human placental DAO were associated with increased complications of pregnancy and fetal wastage (Southern *et al.*, 1966; Weingold and Southern, 1968). Histamine methyltransferase (EC 2.1.1.8) catalyzes the N-methylation of histamine and has been isolated and purified from human placentas (Kapeller-Adler, 1965). Methylation results in inactivation and thus, in view of the potential importance of the role of histamine in the placenta, regulation of the activity of this enzyme assumes considerable importance. The activity appears to increase rapidly during the first half of pregnancy but does not fluctuate considerably after this period.

Catechol-*O*-methyltransferase (EC 2.1.1.6) is an extremely important catalyst for the inactivation of epinephrine and norepinephrine in biological tissues and thus is of interest not only to pharmacologists but to all biologists. Methyl groups are transferred from *S*-adenosyl methionine to the *m*-phenolic hydroxyl group of various catechols. The placental enzyme also attacks several xenobiotic substrates and has been discussed above.

Tyrosine aminotransferase (EC 2.6.1.5) and hydroxytrypophan decarboxylase are also involved in the metabolism of important biogenic amines and have been reported to be present in placental tissues (Hagerman, 1969). Their significance to the physiology or pharmacology of pregnancy, however, is unknown. Dihydroxyphenylalanine (dopa) decarboxylase reportedly is absent from placental tissues.

Several peptidases shown to be present in placental tissues are of considerable pharmacologic interest and may be important determinants of the endocrinology of pregnancy. Renin catalyzes the conversion of angiotensinogen (an α_2-globulin) to angiotensin I, a decapeptide. Angiotensin I subsequently is converted (primarily in the lung) to angiotensin II which stimulates the release of aldosterone from the adrenal cortex. Aldosterone acts upon renal tubules to promote sodium retention and increase blood volume. Whether or not renin produced by placental tissues contributed significantly to this sequence of events, however, remains to be determined. Human amniotic fluid and umbilical cord blood contain renin activity and the enzyme also has been detected in the rabbit placenta (Gross *et al.*, 1964).

The reported presence of oxytocinase in human placental tissues is of special interest because of the fact that oxytocin (Pitocin) is so frequently employed in the management of labor. Cystine aminopeptidase and oxytocinase activities are felt to be equivalent and the research of Mathur and Walker (1968, 1969) tends to indicate that oxytocinase synthesized by syncytiotrophoblast cells is released from the placenta during labor. Since oxytocin is capable of constricting the umbilical vasculature, placental oxytocinase activity may be highly important as a factor in determining pregnancy outcome.

Placental insulinase long has been regarded as a possible factor in the etiology of the decreased glucose tolerance and diabetes of pregnancy although direct evidence for such a role appears to be lacking. According to the researches of Wolf *et al.* (1969), bovine insulin will not pass across the placental membranes from the maternal to fetal bloodstream. These investigators felt that placental insulinase could be a factor in preventing insulin transfer to the fetus. They did not present data which were supportive of that supposition; however, such a view appears to be very logical.

The placenta also contains enzymes which are capable of inactivating vasopressin (antidiuretic hormone, ADH). The enzyme(s) involved have not been purified or characterized. In view of the many active peptidases present in placental tissues, it would appear that other polypeptide hormones (kinins, etc.) likely would undergo degradation within that organ.

Other placental enzymes of pharmacological interest include NADPH cytochrome *c* reductase, reportedly present in placental "microsomes" (Hagerman *et al.*, 1966), a flavoprotein which functions in the hepatic microsomal drug oxidizing electron transport chain, and ATPase, which normally is thought to be involved in active transport systems. Since the placenta is known to actively transport nutrient materials from maternal to fetal tissues, and recently (McNay and Dayton, 1970) has been reported to transfer triamterene (a pteridine compound which has been used as a diuretic agent) from fetal to maternal tissues against a concentration gradient, it seems surprising that more interest in placental ATPases has not been exhibited.

III. Effects of Drugs on Placental Metabolic Functions

It now seems abundantly evident that drugs reaching the fetus are able to produce temporary or permanent alterations on a *multitude* of developmental parameters. With adequate knowledge, certain of these alterations could be beneficial and certain drugs might thus be useful in a variety of therapeutic applications when administered to the fetus. An understanding of fetal and placental biochemical functions and factors affecting such functions is a primary requisite in the pronouncement of judgments of beneficial versus toxic effects in these situations. Recognition of the fetus and placenta as a functional unit and of the fact that drugs are most important regulators of biochemical functions automatically leads to recognition of the need for understanding of the effects of drugs on placental biochemical parameters.

A. Effects of Drugs on Steroid Biotransformation

In the case of drug–steroid interactions, interest has focused on induction–repression mechanisms and on competitive inhibition of biotransformation catalysis. In retrospect, this seems natural because of the very similar types of biotransformation reactions which drugs and steroids undergo. Extremely important in this regard are the mixed-function oxidative reactions for which both drugs and steroids utilize NADPH, molecular oxygen, flavoproteins, and cytochrome P-450. For several years it has been recognized that pretreatment of experimental animals with drugs known to induce hepatic microsomal xenobiotic metabolizing enzymes also would induce hepatic steroid-metabolizing enzymes (Conney, 1967). Steroids also inhibit drug-hydroxylating reactions and, on the basis of kinetic analyses with unpurified liver microsomal preparations, the claim frequently has been made that the inhibition is competitive. Thus, an oversimplified notion that drugs and steroids utilize the same enzymes for biotransformation reactions has received some credence.

It is evident from such studies that drugs can influence markedly the rate of steroid biotransformation and vice versa, and it seems probable that drugs and steroids may utilize the same enzymes for *certain types* of metabolic reactions. Therefore, since steroid biotransformation is a major function of the placenta, the question of the effects of drugs on the reactions involved seems particularly pertinent. The enzymes which catalyze the rate-limiting reactions in the placental conversion of cholesterol to progesterone and androgens to estrogens both are of the mixed-function oxidase type. Since cigarette smoking markedly increased mixed-function drug oxidation (benzo[a]pyrene), it would be highly interesting to determine whether smoking also exerts effects on the rates of biosynthesis of progesterone and estrogens. Juchau (1973), however, has presented evidence which indicates that human placental hydroxylation of benzo[a]pyrene is not catalyzed by the same enzyme systems which catalyze these steroid syntheses.

Certain drugs are known to inhibit cholesterol side-chain oxidation in adrenal cortex mitochondria and might be expected to inhibit the same reaction in the placenta. Aminoglutethimide is a well-known example of such drug inhibitors of progesterone biosynthesis, but its effect on the placental system has been ascertained. Very recently it has been reported that aminoglutethimde is inhibitory to the human placental aromatase system (Thompson *et al.*, 1971). These investigators also reported that certain C_{19} steroids were also inhibitory to the aromatase but that metyrapone, estrone, progesterone, or estriol had no significant effect on the reaction *in vitro*. The possibility that more than one pathway for placental aromatization exists (Milewich and Axelrod, 1971; Megis and Ryan, 1971; Thompson *et al.*, 1971) renders studies with drugs as inhibitors much more complex, however, and inhibitory mechanisms will be difficult to ascertain until the components of the system have been isolated and purified.

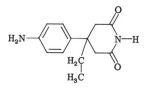

Aminoglutethimide

A practical example of the importance of knowledge of drug–steroid interactions during pregnancy recently has been provided by a demonstration showing that progesterone could suppress the embryotoxic action of actinomycin and Triton WR 1339 (Tuchmann-Duplessis, 1969).

B. Effects of Drugs on Placental Intermediary Metabolism

Systematic investigations of the effects of drugs on metabolic processes of the placenta have not been undertaken. It is to be expected that drugs would exert effects on placental enzymes similar to the effects observed on the same or analogous enzymes in other tissues. However, this assumption may not be justified in many instances, and differences in effects could provide needed clues to the mechanisms of drug toxicity in the fetus or neonate.

Using tissue cultures of trophoblast cells, Uher (1969) studied the effects of six drugs on glucose utilization by the cells in the culture. Sulfamethoxypyrimidine, ketophenylbutazone, and mebrophenhydramine all reduced glucose utilization by the explanted chorionic tissue, and produced an increase in lactate production and in lactate/pyruvate ratios, whereas nitrofurantoin, benzopyrazone, and azauridine did not affect these parameters. It is interesting to note that those drugs which affected carbohydrate metabolism also were reported themselves to be metabolized in the culture medium. Because of the high sensitivity of the fetus to changes in glucose supply during the period of organogenesis, the effects of drugs on placental carbohydrate and lipid metabolism should be studied in much more detail.

C. *Effects of Drugs on the Placental Vasculature*

The subtitle heading may suggest a departure from the original theme of the chapter. The extreme importance of an adequate placental circulation, as well as the occurrence of placental enzymes which catalyze the biotransformation of highly vasoactive endogenous substances, however, appears to justify considerations of such effects. Some of the most interesting effects of drugs on placental vasculature, for example, are produced by drugs which inhibit monoamine oxidase, a catalyst for the biotransformation of serotonin. Serotonin has been observed to produce death of fetal mice when given to the mother. It is capable of reducing the blood supply to the placenta as well as altering placental permeability (Honey *et al.*, 1967). Serotonin also is an extremely effective vasoconstrictor of human umbilical blood vessels (Somlyo *et al.*, 1965) and was found to be more effective than epinephrine or norepinephrine which are also inactivated via monoamine oxidase catalysis. Nevertheless, the roles of placental monoamine oxidase and the vasoactive amines whose degradation it catalyzes have not yet been elucidated.

Approximately 600 ml/minute of blood are required by the human term placenta, all of which is supplied via the spiral arteries to the intervillous spaces. Almost nothing is known concerning the response of these arteries to vasomotor influences, and in view of the presence of several compounds in the placenta which are known to affect vascular elements, it would appear to be important to determine not only the effects of drugs on spiral artery vasomotion but also their effects on the metabolism of endogenous compounds which might influence this vascular system. It is now known, however, that the spiral arteries are practically devoid of the musculoelastic tissues (Dixon and Robertson, 1969) that usually are required for normal vascular responses. It is felt by many that the necessary delicate control of blood supply must be at a more proximal site than the spiral arteries and probably exists at the level of radial arteries of the uterus. The radiospiral artery junction also has been suggested as a site of vasoconstriction. In view of the fact that the commonest cause of stillbirth is intrauterine anoxia it would seem highly important that the physiology and pharmacology of those vessels be well understood. Histamine, oxytocin, and vasopressin all are capable of exerting profound influences on vascular elements, and it is entirely feasible that drugs which could alter rates of metabolism of these substances by placental enzymes might also exert significant influences on the placental circulation.

Lysergic acid diethylamide (LSD), a compound structurally related to serotonin, and mescaline, related structurally to norepinephrine, have been shown to be highly effective agonists for vasoconstriction of umbilical blood vessels (Gant and Dyer, 1971). Other hallucinogens which constrict human umbilical vessels include bufotenine, psilocin, and psilocybin (Juchau and Dyer, 1972). Also, analgesics such as meperidine, morphine, and codeine have been reported to constrict perfused human placental vessels *in vitro*. Whether or not any of these substances can influence vascular responses via influences on placental enzymes, however, is not known at present. Also, it is unknown whether the parent compounds or metabolites thereof are the active vasoconstrictor substances.

IV. Summary and Conclusions

It now seems clear that a large variety of chemical substances, both endogenous and exogenous, will undergo biotransformational changes in the presence of placental tissues from humans as well as other species. Mere recognition of this fact is important in itself, but more importantly, of course, these tissues contain catalysts and catalytic systems which serve to regulate the rates of many of these reactions. With respect to the biotransformation of xenobiotic (drug) substrates in the placenta, it now appears that systems are available within that organ for catalysis of each of the four classic drug-metabolic reaction types: oxidation, reduction, hydrolysis, and conjugation. Nevertheless, only very limited information is available with respect to quantitative comparative data and mechanisms of such biotransformations. In addition, conflicting data have been reported with respect to several reactions. Therefore conclusions can be drawn for only a small proportion of the reactions reportedly catalyzed by placental components.

For placental drug oxidations, only the hydroxylation of benzo[a]pyrene has been studied sufficiently to warrant the drawing of conclusions. Studies from several independent laboratories are in general agreement that particulate fractions of placental homogenates contain enzymes which catalyze the mixed-function oxidation reaction. As in hepatic and other tissues, the system is induced by administration of any of a number of polycyclic aromatic hyrocarbons to the pregnant female. In humans, cigarette smoking results in a marked increase of the enzyme in the placenta during the latter stages of gestation but apparently has little if any influence during the first trimester. Both human and rodent placental hydroxylases display many similarities to the extensively investigated rat hepatic system, but specific activities in placental preparations are one to two orders of magnitude lower than in corresponding rodent hepatic preparations.

Reduction of xenobiotic substrates occurs in the presence of placental tissues but in these cases, the nonenzymatic (heat-stable) components of the reactions are highly important. Only two placental xenobiotic reduction reactions have been examined in any depth, and these have been studied extensively only in soluble fractions of placental homogenates. Rates of azo-linkage reduction in these fractions is dependent entirely upon additions or generation of nucleotide reducing equivalents which are able to reduce the azo compounds spontaneously. The placental hexose monophosphate shunt pathway appears to play a very important role for this reaction. Aromatic nitro group reduction can be catalyzed in placental tissues by a variety of heme-containing compounds including hemoglobin, methemoglobin, and hematin. These catalysts are not inactivated by heating but heat labile catalysts for aromatic nitro group reduction appear to be present in particulate fractions of placental homogenates.

Hydrolytic reactions have not been investigated systematically in placental tissues, thus few generalizations can be made at present. Judging from the extensive hydrolytic capabilities of the placenta with respect to endogenous substrates and the few scattered reports of xenobiotic hydrolyses, however, it appears that a variety of hydrolyzable drugs would undergo extensive metabolism in the placenta.

Extensive conjugation of endogenous or exogenous substrates does not appear to occur in the placenta although reports tend to indicate that certain substrates may be readily conjugated. Acetylation of aromatic amines has been reported by several investigators, and it appears that amino acid conjugation reactions would be catalyzed by placental mitochondria. Glucuronide formation has been reported to occur in rabbit placentas but most attempts to demonstrate the reaction in human placentas have been negative.

The placenta also contains enzymes which catalyze the metabolism of a large number of pharmacologically important endogenous compounds. These include important vasoactive substances such as epinephrine, norepinephrine, serotonin, histamine, and acetylcholine. Also included are highly important polypeptide hormones such as insulin, oxytocin, angiotensin, and vasopressin.

REFERENCES

Aito, A. (1974). *Biochem. Pharmacol.* **23**, 2203.
Autor, A. P., Strobel, H. W., Heidema, J., and Coon, M. J. (1971). *Fed. Proc., Fed. Amer. Soc. Exp. Biol.* **30**, 505.
Bardsley, W. G., Crabbé, M. J. C., and Scott, I. V. (1974). *Biochem. J.* **139**, 169.
Bastide, P., Meunier, S., and Dastugue, G. (1963). *Ann. Biol. Clin. (Paris)* **21**, 265.
Beckman, L., Beckman, G., Mi, M. P., and De Simone, J. (1969). *Hum. Hered.* **19**, 249.
Benzi, G., Berté, F., Crema, A., and Arrigoni, E. (1968). *J. Pharm. Sci.* **57**, 1031.
Bergheim, P., Rathgen, G. H., and Netter, K. J. (1973). *Biochem. Pharmacol.* **22**, 1633.
Berté, F., Manzo, L., De Bernardi, M., and Benzi, G. (1969). *Arch. Int. Pharmacodyn. Ther.* **182**, 182.
Bogdan, D. P., Yaffe, S. J., and Juchau, M. R. (1969). *Fed. Proc., Fed. Amer. Soc. Exp. Biol.* **28**, 676.
Bogdan, D. P., and Juchau, M. R. (1970). *Eur. J. Pharmacol.* **10**, 119.
Bull, G., Hebb, C., and Ratkovic, C. (1961). *Nature (London)* **190**, 1202.
Christie, G. A. (1968). *Histochemie* **12**, 189.
Conney, A. H. (1967). *Pharmacol. Rev.* **19**, 317.
Creaven, P. J., and Parke, D. V. (1965). *Fed. Eur. Biochem. Soc.* **A128**, 88.
De Maria, F. J. (1963). *Amer. J. Obstet. Gynecol.* **87**, 27.
Diczfalusy, E. (1969). *In* "The Foeto-Placental Unit" (A. Pecile and C. Finzi, eds.), Int. Congr. Ser. No. 183, p. 65. Excerpta Med. Found., Amsterdam.
Dixon, H. G., and Robertson, W. B. (1969). *In* "Foetus and Placenta" (A. Klopper and E. Diczfalusy, eds.), p. 1. Blackwell, Oxford.
Dixon, R. L., and Willson, V. J. (1968). *Arch. Int. Pharmacodyn. Ther.* **172**, 453.
Dupré, S., Brunori, M., Wilson, M. T., and Greenwood, C. (1974). *Biochem. J.* **141**, 299.
Dutton, G. J. (1966). *In* "Glucuronic Acid: Free and Combined. Chemistry, Biochemistry, Pharmacology, and Medicine" (G. J. Dutton, ed.), p. 276. Academic Press, New York.
Fahim, I., Robson, J. M., and Senior, J. B. (1966). *Brit. J. Pharmacol. Chemother.* **26**, 237.
Feuer, G. (1973). *Rev. Can. Biol.* **32**, Suppl., 113.

French, A. P., and Warren, J. C. (1967). *Biochem. J.* **105**, 233.

Gant, D. W., and Dyer, D. C. (1971). *Life Sci.* **10**, 235.

Gelboin, H .V. (1969). *In* "Jerusalem Symposia on Quantum Chemistry and Biochemistry" (E. D. Bergmann and B. Pullman, eds.), pp. 175–182. Isr. Acad. Sci. Hum., Jerusalem.

Goodlin, R. C. (1970). *Amer. J. Obstet. Gynecol.* **107**, 429.

Gough, D. E., Lowe, M. I., and Juchau, M. R. (1975). *J. Nat. Cancer Inst.* **54** (in press).

Govier, W. C. (1965). *J. Pharmacol. Exp. Ther.* **150**, 305.

Gross, F., Schaectelin, G., Zeigler, M., and Berger, M. (1964). *Lancet* **1**, 914.

Gugler, R., Knuppen, R., and Breuer, H. (1970). *Biochim. Biophys. Acta* **220**, 10.

Guibbert, D., Duperray, B., Pacheo, H., Tormatis, L., and Turusov, V. (1972). *Therapie* **27**, 907.

Hagerman, D. D. (1969). *In* "Foetus and Placenta" (A. Klopper and E. Diczfalusy, eds.), p. 413. Blackwell, Oxford.

Hagerman, D. D., Smith, O. W., and Day, C. F. (1966). *Acta Endocrinol. (Copenhagen)* **51**, 591.

Hebb, C. O., and Ratkovic, D. (1962). *J. Physiol. (London)* **163**, 307.

Honey, D. P., Robson, J. M., and Sullivan, F. M. (1967). *Amer. J. Obstet. Gynecol.* **99**, 250.

Idapään-Heikkilä, J. E., Jouppila, P. I., Puolakka, J. O., and Vorne, M. S. (1971). *Amer. J. Obstet. Gynecol.* **109**, 1011.

Juchau, M. R. (1969). *J. Pharmacol. Exp. Ther.* **165**, 1.

Juchau, M. R. (1971a). *Fed. Proc., Fed. Amer. Soc. Exp. Biol.* **31**, 48.

Juchau, M. R. (1971b). *Toxicol. Appl. Pharmacol.* **18**, 665.

Juchau, M. R. (1973). *CRC Crit. Rev. Toxicol.* **2**, 125.

Juchau, M. R., and Dyer, D. C. (1972). *Pediat. Clin. N. Amer.* **19**, 65.

Juchau, M. R., and Namkung, M. J. (1974). *Drug Metab. Disposition* **2**, 380.

Juchau, M. R., and Pedersen, M. G. (1973). *Life Sci.* **12**, 193.

Juchau, M. R., and Smuckler, E. A. (1973). *Toxicol. Appl. Pharmacol.* **126**, 163.

Juchau, M. R., and Symms, K. G. (1972). *Biochem. Pharmacol.* **21**, 2053.

Juchau, M. R., and Yaffe, S. J. (1967). *Pharmacologist* **9**, 190.

Juchau, M. R., and Yaffe, S. J. (1969). *In* "The Foeto-Placental Unit" (A. Pecile and C. Finzi, eds.), Int. Congr. Ser. No. 183, p. 260. Excerpta Med. Found., Amsterdam.

Juchau, M. R., and Zachariah, P. K. (1975). *Biochem. Pharmacol.* **24**, 227.

Juchau, M. R., Niswander, K. B., and Yaffe, S. J. (1968a). *Amer. J. Obstet. Gynecol.* **100**, 348.

Juchau, M. R., Krasner, J., and Yaffe, S. J. (1968b). *Biochem. Pharmacol.* **17**, 1969.

Juchau, M. R., Krasner, J., and Yaffe, S. J. (1970). *Biochem. Pharmacol.* **19**, 443.

Juchau, M. R., Pedersen, M. G., and Symms, K. G. (1972). *Biochem. Pharmacol.* **21**, 2269.

Juchau, M. R., Zachariah, P. K., Colson, J., Symms, K. G., Kraser, J., and Yaffe, S. J. (1974). *Drug Metab. Disposition* **2**, 79.

Kappeller-Adler, R. (1965). *Clin. Chim. Acta* **11**, 191.

Keyegombe, D., Franklin, C., and Turner, P. (1973). *Lancet* **2**, (24), 405.

Krasner, J., Juchau, M. R., Niswander, K. G., and Yaffe, S. J. (1971). *Amer J. Obstet. Gynecol.* **109**, 159.

Lake, B. G., Hopkins, R., Chakraborty, J., Bridges, J. W., and Parke, D. V. W. (1973). *Drug Metab. Disposition* **1**, 342.

Levvy, G. A., and Storey, I. D. E. (1959). *Biochem. J.* **44**, 295.

Lu, A. Y. H., Kuntzman, R., and Conney, A. H. (1971). *Fed. Proc., Fed. Amer. Soc. Exp. Biol.* **30,** 1726.

Lust, J., Hagerman, D. D., and Villee, C. A. (1954). *J. Clin. Invest.* **33,** 38.

McNay, J. L., and Dayton, P. G. (1970). *Science* **167,** 988.

Mason, J. I., and Boyd, G. S. (1971). *Eur. J. Biochem.* **21,** 308.

Mathur, V. S., and Walker, J. M. (1968). *Brit. Med. J.* **3,** 96.

Mathur, V. S., and Walker, J. M. (1969). *J. Physiol. (London)* **204,** 59P.

Meigs, R. A., and Ryan, K. J. (1968). *Biochim. Biophys. Acta* **165,** 476.

Meigs, R. A., and Ryan, K. J .(1971). *J. Biol. Chem.* **246,** 83.

Milewich, L., and Axelrod, L. R. (1971). *Fed. Proc., Fed. Amer. Soc. Exp. Biol.* **30,** 1106.

Nebert, D. W., and Gelboin, H. V. (1968). *J. Biol. Chem.* **243,** 6250.

Nebert, D. W., Winker, J., and Gelboin, H. V. (1969). *Cancer Res.* **29,** 1763.

Parke, D. V. (1968). "The Biochemistry of Foreign Compounds." Permagon, Oxford.

Pasqualini, J. R., Cédard, L., Nguyen, B. L., and Alsat, E. (1967). *Biochim. Biophys. Acta* **139,** 177.

Pecile, A., Chiesara, E., Finzi, C., and Conti, F. (1969). *In* "The Foeto-Placental Unit" (A. Pecile and C. Finzi, eds.), Int. Congr. Ser. No. 183, p. 255. Excerpta Med. Found., Amsterdam.

Pelkonen, O., Jouppila, P., and Karki, N. T. (1972). *Toxicol. Appl. Pharmacol.* **23,** 399.

Percy, A. K., and Yaffe, S. J. (1964). *Pediatrics* **33,** 965.

Rane, A. (1973), Berggren, M., Yaffe, S. J., and Ericsson, J. L. E. (1973). *Xenobiotica* **3,** 37.

Ryan, K. J. (1969). *In* "The Foeto-Placental Unit" (A. Pecile and C. Finzi, eds.), Int. Congr. Ser. No. 183, p. 120. Excerpta Med. Found., Amsterdam.

Smith, R. L., and Williams, R. T. (1966). *In* "Glucuronic Acid: Free and Combined. Chemistry, Biochemistry, Pharmacology, and Medicine" (G. J. Dutton, eds.), p. 457. Academic Press, New York.

Somlyo, A. V., Woo, C. Y., and Somlyo, A. P. (1965). *Amer. J. Physiol.* **200,** 748.

Southern, A. L., Kobayashi, Y., Weingold, A. B., and Carmody, N. C. (1966). *Amer. J. Obstet. Gynecol.* **96,** 502.

Symms, K. G., and Juchau, M. R. (1971). *Proc. West. Pharmacol. Soc.* **14,** 104.

Symms, K. G., and Juchau, M. R. (1972). *Biochem. Pharmacol.* **21,** 519.

Symms, K. G., and Juchau, M. R. (1973). *Life Sci.* **13,** 1221.

Symms, K. G., and Juchau, M. R. (1974). *Drug Metab. Disposition* **2,** 194.

Szabo, A. J., and Grimaldi, R. D. (1970). *Advan. Metab. Dis.* **4,** 185.

Thompson, E. A., and Siiteri, P. K. (1974). *J. Biol. Chem.* **249,** 5373.

Thompson, E. A., Bolton, S. B., and Siiteri, P. J. (1971). *Fed. Proc., Fed. Amer. Soc. Exp. Biol.* **30,** 1160.

Traeger, A., Hoffman, H., Franke, H., and Gunther, M. (1972). *Z. Geburtsh. Perinatologie* **176,** 397.

Troen, P., De Miquel, M.. and Alonso, C. (1966). *Biochemistry* **5,** 332.

Tuchmann-Duplessis, H. (1969). *Foetal Autonomy, Ciba Found. Symp.*, p. 245.

Uher, J. (1969). *In* "The Foeto-Placental Unit" (A. Pecile and C. Finzi, eds.), Int. Congr. Ser. No. 183, p. 240. Excerpta Med. Found., Amsterdam.

Uher, J., Dvorak, K., Queissnerova, M., Konickova, L., and Turinova, J. (1966). *Amer. J. Obstet. Gynecol.* **95,** 1005.

Van Petten, G. R., Hirsch, G. H., and Cherrington, A. D. (1968). *Can. J. Biochem.* **46,** 1057.

Walker, R. (1970). *Food Cosmet. Toxicol.* 8, 659.

Weingold, A. B., and Southern, A. L. (1968). *Obstet. Gynecol.* 32, 593.

Welch, R. M., and Harrison, Y. (1967). *Pharmacologist* 9, 202.

Welch, R. M., Harrison, Y. E., Conney, A. H., Poppers, P. J., and Finster, J. (1968a). *Science* 160, 541.

Welch, R. M., Poppers, P. J., Harrison, Y. E., and Conney, A. H. (1968b). *Fed. Proc., Fed. Amer. Soc. Exp. Biol.* 27, 301.

Welch, R. M., Harrison, Y. E., Gomni, B. W., Poppers, P. J., Finster, M., and Conney, A. H. (1969). *Clin. Pharmacol. Ther.* 10, 100.

Wicksell, F. (1949). *Acta Physiol. Scand.* 17, 295.

Wolf, H., Sabata, V., Frerichs, H., and Stubbe, P. (1969). *Horm. Metab. Res.* 1, 274.

Yaffe, S. J., and Juchau, M. R. (1974). *Annu. Rev. Pharmacol.* 14, 219.

Zachariah, P. K., and Juchau, M. R. (1974). *Drug Metab. Disposition* 2, 74.

Zachariah, P. K., and Juchau, M. R. (1975). *Life Sci.* 16, 1689.

Zacks, S. I., and Wislocki, B. G. (1953). *Proc. Soc. Exp. Biol. Med.* 84, 438.

3

Disposition of Drugs in the Fetus

William J. Waddell

G. Carolyn Marlowe

I. Anatomic and Histological Considerations

In order to discuss the distribution and metabolism of drugs in fetal tissues, a brief review of the developmental anatomy of these tissues should be useful. Emphasis will be placed on the early part of gestation when the embryo is differentiating, the fetal membranes are forming, and the embryo is susceptible to teratogenic agents. It is surprising how few

119

studies have been made on the physiology of these tissues in early gestation. The attachment and relative position of these membranes to maternal tissues differs greatly among the species. Primary comparison will be made here, however, between the human in the first trimester and mouse in the first 2 weeks of gestation with occasional correlations with other species. The mouse has been used so extensively in experimental studies on the localization and metabolism of drugs that an understanding of the relative rates of formation of these embryos is important. The morphology and physiology of the placenta near term has been covered well in recent publications (e.g., Assali, 1968) so that no discussion of the placenta in late gestation will be attempted. Figures 1–4 show the relative growth of the human and mouse embryos and their membranes

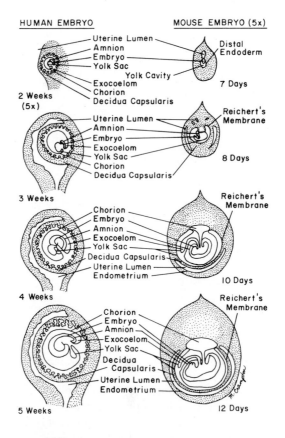

FIG. 1. The developmental stages are depicted from the formation of the primitive streak up to the beginning of chondrification. (Drawings reduced to 0.6 of original.)

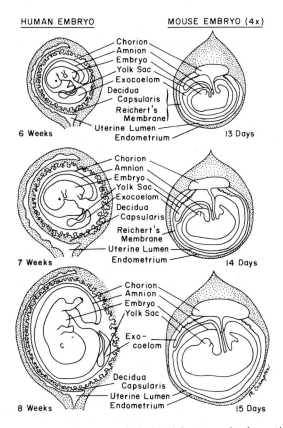

FIG. 2. The developmental stages are depicted between the formation of the primary lid fold and closure of the palate. (Drawings reduced to 0.6 of original.)

in early gestation. Each pair of drawings is for approximately the same stage of embryonic development in the two species. The drawings were originally life-size except where indicated. Note that in the human, the yolk sac is an appendage between the amnion and chorion; in the mouse the yolk sac surrounds the amnion, and the chorion is confined to a small area on the uterine wall. The time interval is depicted during which differentiation is occurring and susceptibility to teratogenic agents exists. The drawings and following discussion are summarized from several sources (Snell, 1941; Hamilton and Boyd, 1960; Hamilton *et al.*, 1964, 1972; Snell and Stevens, 1966; Patten, 1968; Rugh, 1968; Balinsky, 1970). Figure 5 shows the crown–rump (CR) length of the human fetus during gestation so that correlations with size can be made. Data were assembled from the sources indicated on the figure.

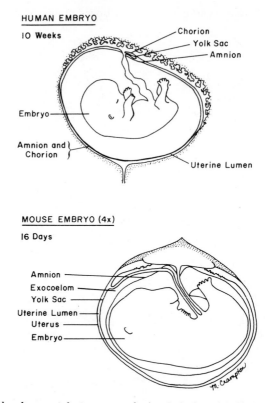

HUMAN EMBRYO

IO Weeks

Chorion
Yolk Sac
Amnion

Embryo

Amnion and
Chorion

Uterine Lumen

MOUSE EMBRYO (4x)

16 Days

Amnion
Exocoelom
Yolk Sac
Uterine Lumen
Uterus
Embryo

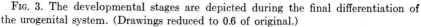

FIG. 3. The developmental stages are depicted during the final differentiation of the urogenital system. (Drawings reduced to 0.6 of original.)

A. Fertilization and Implantation

In mammals, the ova are fertilized in the uppermost part of the oviduct. Cleavage of the egg occurs during its passage through the oviduct to the uterus. Repeated cleavage produces a solid mass of cells commonly referred to as the morula (little mulberry). The morula is rather arbitrarily divided into what is referred to as an inner cell mass and an enveloping layer of cells. The cells of the inner cell mass have a more basophilic cytoplasm and are those which differentiate into the embryo itself. The cells of the enveloping layer stain poorly with basic dyes; the enveloping layer of cells gives rise to the embryonic membranes.

The blastodermic vesicle or blastula is formed by a partial separation of the inner cell mass from the remainder of the cells (trophoblasts) to create a roughly spherical cavity referred to as the blastocoele. The blastocoele is bound by the inner cell mass and, to a greater extent, by tropho-

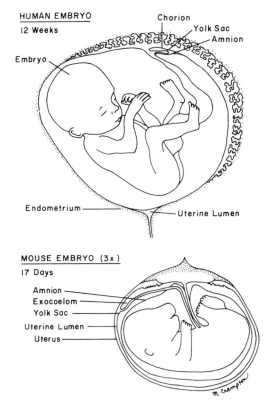

FIG. 4. The embryos and their membranes are shown at the time when organ differentiation is essentially complete. (Drawings reduced to 0.6 of original.)

blastic cells. It is at this stage that the developing embryo attaches itself to the uterine wall. This developing embryo burrows into the uterine mucosa with rapid proliferation of the trophoblasts or trophectoderm. The inner cell mass develops more slowly; it is as though the expanding trophectoderm was preparing for exchange of nutrients to the embryonic disc before proliferation of the embryo.

B. Formation and Development of Membranes

1. HUMAN

During the time interval in which the embryo is becoming implanted in the mucosa of the uterus, the trophoblasts have eroded a cavity in the endometrium, and the blastocoele has enlarged to produce a fluid-filled cavity referred to as the exocoelom. The inner cell mass or embry-

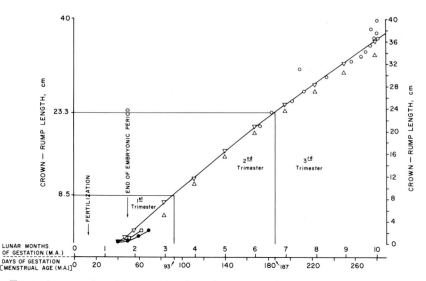

FIG. 5. A composite of information from five sources shows the crown–rump length in centimeters of the human fetus at different times from the beginning of the mother's last menstrual period. The lines were drawn by simple inspection. ○: Potter, 1961; △: Streeter, 1920; △: Scammon and Calkins, 1929; ●: Witschi, 1956; □: Iffy et al., 1967.

onic disc differentiates during this week of implantation to form a small cavity on either side of the disc. The cavity, formed by ectoderm, which is oriented toward the uterus, is referred to as the amnionic cavity. The cavity, formed from endoderm, which is oriented toward the uterine lumen is referred to as the yolk sac. The situation then is one of an embedded cyst, the walls of which were formed from trophectoderm which contains a tiny double sac (amnionic cavity and yolk sac) separated by the embryonic disc. The amnion is connected to the trophectoderm at the site at which the inner cell mass was connected to the enveloping cell layer.

It is from this point that the relative growth of these membranes surrounding the embryonic disc in various species accounts for some of the different types of placental attachments. Since many teratogenic agents are able to effect their action this early in gestation, a selective distinction between the embryonic membranes and the embryonic disc is perhaps already possible chemically. Most of the embryonic differentiation occurs during the next month, and virtually all of it has occurred by the end of the third month.

Although no yolk is present in the human ovum, the yolk sac is a prominent part of the early developing human embryo. The cells lining the yolk sac are continuous with those that form the gut and the yolk sac may be thought of as an out-pouching from the midgut region. It continues to grow up until about 6 or 8 weeks of gestation when it may reach a diameter of greater than $\frac{1}{2}$ cm. After that time it regresses slightly but persists throughout pregnancy. It can be found at term between adherent amnion and the chorion near the insertion of the umbilical cord into the fetal side of the placenta. The yolk sac is as large as the remainder of the developing embryo for at least the first 4 weeks of its life and is a prominent part of the developing embryo during the first 2 months.

The cavity that forms on the top of the embryonic disc becomes the amnionic cavity and is composed of ectoderm. The amnion continues to develop until it completely surrounds the embryo and covers the body stalk. Enclosed within the body stalk are the original attachment of the embryonic disc to the trophectoderm, the yolk sac stalk, and the blood vessels connecting the embryo to the chorion.

The ventral diverticulum from the gut or primitive bladder which is called the allantois continues for some distance into the body stalk. Later, blood vessels from the allantois fuse with the chorion to form the rich plexus of blood vessels that become the placenta. The blood vessels from the allantois furnish an important blood supply to the chorion because the developing amnion pinches off most of the blood vessels from the embryo to the chorion. The chorion then is formed from the developing allantois and the serosa or trophectoderm, i.e., the cells lining the blastocystic cavity. The space between the amniotic cavity and the chorion is called the extraembryonic coelom which in late gestation is virtually nonexistent because of the expansion of the amnion to lie directly against the chorion.

The part of the uterine wall that is between the blastocyst and the uterine lumen is pushed into the lumen as the embryo enlarges; this becomes the decidua capsularis. Numerous chorionic villi are in the decidua capsularis in the beginning. By the twelfth week, the decidua capsularis has thinned completely leaving only chorion and amnion covering the fetus toward the uterine lumen. There is truly a meager amount of information in the literature on the membranes at this stage of gestation. Details on the amount of decidua capsularis existing at 10 weeks of gestation could not be found.

2. Mouse

At about the time of implantation, on the fifth postconception day, the blastula differs from that described for the human; the inner cell mass is separated from the blastocystic cavity by differentiating cells which become the proximal endoderm of the yolk sac. Between the proximal endoderm and the trophectoderm is the yolk cavity; the trophectoderm differentiates into the distal endoderm. The inner cell mass begins to cavitate to form the egg cylinder. With the formation of the primitive streak in the embryonic area, mesoderm is formed which grows into the middle of the egg cylinder and ultimately forms two separate cavities. The end distal to the ectoplacental cone will become the amnion and developing embryo while the proximal portions of this cell mass (the ectoplacental cone) will form the chorion. The ingrowth of mesoderm cavitates to form the exocoelom. The exocoelom is separated from the lower cavity (the amniotic cavity) by a membrane composed of mesoderm and ectoderm; this becomes the amnion. The exocoelom is separated from the ectoplacental cavity by a similar set of cells which are the chorion. These two cavities, the amniotic cavity and the exocoelom, continue to enlarge with further differentiation of the distal cell mass to become the embryo. The allantois grows out from the distal end of the primitive streak into the exocoelom toward the chorion. With attachment to the chorion on about the eighth day, the ectoplacental cavity is obliterated and a continuous structure, the chorioallantois, is formed. This provides an avenue for embryonic blood vessels to make contact with the maternal blood supply.

By the eighth day, when organ differentiation commences, the embryo consists of the differentiating primitive streak surrounded outside by proximal endoderm which is the continuation of the midgut. This proximal endoderm completely surrounds the cell mass up to the ectoplacenta; it then folds and continues as distal endoderm to enclose within the space the yolk sac cavity. Inside the developing embryo is the amniotic cavity which is separated from the exocoelom by the amnion. The peculiar situation then is that of endoderm continuous with the midgut surrounding the entire differentiating cell mass which then folds back upon itself at the chorion to form a continuous lining for the blastocystic cavity, the yolk cavity. It is analogous to the way that a fist pushed into a partially filled balloon would be enclosed by two layers of balloon; the interior of the balloon would correspond to the yolk cavity. The embryo is inside out; the ectoderm which will give rise primarily to neural structures and the integument is deep within the embryo.

With growth of the embryo, the ectoderm expands while the gut is closing. The gut is formed by invagination of the endoderm into the embryo in the foregut and hindgut regions; then, in zipperlike fashion from the foregut and hindgut, the endoderm encloses a tube which becomes the intestine. This cavity and its lining remain continuous with the proximal yolk sac through a stalk at the midgut region. The closing of the gut and expansion of the ectoderm requires a complete turning of the embryo. Imagine the embryo as a "U" with the inside surface of the "U" as ectoderm and the outside as endoderm. Then, after the zippering of the gut, the "U" has twisted completely so that ectoderm now is on the outside and the gut on the inside. A stalk runs from the midgut to the yolk sac. The vitelline vessels are in this stalk. The allantois grows out from the posterior end of the embryo between the yolk cavity and the amniotic cavity. Eventually, the amnion surrounds both, and compressed together, the vitelline and allantois stalks form the umbilical cord at the embryo. In late gestation the umbilical cord may be identified as a single structure near the embryo which bifurcates about midway to the chorioallantoic placenta into two almost equal-sized cords: the chorioallantoic cord and the yolk sac (or vitelline) cord. Further details and diagrams of the rotation of the embryo may be found in Snell and Stevens (1966, pp. 230 and 231).

The formation of the membranes in the mouse (and other rodents) is rather different from most other vertebrate embryos. The cell layers in the mouse embryo are reversed; by the time organ differentiation begins on about the eighth day, the inner cell mass is ectoderm with the endoderm constituting a thin outer layer of cells which gives rise to the gastrointestinal lining. It is somewhat analogous to the whole embryo arising from the interior of an inverted gastrointestinal tract.

As the embryo grows it pushes into the amniotic cavity which in turn pushes into the exocoelom. This coincides with a collapse of the yolk sac cavity as the proximal and distal endoderm of the yolk sac become contiguous. Although it appears that the distal endodermal cells are essentially continuous with the trophectoderm, there is evidence that Reichert's membrane is secreted by the distal endodermal cells as a thin, noncellular, pink-staining membrane immediately over the inner surface of the trophectoderm. Reichert's membrane ruptures on about the fifteenth day in the mouse and the proximal endodermal cells then face the uterine lumen directly.

The decidua capsularis is clearly present in the mouse up to the twelfth day; thereafter, it rapidly becomes very thin.

3. OTHER SPECIES

Recent reports of the comparative embryology of the membranes of several species include Balinsky (1940), Bellairs (1971), and Bryden *et al.* (1972). Virtually every conceivable arrangement of fetal membranes for attachment to the mother may be found among the vertebrates. The most complete review of these types of placental attachments is Mossman's (1937). The two major placentas, the chorioallantoic and the yolk sac, may each predominate at different times during gestation for one species. Therefore, an arbitrary comparison of attachments was made at the stage of limb bud development. Organogenesis is occurring and the embryo is susceptible to teratogenic agents at this time. Table I summarizes Mossman's review at the stage of limb bud development into the three categories of species, viz., those with primarily or solely a chorioallantoic attachment, those with primarily or solely a yolk sac attachment, and those that have extensive attachments of each. Of those with considerable development of both types, the dog and raccoon have a yolk sac that is adjacent to the uterine lumen. Only in these would a secretion by the yolk sac have direct access to the uterine lumen.

TABLE I   Species of Animals Grouped According to the Type of Placental Attachment Existing at the Time of Limb Bud Development[a]

Primarily or solely chorioallantoic	Chorioallantoic and yolk sac	Primarily or solely yolk sac
Man	Rabbit	Tree shrew
Pig	Beaver	Kangaroo rat
Sheep	Dog	Mouse
Three-toed sloth	Muskrat	Guinea pig
Tenrec	Ferret	Pocket gopher
Tarsius	Horse	Rat
Macaque	Raccoon	
	Ground squirrel	
	Coney	
	Cape golden mole	
	Hedgehog	
	Shrew	
	Mole	
	Flying fox	
	Bat	
	Loris	
	Golago	
	Flying lemur	
	Armadillo	
	Scaly anteater	

[a] Mossman, 1937.

C. Histology and Histochemistry of Membranes

1. HUMAN

The human chorion arises from mesoderm in the blastocyst and during early gestation is well vascularized. Some time during the third month of gestation, the fetal circulation on the interior of the chorion as well as the maternal circulation through the decidua capsularis both disappear. Vessels are seen in specimens taken during the second month, but only rarely in those taken in the third month (Hoyes, 1971). However, some vascular structures have been described in material taken at term (Lister, 1968). The layers of the chorion in its final definitive form (Bourne, 1960, 1962) after degeneration of the blood vessels are, from the fetal side out: (1) a cellular layer of loosely interlacing fibroblasts, (2) a thick network of mostly parallel fibers, (3) a pseudobasement membrane for the trophoblast consisting of dense argyrophil connective tissue firmly adherent to both the reticular layer and the trophoblast, and (4) finally, a trophoblast layer that varies considerably in thickness. There is no cell layer or type in the human chorion to suggest that it has a secretory or absorptive function.

The amnion is a continuation of the skin of the embryo and consists of the following layers (Bourne, 1962) from the fetal side out: (1) An epithelium of a single layer of cells which varies from cuboidal to columnar. These cells are closely packed to form a continuous sheet which could very well function to transport water or solutes. There seems to be some controversy over the brush border on these cells. Bourne (1960, 1962) states that the brush border is on the exposed surface of these cells facing the amniotic fluid. Sinha (1971) also found the microvilli on the surface facing the amniotic fluid. However, Danforth and Hull (1958) found the brush border only on the opposite side of the cells where they are attached very tightly to a basement membrane. One possible interpretation for the brush border on the side facing the membrane is that the cell transports in this direction and that the transported material diffuses through the remaining layers of amnion and those of the chorion. Another possibility is that this brush border consists of invaginations which account for the very firm attachment to the basement membrane. Further studies of this cell layer would be highly desirable. (2) The next outer layer is a thin network of reticular fibers which serve as a basement membrane for the epithelial cells. (3) A relatively dense complex of reticular fibers devoid of cells is the next and probably the strongest of the layers of the amnion. (4) A loose fibroblast network embedded in a mass of reticulum constitutes the thickest layer. (5) A spongy layer containing the compressed elements of extraembryonic coelom is adjacent to the chorion and allows lubrication for sliding of the two membranes against each other.

Throughout both the amnion and chorion are Hofbauer cells which are vacuolated macrophages, which probably have an unusual capacity for fluid ingestion, and perhaps serve in some regulatory capacity (Enders and King, 1970). Another view is that they are degenerated elements of the mesenchyme (Hoyes, 1970).

The human yolk sac has been studied by electron microscopy in two laboratories (Hoyes, 1969; Hesseldahl and Larsen, 1969). These add much detail to the histology of this tissue described earlier. It consists, between the fourth and sixth weeks of gestation, of proliferating endoderm to form cords of cells projecting into the mesenchyme. Abundant endoplasmic reticulum, glycogen, and iron-containing material is apparent in these endodermal cells. Both surfaces of the sac possess cells with microvilli and pinocytotic vesicles. Some of the endodermal cells resemble hemocytoblasts and others megakaryocytes.

Several possible functions of the human yolk sac are suggested from the morphological studies. These include synthesis of protein and hemoglobin as well as other hemopoietic activity. It has been recognized as the principal site of hemopoietic activity between the fifth and ninth weeks of gestation (Bloom and Bartelemez, 1940). Since both surfaces of the sac contain a brush border and microvilli, it may be responsible for at least part of the production of the fluid in the extraembryonic coelom; the disappearance of the coelom and the decline in the activity of the yolk sac coincide.

The possibility should not be overlooked that metabolic and secretory activities of the yolk sac for waste material could exist. Compounds metabolized and secreted by the yolk sac into the exocoelom could diffuse through the layers of chorion into the uterine lumen. The tight cell layer on the inside of the amnion could prevent reentry of these compounds back into the fetus. In this manner it could have a role similar in function to that of the rodent yolk sac.

2. RODENTS

There are numerous descriptions of the histology of fetal membranes of rats and mice. Lucid accounts are to be found in recent texts on the mouse (Snell and Stevens, 1966; Rugh, 1968). Since the chorion in the mouse is restricted to the base of the chorioallantoic placenta, the only membranes existing by the eighth day when organ differentiation begins are the amnion and the yolk sac.

The amnion is composed of a cellular layer of ectoderm and one of mesoderm. The ultrastructural features of this membrane have been described for the rat by Wynn and French (1968).

The yolk sac serves as the primary organ of nourishment of the embryo in early gestation and as a major contributor throughout gestation. The endodermal cells, by day 7, are mature and have microvilli, coated invaginations and vacuoles, an apical canalicular system, and an abundance of absorptive droplets and vacuoles (Haar and Ackerman, 1971b). They are attached to a basement membrane on the proximal side, and the microvilli face the yolk cavity. Basophilia increases in these cells between days 8 and 12 of gestation and corresponds with the development of a highly organized rough endoplasmic reticulum by 12 days. This largely converts to a smooth endoplasmic reticulum by 18 days. Apparently, emphasis is on synthetic mechanisms in earlier gestation and on absorption in later gestation, although both processes occur throughout (Calarco and Moyer, 1966).

The endodermal cells which grow out from the inner cell mass to line the trophectoderm become the pareital wall of the yolk sac. These cells secrete the thin, noncellular, pink-staining membrane called Reichert's membrane (Pierce et al., 1962; Midgley and Pierce, 1963). Straining properties of this membrane suggest that it consists of a carbohydrate–protein complex. The protein contains basic amino acids and those typical of proteins of epithelial origin (Wislocki and Padykula, 1953; Kulay and Fava De Moraes, 1965). The membrane ruptures on the fifteenth day leaving the proximal endodermal cells directly exposed to the uterine lumen.

Histochemical studies on fetal membranes of the mouse reveal 3β-hydroxysteroid dehydrogenase activity in the endodermal cells of the yolk sac when dehydroepiandrosterone is the substrate. Both 17α- and 17β-hydroxysteroid dehydrogenase activity, NAD-dependent, was present with a variety of substrates. Activity of 17β-hydroxysteroid dehydrogenase, NADP-dependent, was demonstrated in the yolk sac only with estradiol-17β (Botte et al., 1968). The visceral yolk sac endoderm of the rat is histochemically positive for ethanol dehydrogenase, furfuryl alcohol dehydrogenase, glutamate dehydrogenase, and sorbital dehydrogenase (Christie, 1968).

Injection of teratogenic doses of trypan blue into pregnant mice decreased the acid phosphatase activity in yolk sac endodermal cells and disrupted their Golgi apparatus (Greenhouse et al., 1969). However, since only 25% of these fetuses were malformed, this was not considered to support the theory of Beck et al. (1967) that the teratogenic action of trypan blue is mediated via the yolk sac. The need for the integrity of the membranes was ascertained by Payne and Deuchar (1972) in 10-day-old rat embryos cultivated *in vitro* following removal of each of the fetal membranes. Less ^{14}C-leucine was taken up by the embryos as the parietal yolk sac, visceral yolk sac, and amnion were removed in succession. Development and survival of the embryos was greater with higher leucine uptake. Anti-yolk sac antibodies retarded growth and differentiation of 10-day-old rat embryos *in vitro*, apparently from specific interaction with the visceral yolk sac endoderm (New and Brent, 1972). Inhibition of the selective exclusion of ^{14}C-valine by the yolk sac of 12-day-pregnant rats was effected by treatment with chlorambucil (Kernis, 1971) which further indicates the pivotal role of the yolk sac in embryonic nutrition.

The yolk sac apparently is the source of the blood cells for the embryo. A sheet of mesoderm inside the endodermal epithelium differentiates into angioblastic cords from which the blood cells and vessels are derived (Haar and Ackerman, 1971a). Several hemoglobin components which are formed in the yolk sac have been identified; their production is not influenced by erythropoietin (Hunter and Paul, 1969). Although Moore and Metcalf (1970) interpret their experiments to indicate that cells from the yolk sac colonize hemopoietic organs of the embryo before it can produce its own red blood cells, Marks and Rifkind (1972a,b) disagree. Apparently there is some question concerning the ability of the colony-forming cells to differentiate into erythrocytes.

3. OTHER SPECIES

The placentation of the baboon (*Papio* sp.) appears to be similar in many respects to that of the human except that implantation is superficial and no decidua capsularis exists (Wynn *et al.*, 1971; Houston, 1969a,b). The amnion consists of a single layer of ectoderm, and the chorion is a mesodermal network with an epithelial cell cover. When amnion and chorion fuse with the decidua parietalis, the combined amnion and chorion is mesoderm with an epithelial cover on each side.

Comparison of the ultrastructure of the amnion of rats, guinea pigs, macaque, and man (Wynn and French, 1968) showed these membranes to be similar with a single cell epithelium and acellular connective tissue layer. The lateral and basal specializations of the plasma membrane were better developed in the primate; rodent amnion had more apical cytoplasmic projections. Evidence for pinocytosis was seen in stromal as well as epithelial cells.

Beautiful, scanning electron microscope pictures by King and Enders (1970) of the visceral yolk sac of the guinea pig show the fantastic similarity of this tissue to the intestinal epithelium. The villi and crypts must indicate that this surface is active in absorption and secretion.

The yolk sac of the bat, *Tadarida brasiliensis cynocephala*, very early in gestation forms a placental relationship with the maternal uterus. Later the allantoic tissues displace the yolk sac, which collapses, and a chorioallantoic placenta is established. The yolk sac in this species is very active in the synthesis and storage of lipid and glycogen (Stephens and Easterbrook, 1968, 1969). These activities are carefully sequenced during gestation. This yolk sac is also involved in hemopoietic activity and the epithelial cells differentiate into the form typical of those active in absorption and secretion (Stephens and Easterbrook, 1971; Stephens and Cabral, 1971).

Observations by electron microscopy of the yolk sac of the spiny dog-fish *Squalus acanthias* suggested a sequential pattern of functional activity by this tissue (Jollie and Jollie, 1967). Animals were observed at different intervals throughout the 2-year gestation. Yolk sacs in the middle of the first summer functioned both in nutritive and respiratory transport; those in the late first summer were involved in only nutritive transport. During the second summer, neither type of transport function was apparent.

II. Transfer of Drugs between Mother and Fetus by Routes Other than the Chorioallantoic Placenta

Although molecules of many sizes and physical properties are capable of being exchanged between the maternal and fetal compartments, the route of transfer is frequently unknown. It is all too common to assume that the chorioallantoic placenta is the organ responsible for the exchange of all molecules. The physical and chemical properties of molecules which determine the rate and extent of their transfer across the chorioallantoic placenta are discussed in detail elsewhere in this volume. It is the purpose of this section to consider routes other than the chorioallantoic placenta which are known to account for the exchange of material between the mother and fetus.

A. Movement of Drugs into the Fallopian Tube, Uterine Fluid, and Their Penetration into the Blastocyst

The composition, production, and accumulation of the fluid in the oviduct is controlled by the stage of the cycle, pregnancy and steroid hormone treatment in the mother (Bishop, 1956; Mastroianni *et al.*, 1961; Hamner and Fox, 1969; Conner and Miller, 1973a; Mastroianni and

Wallach, 1961). The pH value of fluid collected from rabbit oviducts is higher than that of plasma (Vishwakarma, 1962), and there is active secretion of chloride into the rabbit oviduct (Brunton and Brinster, 1971). Furthermore, amino acids are secreted into the endometrial cavity which apparently facilitates their penetration into the blastocyst during the time interval between fertilization and implantation in the rabbit (Jaszczak et al., 1970).

These secretory mechanisms for normal constituents of biological fluids may account for some of the observations seen on apparent secretion of drugs into the fallopian tube and uterine fluid. For instance, one would expect basic drugs to be found in lower concentrations and acidic drugs in higher concentrations in this fluid if the pH is higher than that of plasma. Deviations from this distribution pattern could be accounted for by specific, active secretory mechanisms, or active reabsorption of water from the oviduct. The distribution of ^3H_2O, barbital, tetraethylammonium bromide, α-aminoisobutyric acid, dimethyloxazolidinedione, ouabain, inulin, and antipyrine into uterine luminal fluid of nonpregnant rats failed to reveal any special transport systems and correlated with the distribution of drugs across lipid barriers at pH 7.4 (Conner and Miller, 1973b).

Six hours after treatment of pregnant rabbits with 1-methyl-^{14}C-caffeine there was approximately 50% more radioactivity in the uterine secretion than in the plasma. One hour after the administration of ^{3}H-nicotine high concentrations of radioactivity were found in the uterine secretion. The radioactivity in the uterine secretion was not found in nonpregnant rabbits under the same experimental conditions (Fabro and Sieber, 1969b).

The blastocysts of rabbits on day 6 of gestation were found to contain significant amounts of 1-methyl-^{14}C-caffeine, ^{3}H-nicotine, ^{14}C-DDT, ^{14}C-barbital, ^{14}C-thiopental, or carbonyl-^{14}C-isoniazid 1–6 hours after the mothers had received the drugs (Fabro and Sieber, 1969a; Sieber and Fabro, 1971; Fabro, 1973). Water and glutethimide attain the same concentration in the blastocyst as that found in the medium (Keberle et al., 1966). The pH value of the fluid inside the blastocyst was reported to be 9.0 (Gottschewski, 1962) which accounts for the accumulation of acidic drugs in this fluid. Furthermore, the rate of uptake by the blastocyst for salicylate, sulfanilamide, antipyrine, and hexamethonium correlated with lipid solubility and the degree of ionization of the drugs (Sieber and Fabro, 1971). The transfer of compounds from the plasma into the uterine secretion has been shown to occur not only in the rabbit but also in other species including mice and rats (McLachlan et al., 1969).

The large size of the rabbit preimplantation blastocyst (3–4.5 mm diameter at 6.5 days and 1 cm at 8 days after fertilization) has attracted the attention of those studying early gestation. The much smaller size of the human, mouse, and rat blastocyst hinders their use. Simple and rapid techniques for observing the effects of potential teratogenic agents on the rabbit blastocyst have been published (Lutwak-Mann and Hay, 1962; Lutwak-Mann, 1973).

Early studies on the penetration of the blastocyst by maternal antibodies by Brambell et al. (1951) demonstrated that some antibodies penetrate the blastocyst wall; furthermore, serum proteins were demonstrated immunofluorescently to penetrate mouse eggs, in vivo (Glass, 1963). A dividing line for molecular size was suggested from the in vitro studies with 6-day rabbit blastocysts (Sieber and Fabro, 1971) which revealed that dextran with a molecular weight of 60,000 to 90,000 did not penetrate, but dextran with a molecular weight of 16,000 to 19,000 did penetrate. This is in slight disagreement with an earlier study with rat, hamster, and rabbit eggs which were permeable to toluidine blue, digitonin, and alcian blue but not to heparin which has a molecular weight of less than 20,000 (Austin and Lovelock, 1958).

Lutwak-Mann (1954) found negligible penetration of the blastocyst by glucose, fructose, and sucrose before implantation. Following implantation, however, the permeability increased considerably. Trypan blue and Congo red were shown to appear in the fluid in rabbit blastocysts on days 7, 8 and up to the middle of the ninth day of gestation (Ferm, 1956). The permeability declines rapidly after day 9 and curiously enough, so does the teratogenic activity of these dyes in the rabbit. Perhaps completion of the integrity of the yolk sac accounts for the decline in the permeability of the blastocyst to these dyes on day 9. Ferm suggested that the change in permeability of the blastocyst to dye in the middle of the ninth day of gestation represents a change from the embryotrophic type of nutrition to that of the histotropic stage. Adams et al. (1961) confirmed the permeability of the rabbit blastocyst to trypan blue as well as its teratogenic effect on the rabbit embryo.

The teratogenic effect of insulin injected into the pregnant rabbit (Brinsmade and Rubsaamen, 1957) might be due to the induced hypoglycemia which Curry and Ferm (1962) reported within the rabbit blastocyst fluid. This is in contrast, however, to the report by Lutwak-Mann (1962) that treatment of mothers with insulin to lower their blood glucose did not lower the glucose in the blastocyst below that in maternal blood. Other maneuvers to alter maternal glucose concentrations were slow to produce changes in the concentration in the blastocyst (Curry and Ferm, 1962).

The ability of the rabbit blastocyst to actually regulate the concentration of glucose, lactic acid, and bicarbonate in its fluid seems to be considerable (Lutwak-Mann, 1962). Treatment of pregnant rabbits with several drugs did not greatly alter the concentration of these metabolites in the unimplanted blastocyst; however, implantation coincided with large changes in the concentration. Salicylate was said to penetrate rapidly both unimplanted and implanted blastocysts and persist in them for hours after it had disappeared from maternal fluids. The effect of ouabain and acetazolamide on the rate and extent of transport of Na^+, K^+, Cl^-, HCO_3^-, and H_2O into the rabbit blastocyst has recently been reported (Smith, 1970).

^{14}C-Thalidomide and its polar metabolites were still present in rabbit embryos 58 hours after administration of the drug to the mother on the eighth day of gestation (Fabro et al., 1965). This may account for the teratogenic action of the drug when given only while the blastocyst is in the preimplantation stage (Hay, 1964). Keberle et al. (1965) reported that ^{14}C-thalidomide was able to penetrate into the blastocyst of preimplantation, implanting, and postimplantation blastocysts but that two of the ^{14}C-metabolites were not able to penetrate until implanation had occurred. ^{14}C-Thalidomide and its polar metabolites were much more concentrated in the embryos of hamsters when given to the mothers at 8.5 days of gestation (Fabro et al., 1967). Lack of penetration into the blastocyst, therefore, cannot explain the difficulty in obtaining a teratogenic action in this species.

Skalko and Morse (1969) demonstrated that the teratogen actinomycin D affected blastocyst formation as well as blastocyst survival and differentiation when mouse blastocysts were cultured in media containing this compound. Studies on the effects of actinomycin D and puromycin at different stages of cell division suggested that cleavage is regulated by RNA and protein molecules which need to be synthesized during each cell cycle (Molinaro et al., 1972).

Ferm et al. (1969) found that cadmium-109 penetrated the implanting hamster blastocyst and that the simultaneous administration of zinc does not prevent the transfer of the teratogen to the embryo. Simultaneous administration of zinc inhibits the teratogenic effect of cadmium, in producing cleft lip and palate, in hamster embryos (Ferm and Carpenter, 1968).

The single injection of an inhibitor of 3β-hydroxysteroid dehydrogenase during the preimplantation stage of the rat blastocyst or even before ovulation produces the adrenogenital syndrome in rats (Goldman, 1969). The extreme persistence of this inhibitor perhaps accounts for its action

DISTALGESIC
INFORMATION FOR PATIENTS

YOUR PRESCRIPTION FOR DISTALGESIC
(Dextropropoxyphene 32.5mg with Paracetamol 325mg)

Your doctor has prescribed Distalgesic tablets for the relief of your pain. Please read this leaflet carefully before you start to take the tablets.

1. **Alcohol**
   The consumption of alcohol whilst taking medicine may be dangerous therefore;

   AVOID ALCOHOL WHILST TAKING DISTALGESIC

2. **Working**
   Some people find that Distalgesic tablets make them drowsy or dizzy at first, especially if they are taking tranquillisers or sleeping pills as well. You should be careful when driving or operating machinery until you know your reaction to Distalgesic.

3. **Dosage**
   TAKE NO MORE THAN TWO TABLETS AT A TIME
   TAKE NO MORE THAN EIGHT TABLETS A DAY

4. **Pregnancy**
   You should not take Distalgesic or any other drugs during pregnancy unless your doctor knows you are pregnant and specifically prescribes them.

5. **Overdosage**
   IF YOU SUSPECT THAT YOU, OR ANYONE ELSE, HAS TAKEN TOO MANY DISTALGESIC TABLETS DON'T DELAY, DIAL 999 FOR AN AMBULANCE IMMEDIATELY, THEN PHONE YOUR DOCTOR

6. **Remember**
   These tablets have been prescribed for YOUR USE ONLY. Keep them in a safe place and do NOT allow anyone else to take them. Destroy unused tablets at the end of treatment. If you have any questions ask your doctor or pharmacist.

DISTA PRODUCTS LIMITED
Kingsclere Road, Basingstoke, Hampshire RG21 2XA

'Distalgesic' is a trade mark

DAL 189/Feb. 1984

Intra fetal Transfusion

Fetal umbilical
fetal liver   } circulation
Drugs + Penicillin

Dry Biotransfusion
~~~~~~~~~

Gestation → embryo is differentially
foetal membranes develop

at later dates in gestation. Other substances which have been found to be lethal in very low concentrations to the early mouse embryo include salicylate (Young *et al.*, 1972) and Cu^{2+} (Brinster and Cross, 1972). The significance of these *in vitro* effects needs to be assessed more carefully since salicylate had no apparent effect on rabbit blastocysts *in vivo* (Fabro, 1973).

In summary, the movement of some substances into the fallopian tube, uterine fluid, and blastocyst has been studied. Most of these have been in the rabbit. However, it is clear that penetration into the blastocyst by a teratogenic agent is not necessary to effect the teratogenic action. More studies on the blastocyst should provide additional knowledge of the process of early differentiation, but probably would have limited value for the mechanism of teratogenic action of drugs.

B. Transfer across the Wall of the Yolk Sac

The tremendous importance of the inverted yolk sac in the transmission of intact proteins from the mother to the fetus was elegantly demonstrated by Brambell and his colleagues. A series of experiments were designed to determine the route by which passive immunity is conferred on the fetus (Brambell, 1958). Antibodies from the uterine lumen or from the maternal circulation were absorbed by the yolk sac endodermal cells and transferred to the fetus through the vitelline circulation in rabbits, rats, and guinea pigs. Ligation of the vitelline circulation stopped the transmission of antibodies to the fetus. Some antibodies that reached the fetus in the absence of the yolk sac were thought to have been absorbed in the endodermal sinuses of Duval in the rat and transported by the allantoic circulation (Brambell and Halliday, 1956). The yolk sac was shown in early electron microscope studies to have the features consistent with absorptive functions; a layer of columnar cells with surface microvilli and apical vacuoles rests on a basement membrane beneath which is a mesenchyme containing a good supply of vitelline vessels. The yolk sac of the guinea pig (Dempsey, 1953), rat (Wislocki and Dempsey, 1955), and rabbit (Luse, 1957) are all morphologically very similar.

The importance of the rodent yolk sac as an organ of nutrition was recognized by Everett (1935) who described the localization of trypan blue and other dyes in the endodermal cells. Reichert's membrane allowed the ready passage of the dye from maternal fluids to the visceral yolk sac. Recent studies (Kernis and Johnson, 1969) reveal that trypan blue and niagara blue 2B both significantly increase the absorption of $^{45}Ca^{2+}$,

$^{35}SO_4{}^{2-}$, and $^{22}Na^+$ by the yolk sac of the rat on days 12, 13, and 14 of gestation. This suggests that these dyes have an effect on the function of the yolk sac which may bear a relationship to the induction of congenital abnormalities.

The accumulation of ^{14}C-inulin in the yolk sac of the mouse may be seen in Fig. 6. The ^{14}C-inulin was given to the pregnant animal 4 hours before sacrifice. It is likely that the isotopic material was phagocytized by the yolk sac endodermal cells in a manner similar to that for antibodies and other large molecules.

The absorption of lipid and Thorotrast from the yolk sac of chick specimens by phagocytosis through the endodermal cells (Lambson, 1970) is no surprise. But the clarification of the exact nature of this mechanism in the yolk sac of mammals is still not completely understood. Ferritin molecules have been traced by electron microscopy after injection into pregnant rats or after placing the material directly in the uterine cavity (Lambson, 1966). The material appears to enter the endodermal cells through an apical canalicular system to become localized in large vacuoles. Later in pregnancy, small vacuoles appear to migrate away from the apical storage vacuoles and proceed to the basement membrane where they appear to pass either directly into vitelline capillaries or through mesothelial cells into the exocoelom. These vacuoles contain acid phosphatase and other esterases which may account for the occasional

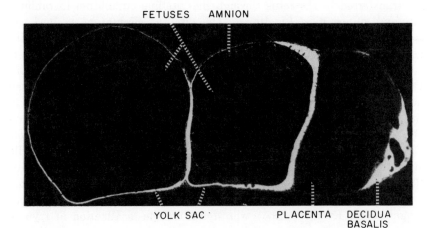

FETUSES   AMNION

YOLK SAC   PLACENTA   DECIDUA
                             BASALIS

FIG. 6. A detail of a print of an autoradiogram of a 20-μm section from a NMRI mouse injected intravenously with ^{14}C-inulin a few days prior to term and frozen 4 hours later. Two fetuses are shown with a high concentration in the yolk sacs. White areas correspond to radioactivity.

presence of ferritin lying free in the cytoplasm (Krzyzowska-Gruca and Schiebler, 1967).

The transfer of ferritin by this same process was confirmed in guinea pig yolk sac by King and Enders (1970). Horseradish peroxidase was transported even more rapidly than ferritin, but Thorotrast was not transported although it was taken up into vacuoles. Hamster yolk sacs also avidly phagocytized Thorotrast but did not transport the material; the connective tissue spaces, blood vessels, and fetal compartments were free of tracer particles at all time intervals after injection (Carpenter and Ferm, 1969).

Further studies on the selective nature of the uptake and transport of large molecules by the visceral yolk sac of rabbits have recently been completed (Slade, 1970; Wild, 1970). By carefully tracing the ferritin in the vacuoles, the notion arose that most of the ferritin is degraded within endodermal cells, but that some is protected by adsorption onto the vesicular membrane. The undegraded ferritin may be within smaller secondary vacuoles which transport the material to the fetal vessels. Fluorescent-labeled proteins were transmitted across the visceral endoderm by pinocytotic vesicles to the fetal circulation. The route for labeled proteins to reach the exocoelom was by diffusion through the paraplacental chorion. Electron microscopic studies failed to clarify the selective nature of the transport process for proteins in the rabbit yolk sac (Wild et al., 1972). The many factors influencing the pinocytosis, degradation, and transfer to fetal circulation of large molecules are still not completely known.

Rat (Padykula et al., 1966) and rabbit (Deren et al., 1966a) visceral yolk sacs have a tremendous capacity to accumulate vitamin B_{12}. The yolk sac had a higher affinity than fetal ilium of the same gestational age. Curiously, the capacity decreases with increasing gestational age.

Rabbit yolk sacs of more than 20 days gestation actively accumulate L-valine, L-isoleucine, L-phenylalanine, L-alanine, and L-methionine; other amino acids are not actively accumulated (Deren et al., 1966b). The membrane was capable of effecting a transfer of L-valine across its full thickness against a concentration gradient. Two separate transport systems were identified for amino acids in the guinea pig yolk sac (Butt and Wilson, 1968). The development of these transport systems was sequenced during gestation, and they preceded the development of amino acid transport systems in the fetal intestine.

Secretion of substances by the yolk sac into the uterine lumen affords an independent mechanism for elimination of drugs. Although very few investigators have been concerned with this possible excretory route, evidence for excretion by the yolk sac was presented by Waddell (1971a,

1972a). Cortisone and other drugs appeared to be secreted by the yolk sac and flow out the vagina of pregnant mice. The significance of this possible route of excretion could be tremendous in animals who have yolk sac placentas directly adjacent to the uterine lumen. Further experiments clarifying this function would be highly desirable. Even in animals whose yolk sac placentas are not exposed to the uterine lumen, metabolism of drugs by this highly active tissue could have a significant effect on fetal growth and differentiation.

The human yolk sac has been demonstrated to be capable of the synthesis of prealbumin, albumin, α-fetoprotein, α-antitrypsin, and transferrin at $5\frac{1}{2}$ weeks of gestation (Gitlin and Perricelli, 1970). These synthetic capabilities decreased at $8\frac{1}{2}$ weeks of gestation and were essentially nonexistent at $11\frac{1}{2}$ weeks. However, production of α-fetoprotein by the human yolk sac, liver and, to a small extent, gastrointestinal tract was demonstrated in fetuses between 4.2 and 18 weeks of gestation (Gitlin et al., 1972). Synthesis of α-fetoprotein was found to occur only in the liver and yolk sac of fetal rabbits (Branch and Wild, 1972; Slade and Budd, 1972).

C. Transfer across the Chorion and Amnion

The transmission of human γ-globulin by intercellular diffusion through the paraplacental chorion of the rabbit (Slade and Wild, 1971) and the gray squirrel (Wild, 1971) has been proposed. This apparently is a nonselective process as opposed to that occurring across the yolk sac. Bovine serum albumin has been reported to cross the human chorion and amnion when deposited in the uterine lumen of women near term (Kulangara et al., 1965). The human chorion laeve is very freely permeable to water and is also permeable to Na^+, Cl^-, urea, glucose, and sucrose; the amnion is rather freely permeable to these substances also (Seeds, 1970; Brame, 1972).

The permeability of the guinea pig amnion to monovalent ions changed with changes in pH of the solutions. Decreased permeability to Na^+ and K^+ at low pH values and decreased permeability to Cl^- at high pH values suggested an effective isoelectric point of 4.2 for the membrane (Foreman and Segal, 1972).

Young human chorion in tissue culture acetylated sulfomethoxypyridine and hydroxylated ketophenylbutazone, benzopyrazone, and mebrophenydramine (Uher, 1969). This raises the possibility for conversion of drugs by the chorion to toxic metabolites which are transferred to the fetus. Alkaline phosphatase, acid phosphatase, 3β-hydroxysteroid dehydrogenase, PAS-positive, esterase, and lactic dehydrogenase activities were also demonstrated histochemically in these cultures.

III. Distribution of Drugs in the Fetus

A search, which was concluded in mid-1973, was made of studies of the distribution of substances in fetal tissues. Emphasis was placed on those which employed autoradiography; although others which attempted discernment in specific fetal tissues were included. Several recent reviews on the distribution of drugs in fetal tissues have appeared (Mirkin, 1973; Ullberg, 1973; Waddell, 1973a). The autoradiographic studies are summarized in the tables on distribution in the following sections.

A. Distribution of Elemental Ions

The elements which have been studied are shown in Table II, and a summary of their distribution patterns is listed in Table III.

The alkali metal ions gain ready access to the fetus—sodium (Huggert *et al.*, 1961) apparently more rapidly than rubidium (Olsson *et al.*, 1969) or cesium (Nelson *et al.*, 1961); the distribution of radiopotassium has not been studied in pregnant animals. A few days prior to term in the mouse, the only fetal tissues to show any specific accumulation of these isotopes were cartilage and bone. However, ^{22}Na (but not ^{86}Rb or ^{137}Cs) was found in higher concentration in fetal brain than in maternal brain. Since thiocyanate (Clemedson *et al.*, 1960), iodide (Ullberg and Ewaldsson, 1964), and bromide (Söremark, 1960) were all found in higher concentration in fetal brain than maternal, the most likely explanation is

TABLE II   Periodic Table of the Elements with Those Circled Whose Isotopes Have Been Studied by Whole-Body Autoradiography in Pregnant Animals

Period	IA	IIA	IIIB	IVB	VB	VIB	VIIB	XIII			IB	IIB	IIIA	IVA	VA	VIA	VIIA	Inert gases
1	H																	He
2	Li	Be											B	(C)	N	O	(F)	Ne
3	(Na)	Mg											Al	Si	(P)	(S)	Cl	Ar
4	K	(Ca)	Sc	Ti	(V)	Cr	Mn	(Fe)	(Co)	Ni	Cu	(Zn)	Ga	Ge	As	(Se)	(Br)	(Kr)
5	(Rb)	Sr	(Y)	(Zr)	(Nb)	Mo	Tc	(Ru)	Rh	Pd	Ag	(Cd)	In	Sn	Sb	Te	(I)	Xe
6	(Cs)	Ba	La*	Hf	Ta	W	Re	Os	Ir	Pt	Au	(Hg)	(Tl)	Pb	Bi	(Po)	At	Rn
7	Fr	Ra	Ac**															

*	(Ce)	Pr	Nd	(Pm)	Sm	Eu	Gd	(Tb)	Dy	(Ho)	Er	Tm	(Yb)	Lu
**	Th	Pa	U	Np	(Pu)	(Am)	Cm	BK	Cf	Es	Fm	Md	No	(Lw)

TABLE III   Distribution of Elemental Ions in Maternal and Fetal Tissues of Mice near Term

Isotope	Conjugate ion	Principal maternal tissues	Principal fetal tissues	Reference
$^{22}Na^+$	Cl⁻	Bone, cartilage	Yolk sac, bone, cartilage	Huggert et al., 1961
$^{86}Rb^+$	Cl⁻	Liver, cartilage, forming bone, skeletal muscle	Bone, cartilage	Olsson et al., 1969
$^{137}Cs^+$	Cl⁻	Skeletal muscle, cartilage, salivary gland, intestine	Bone, cartilage	Nelson et al., 1961
$^{45}Ca^{2+}$	Cl⁻	Bone, some muscle groups, intestinal contents	Bone	Appelgren et al., 1961; Ericsson and Hammarström, 1964
$^{91}Y^{3+}$	Cl⁻	Bone, cartilage, renal cortex, gastric mucosa	Yolk sac, bone	Appelgren et al., 1966
$^{95}Zr^{4+} + {}_{95}Nb^{5+}$	Oxalate	Bone, connective tissue, liver	Yolk sac, bone, liver, blood	Bäckström et al., 1967
$^{95}Nb^{5+}$	Oxalate	Bone, connective tissue, liver	Yolk sac, bone, liver, blood	Bäckström et al., 1967
$^{59}Fe^{3+}$	Citrate	Bone marrow, choroid plexus, red pulp of spleen, liver, gastrointestinal tract	Liver, blood, bone, choroid plexus	Ullberg et al., 1961
$^{103}Ru^{3+}$	Cl⁻	Connective tissues, renal cortex, red pulp of spleen, liver	Yolk sac	Nelson et al., 1962
$^{60}Co^{2+}$	Cl⁻	Cartilage, liver, kidney, pancreas	Yolk sac, bone, liver	Flodh, 1968a
$^{65}Zn^{2+}$	Cl⁻	Liver, kidney, bone, mammary gland, gastric and intestinal mucosa	Yolk sac, bone, liver, kidney	Bergman and Söremark, 1968
$^{109}Cd^{2+}$	Cl⁻	Liver, kidney, pancreas, bone marrow	Yolk sac	Berlin and Ullberg, 1963d; Forberg et al., 1964
$^{203}Hg^{2+}$	Cl⁻	Renal cortex, liver, spleen, bone marrow, placenta	Yolk sac, liver, kidney, spleen	Berlin and Ullberg, 1963a; Berlin and Lewander, 1965; Ukita et al., 1969

$^{210}Po^{4+}$	NO_3^-	Blood, kidney, spleen, liver, lung, placenta, mammary gland	Yolk sac	Söremark and Hunt, 1966
$^{18}F^-$	Na^+	Bone, kidney, areas of placenta	Bone	Ericsson and Ullberg, 1958; Appelgren et al., 1961; Ericsson and Hammarström, 1964
$^{82}Br^-$	NH_4^+	Gastric mucosa and contents, urine, retina, blood, bone	Yolk sac, bone, CNS	Söremark, 1960; Söremark and Ullberg, 1960
$^{125}I^-$, $^{131}I^-$	Na^+	Thyroid, salivary gland, gastric mucosa, ovarian follicles, mammary glands	Yolk sac, thyroid, gastric mucosa, thymus	Forberg et al., 1964; Ullberg and Ewaldsson, 1964; Ullberg et al., 1964
$^{144}Ce^{3+}$	Cl^-	Liver, kidney, bone, adrenal cortex	Yolk sac, bone	Ewaldsson and Magnusson, 1964a
$^{147}Pm^{3+}$	Cl^-	Liver, bone, kidney	Yolk sac, bone	Ewaldsson and Magnusson, 1964a
$^{160}Tb^{3+}$	Cl^-	Liver, bone marrow, spleen, adrenal cortex, kidney, cartilage	Yolk sac, bone	Ewaldsson and Magnusson, 1964b
$^{166}Ho^{3+}$	Cl^-	Liver, bone marrow, spleen, kidney, adrenal cortex	Bone, intestine	Ewaldsson and Magnusson, 1964b
$^{169}Yb^{3+}$	Cl^-	Liver, bone marrow, spleen, kidney	None	Ewaldsson and Magnusson, 1964b
$^{239}Pu^{6+}$	Citrate	Liver, bone, mammary gland, ovarian follicles	Yolk sac	Ullberg et al., 1962
$^{241}Am^{3+}$	NO_3^-	Liver, bone, adrenal cortex, ovarian follicles	Yolk sac, bone	Hammarström and Nilsson, 1970
^{85}Kr		Not studied	Yolk sac	Bergeron et al., 1973

the larger extracellular space of fetal brain. Although ^{22}Na had attained its specific distribution pattern in the fetus by 4 hours after administration to the mother, ^{86}Rb and ^{137}Cs concentrations were still much lower in fetal bone and muscle than in maternal 6 hours after administration. Several days were required for fetal concentrations of ^{86}Rb and ^{137}Cs to approximate those in the mother. The very rapid equilibrium of ^{22}Na in cartilage suggests a high mobility of these ions in this tissue since blood vessels are sparse. Oral administration of ^{134}CsCl to pregnant mule deer that were shot 12 and 18 days later revealed that about 5% of the radioactivity was deposited in 24- and 27-week-old fetuses. Fetal muscle contained less activity than maternal muscle while fetal bone marrow and calcified bone contained more activity than the corresponding maternal tissues (Hakonson and Whicker, 1971).

The effect of gestational age on the distribution of ^{134}Cs in the fetal rat was studied by Wykoff (1971a). Pregnant rats were injected with ^{134}Cs on days 12, 14, or 16 of gestation; every 24 hours for the following 5 days the Cs concentration in whole fetuses was determined by direct counting. Rats were also injected on day 18 and fetuses removed for the following 3 days. The concentration (% of dose/gm) in placenta was almost three times higher when mothers were dosed on days 12 and 14 than near term. The highest fetal concentration (% maternal dose/gm fetus) was observed on dose day 14; it was lower on day 12 and much lower on days 16 and 18. There was little Cs observed in fetal fluids.

The only alkaline earth whose distribution has been studied in pregnant animals by whole-body autoradiography is ^{45}Ca (Appelgren et al., 1961; Ericsson and Hammarström, 1964). At 2 minutes after intravenous injection in mice only 2 days prior to term, radioactivity was discernible in the fetal yolk sac, but not in other fetal tissues. By 30 minutes after either intravenous or oral administration, there was a heavy and specific accumulation in the fetal skeleton. By comparison, ^{18}F was barely discernible in the fetal skeleton at the same time interval. Maternal tissues which accumulate ^{45}Ca include skeleton, some muscle groups, and intestine. It was suggested that since ^{45}Ca-negative muscle bundles are observed which cross ^{45}Ca-rich bundles, the uptake of ^{45}Ca in certain muscles may be those which contracted during freezing. Quantitative analyses indicated that at time intervals of up to 4 hours about ten times as much of the dose of ^{45}Ca was found in the fetus as was the dose of ^{18}F, in spite of a more complete maternal absorption of ingested ^{18}F. There were discrete spots of accumulation in the placenta for both ^{18}F and ^{45}Ca; these were thought to be areas of degenerative calcification often present adjacent to the trophoblastic layers. Braithwaite et al. (1972) injected ^{45}Ca into fetuses of pregnant ewes at three stages of gestation and found the Ca still present in the fetus 5–6 hours later. Since there was no detectable radioactive Ca in the mother or in a twin fetus they concluded calcium transfer was one way. It is also possible that rapid sequestration by the injected fetus did not leave sufficient ^{45}Ca in the blood for transfer to the mother. Avid sequestration of F by maternal tissues which lowers the concentration in maternal blood available for transfer to the fetus is a likely explanation for the minimal distribution of F into the fetus.

Wykoff (1971b) found that as much as 60% of the ^{85}Sr in rat conceptus was in fetal fluids and placenta 1–3 days after administration to the mother; 5 days after administration most of the ^{85}Sr had been transferred to the fetus. When pregnant pigs received single, daily doses of ^{89}Sr orally for 105 days, a high uptake of radiostrontium was found in the fetal bones; this fetal uptake was lower than the maternal (Werner, 1971a,b). This affinity by the maternal skeleton affords a protective action against the transfer of strontium to the fetus.

Isotopes of yttrium, zirconium, and niobium account for a significant fraction of the products from nuclear fission. Since ^{90}Y is a daugher of ^{90}Sr it was of interest to find out whether ^{90}Y is localized at or away from strontium deposition sites. The patterns of distribution of these elements have been studied by whole-body autoradiography in pregnant mice a few days prior to term. The isotopes ^{91}Y (Appelgren et al., 1966), ^{95}Zr + ^{95}Nb, and ^{95}Nb alone (Bäckström et al., 1967) concentrate in maternal and fetal bone; ^{95}Zr + ^{95}Nb more so than ^{95}Nb alone. These isotopes were not selective for hard tissues. There was some uptake in maternal soft tissues; ^{95}Zr + ^{95}Nb and ^{95}Nb accumulated in fetal liver and blood. The yolk sac epithelium had an intense activity with a concentration similar to that of bone. The only suggestion offered by the authors for this tremendous concentration was that the yolk sac somehow functions as a protective organ for the fetus. It could also be secretion by the yolk sac. A few localized areas in the placenta with strong uptake of radioyttrium were observed perhaps corresponding to sites of degenerative calcification. In the nonpregnant females there was a high concentration of ^{91}Y in the walls of some, but not all, follicles in the ovary. No explanation was apparent. Atomic dimensions and bonding energies for these ions must be such that they interact with sites which ordinarily are available for other molecules.

Isotopes of iron (Ullberg et al., 1961), cobalt (Flodh, 1968a), and ruthenium (Nelson et al., 1962) have been studied by whole-body autoradiography in pregnant mice. As early as 5 minutes after intravenous administration of ^{59}Fe to mice at what appears to be late gestation, activity was observed in fetal blood, liver, and bone; by 20 minutes the fetal blood concentration was higher than that in maternal blood. In addition, ^{59}Fe uptake in fetal liver and central nervous system, including choroid plexus, was greater than that in the corresponding maternal tissues.

Whereas maternal bone marrow had more radioactivity than fetal marrow, these distributions may reflect differences in red cell production between mother and fetus. In those pregnant mice which received the radioiron perorally or subcutaneously the fetal liver still showed a high uptake but the maternal liver was surprisingly very low. At early times after administration (20 minutes) there was more ^{59}Fe in the chorioallantoic placenta than in the yolk sac placenta; however, at 4 and 24 hours after administration the yolk sac placenta had much more activity.

A curious absence of radioactivity was seen in some fetuses. Fetuses that did not contain any radioactivity were connected to placentas that had a very high accumulation of ^{59}Fe. Fetuses that had radioactivity with the distribution pattern described above were connected to placentas which had distinctly less radioactivity. There was no apparent explanation for this peculiar observation. The histological quality of the tissues of the fetuses with no radioactivity was not discernibly different from that of fetuses with radioactivity, suggesting that there was no difference in the viability of the fetuses. Estradiol-17β (W. J. Waddell, unpublished) has been seen to have this same pattern (Fig. 7). It was originally thought that the explanation for the estradiol pattern was a difference in affinity between male and female fetuses. However, it was not possible to distinguish between male and female fetuses in the sections. Bowman *et al.* (1964) also found this same curious distribution phenomenon for cotinine. In a 19-day pregnant mouse which received vitamin B$_{12}$, only one of the two fetuses contained radioactivity (Flodh, 1968a; Ullberg *et al.*, 1967). Since this phenomenon has been seen with such a wide vari-

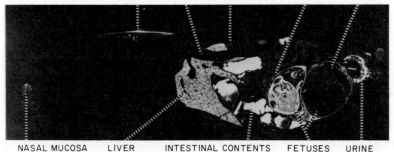

SITE OF INJECTION   BLOOD   ADRENAL CORTEX   YOLK SAC   PLACENTA

NASAL MUCOSA   LIVER   INTESTINAL CONTENTS   FETUSES   URINE

FIG. 7. A print of an autoradiogram of a 20-μm section from an A/JAX mouse injected subcutaneously with ^{14}C-estradiol-17β and frozen 3 hours later. Note the high concentration (white areas) in one fetus and the absence of radioactivity in an adjacent fetus.

ety of substances, it must be that the fetuses are dead which do not show any accumulation of the administered material.

Rats in late gestation given $^{59}FeSO_4$ by stomach tube were killed 1 and 3 days after administration (Past, 1963). The tissues were processed in fixing solutions; consequently, only iron incorporated covalently into large molecules was seen in the autoradiograms. Radioactivity was seen in tissues with active osteogenesis and hemopoiesis. The choroid plexus had activity suggesting that the uptake seen in mouse fetuses at this site is iron incorporated into some protein, perhaps an enzyme active in transport processes. However, some radioactivity in the yolk sac epithelium, kidney, and pancreas might indicate merely that the element was trapped in each of these tissues by some pinocytotic process. Interpretation of the results of Kalberer (1966a,b) on the distribution of $^{59}FeCl_3$ in pregnant rats was difficult since thick sections of frozen animals were taken at room temperature. However, after 30 minutes pronounced accumulation was seen in maternal skeleton and fetuses; specific fetal tissues were not identified.

Placental transfer of ^{59}Fe was studied in sheep (Dyer *et al.*, 1973) and sows (Douglas *et al.*, 1972). Twenty-five minutes after a 100-day-pregnant sow received the ^{59}Fe only very low levels of radioactivity were found in the placenta and fetal tissues. However, significant uptake was found in the placenta, fetal red blood cells, liver, heart, kidney, and spleen when the sow was sacrificed 14 days after injection. Fetal sheep liver at 130–135 days of gestation accumulated about one-fourth of the iron that reached the fetus.

The gestational age of mice given $^{60}CoCl_2$ was not stated (Flodh, 1968a). However, in mice sacrificed 4 days after injection, there was marked accumulation of the isotope in fetal skeleton which was as great as the uptake in maternal cartilage. Radioactivity was also observed in fetal liver but this was lower than maternal liver. There was a marked accumulation of ^{60}Co in the yolk sac epithelium. In fetuses whose mothers were given the isotope 16 days prior to sacrifice, there was no visible accumulation of cobalt in the placenta or fetuses. The lack of correlation of the distribution in the fetuses with that in the soft tissues of the mother (kidney, pancreas, intestine, choroid plexus, etc.) may be due to the younger gestational age of the fetuses in this study compared with that of ^{59}Fe.

Radioruthenium is another element occurring in relatively high yield from nuclear fission. Although ruthenium is poorly absorbed, it is present in animal tissues and foods. Complexes of iron, ruthenium, and osmium should have certain similarities. Mice in late gestation had no accumulation of ^{103}Ru in fetal tissues although there was intense radioactivity in the yolk sac epithelium (Nelson et al., 1962). When the isotope was administered to the mothers on the third day of gestation, no activity was seen in the fetus or yolk sac when the animals were killed 16 days later. Apparently the element had been eliminated or sequestered before the yolk sac had formed. There was some correlation in the mother between the distribution of radioactivity and the presence of collagen which was revealed by Van Gieson's stain. Areas of accumulation which did not stain, however, with Van Gieson's, were the fetal membranes, renal cortex, liver, and red pulp of the spleen.

Zinc-65 was administered to pregnant mice apparently a few days before term and studied by whole-body autoradiography (Bergman and Söremark, 1968). In most tissues the isotope accumulated rapidly; exceptions were the hard tissues, central nervous system, and fetus where it was relatively slow. At 1 hour after administration some activity was observed in the fetus and within 4 hours fetal bone, liver, kidney, and yolk sac had a high uptake. The same maternal tissues had high affinities in addition to pancreas, mammary gland, and spleen. Since the main route of excretion of zinc is the feces, the high accumulation in the maternal intestinal mucosa and contents is not surprising.

The ability of the human fetal liver to accumulate Cu, Zn, Mn, Cr, and Co was studied by Widdowson et al. (1972). From the twentieth week of gestation, the concentration of Cu and Zn was higher in the fetus than in the adult. The concentration of Zn in human fetuses increased abruptly between the thirty-first and thirty-fifth day of gestation to 7X the concentration prior to that time. Perhaps this corresponds to the onset of fetal synthesis of a Zn-containing enzyme, such as carbonic anhydrase (Chaube et al., 1973). No uptake of Mn, Cr, or Co was seen in the human liver before birth (Widdowson et al., 1972). The administration of sodium nitrilotriacetate, a substitute for trisodium phosphate in detergents, had no effect on the accumulation of Cd in rat fetuses (Scharpf et al., 1972).

$^{109}CdCl_2$ has been studied by whole-body autoradiography (Berlin and Ullberg, 1963d; Forberg et al., 1964) in pregnant mice because of the increasing occupational poisoning after chronic exposure to cadmium. No accumulation of radioactivity was seen in the fetal tissues in late gestation, although the yolk sac and placenta showed high activity. No transfer to the fetus was apparent in mice frozen at time intervals ranging from 5 minutes to 4 days after injection.

$^{203}HgCl_2$ administered to 14- and 18-day-pregnant mice (Berlin and Ullberg, 1963a) and sacrificed on day 18 of gestation showed minimal penetration to the fetus. The slight amount of radioactivity that does appear in the fetuses was also found in the same organs of the mother, i.e., liver, kidney, and spleen. There was also a pronounced accumulation in the placenta and fetal membranes. Even when the isotope was given on the second day of gestation and the pregnant animal examined 16 days later, the yolk sac had a high concentration of radioactivity. Treatment with 2,3-dimercaptopropanol (BAL) changed the distribution pattern of ^{203}Hg in maternal tissues but had little effect on fetal tissues (Berlin and Lewander, 1965). The high concentration in fetal membranes and placenta with virtually no radioactivity in the fetuses in mice 48 hours after injection was confirmed by Ukita et al. (1969). Takahashi et al. (1971) found a similar pattern of distribution when 15-day-pregnant rats were given ^{203}HgCl$_2$; high activity was observed in placenta and fetal membranes and low activity in the fetus. An experiment which may have great potential significance on the mechanism by which the yolk sac accumulates ^{203}Hg was done by Garrett et al. (1972). The visceral yolk sac of rats on day 16 of gestation was exposed by incising the uterine wall and allowing it to retract to the base of the chorioallantois. Consequently, the only blood supply to this yolk sac was the vitelline circulation from the fetus. When ^{203}HgCl$_2$ was given to the mothers, radioactivity accumulated in this exposed yolk sac to the same, high concentration as that found in yolk sacs in contact with endometrium. The only interpretation is that ^{203}Hg reached the yolk sac after having gone through the chorioallantoic placenta and the fetus. Since none of the fetuses accumulated much radioactivity, the high concentration in the yolk sac must have been due to specific binding.

Although these studies show little accumulation of ionic Hg in fetal tissues, recent reports (Clarkson et al., 1972; Greenwood et al., 1972) showed high fetal levels of Hg despite much lower maternal blood levels in rats after injection of elemental mercury or inhalation of mercury vapor. The fetal content of Hg was approximately 10 times higher after injection of elemental Hg and 40 times higher after exposure to Hg vapor when compared to the Hg level after injection of ionic Hg.

Quail given ^{203}Hg(NO$_3$)$_2$ had pronounced accumulation in kidney, yolk of ovarian follicles, and pituitary gland; males showed significantly less uptake in kidneys (Bäckström, 1969). Fifty percent of ^{203}Hg was excreted via the eggs when a dose of 50 μg was given; the peak excretion was on the third day after injection and little was excreted after the first week. The chick accumulated ^{203}Hg from the earliest stages of development; highest concentrations were seen in internal yolk sac and intestine. Moderate uptake was found to occur in kidney, liver, and bone. Autoradiographic studies of laying quail injected with ^{203}Hg(NO$_3$)$_2$ showed the principal sites of uptake to be liver, kidney, and ova. While there was a high accumulation in the yolk, there was none detectable in albumin and shell (Nishimura et al., 1971).

Thallium poisoning and intoxication have occurred through its industrial, clinical, and rodenticidal uses. Although $^{204}(Tl)_2SO_4$ was studied in
pregnant mice (André et al., 1960), the fetal distribution was not presented. Significant amounts of ^{204}Tl were found in maternal bone, hyaline
cartilage, renal medulla, intestine, salivary gland, and pancreas and in
epididymis in the male.

Radiopolonium (Söremark and Hunt, 1966) was studied in pregnant
mice by whole-body autoradiography. These studies were limited to the
first 5 days after administration to decrease the likelihood of tissue damage. A high concentration of ^{210}Po remained in maternal blood for the
entire 5 days studied. Also maternal kidney, spleen, liver, and lung had
a marked accumulation. Polonium did not appear in the fetuses up to
4 days after administration, although the placenta had a marked accumulation and a slight concentration was found in fetal membranes. Mi-
croautoradiographic studies on mice receiving the ^{210}Po on day 13 of gestation and sacrificed 5 days later revealed a small uptake in the fetuses.
Bone was the only fetal tissue with a high concentration. The authors
observed some placental damage and destruction of tissue.

Radiotellurium (Duckett and Ellem, 1971, Scott et al., 1971; Agnew,
1972) was given to pregnant rats but the fetuses were removed and fixed
in solutions which could translocate or remove any unbound isotope before taking sections for auotradiography. Tellurium has a high affinity
for certain fetal and maternal proteins (Agnew and Cheng, 1971); consequently the distribution patterns seen in these studies merely reveals
this binding. Accumulation of radioactivity was found in fetal brain,
liver, kidney, and cardiovascular system; however the placenta and yolk
sac had tremendous concentrations of isotope. Because of the technique,
this clearly indicates binding substances in placenta and yolk sac for
tellurium. Perhaps the same substances are binding other elements such
as mercury to account for their high accumulation at these sites. A high
uptake in the choroid plexus was suggested as possibly related to the
hydrocephalus produced by tellurium (Agnew, 1972).

^{18}F has been studied alone (Ericsson and Ullberg, 1958) and in combination with ^{45}Ca (Appelgren et al., 1961; Ericsson and Hammarström,
1964). All of these reports were of whole-body autoradiography in pregnant mice a few days before term. Because of the short half-life of ^{18}F,
the longest survival times after either intravenous or oral administration
were 1 hour. The only fetal accumulation of ^{18}F was in the skeleton,
and this was observed within 30 minutes after injection. High concentrations were seen in maternal bone as early as 2 minutes. This activity
was lower in fetal than in maternal bone; however, the short survival
times after single doses may be deceptive. It is certainly possible that

an entirely different distribution pattern between mother and fetus could exist if autoradiography were possible several days after receiving the isotope.

In contrast to fluoride, the other two halides studied in mice in late gestation by whole-body autoradiography distributed much more uniformly in the fetus. Most of the ^{82}Br was localized in fetal bone, but the concentration in maternal cartilage was higher. However, fetal brain and spinal cord concentrations were higher than the corresponding maternal tissues (Söremark, 1960; Söremark and Ullberg, 1960). Maternal blood activity remained high throughout all time intervals studied; the only tissues with greater affinity for the ^{82}Br were gastric mucosa, contents of stomach and urinary bladder, blood vessel walls, and retina. A relatively high concentration was also found in the placenta, especially close to the attachment of the fetal membranes. Radioiodide was high in fetal thyroid, salivary gland, stomach, and thymus (Ullberg and Ewaldsson, 1964; Forberg et al., 1964; Ullberg et al., 1964). Secretion of iodide by maturing stomach and salivary gland in the fetus near term undoubtedly accounts for this selective accumulation. Except for the thymus, the maternal concentration in these selective tissues was higher than the fetal concentration; accumulation in the thymus was seen in only a few of the mothers. Since fluoride and iodide have selective affinities, bromide (and chloride?) is (are) more closely representative of the extracellular space. The higher concentration of bromide in the fetus after 1 hour is most likely due to the kinetics of distribution between mother and fetus of this substance which, like urea, crosses the placenta, distributes in fetal and maternal water, and is rapidly eliminated from the mother (Waddell, 1968). Although thiocyanate should also give an indication of extracellular space, it is found in very high concentration in gastric mucosa and gastric contents of mother and fetus near term (Clemedson et al., 1960). The explanation for this observation is not clear.

Several isotopes of the rare earths have been studied by whole-body autoradiography in pregnant mice in late gestation. The light lanthanides—cerium and promethium (Ewaldsson and Magnusson, 1964a), the heavy lanthanides—terbium, holmium, and ytterbium (Ewaldsson and Magnusson, 1964b), as well as the actinides plutonium (Ullberg et al., 1962) and americium (Hammarström and Nilsson, 1970) all had similar distribution patterns in fetal tissues. After 24 hours a slight amount of radioactivity was seen in the fetal skeleton when ^{144}Ce, ^{147}Pm, ^{160}Tb, ^{166}Ho, and ^{241}Am were injected. Also a trace amount of ^{166}Ho was found in fetal intestine. Radioplutonium was not seen in the fetus but the fetal membranes had the highest concentration, except for maternal skeleton, in the body. This marked accumulation persisted even when there was a long interval between injection and sacrifice. No uptake of [166]Ho and [169]Yb in yolk sac was observed; by 24 hours the other rare earths were localized in the yolk sac. Maternal tissues in which rare earths frequently accumulated were liver, adrenal cortex, ovary, and bone. It is difficult to interpret these affinities because so little is known about the biological actions of these elements.

Naharin et al. (1969) found 0.23% of the mother's body burden in each fetus when pregnant mice were injected with [144]Ce citrate 2 days before expected delivery and the fetuses analyzed at delivery. Administration of the isotope at or before mating decreased markedly the amount of [144]Ce that appeared in the fetuses; however, large amounts of radioactivity were transferred to the newborn via the milk of the mothers.

Hammarström and Nilsson (1970) found radioamericium concentrated in the zona glomerulosa of the adrenal cortex; it exceeded that of the other zones of the cortex in male mice. In females the concentration was uniform in the adrenal cortex. They also reported no accumulation in the adrenal cortex of neonatal rats. In the ovary, Tb, Ho, Yb, and Ce isotopes were found to be highest in the corpora lutea while the ovarian follicles selectively accumulated Am, Pu, and, to a lesser extent, Pm. The relationship of this accumulation to the occurrence of tumors in these soft tissues is obvious; however, the possible correlation with steroid hormone metabolism and action is an intriguing enigma.

The inert gas krypton-85 has been used for studies of blood flow to various organs in patients including pregnant women. Bergeron et al. (1973) investigated the extent of transfer of [85]Kr to fetal rats in late gestation during the first 60 seconds after administration of the isotope into the iliac artery. Very little radioactivity was found in the fetus with relatively high amounts of radioactivity in the placenta and fetal membranes.

B. Distribution of Inorganic Ions

Table IV lists the inorganic ions whose distribution patterns have been studied by whole-body autoradiography in pregnant animals.

Bicarbonate, labeled with ^{14}C, will distribute according to pH gradients in the body and will also be incorporated into larger molecules. The distribution pattern in pregnant mice a few days prior to term by whole-body autoradiography (Waddell et al., 1969) revealed both incorporated and unincorporated radiocarbon. Radioactivity in bone was intense and most likely due to trapping of the $^{14}CO_3^{2-}$ ion. The large amount of radioactivity seen in maternal liver, pancreas, salivary gland, kidney, bladder, and intestine was apparently in molecules synthesized from [14]C. At 3

TABLE IV Distribution of Inorganic Ions in Maternal and Fetal Tissues of Mice or Rats near Term

Isotope	Conjugate ion	Principal maternal tissues	Principal fetal tissues	Reference
$^{14}CO_3{}^{2-}$	Na^+	Bone, liver, pancreas	Yolk sac, bone	Waddell et al., 1969
$^{14}CN^-$	K^+	Gastric mucosa and contents, submaxillary gland, thyroid	Yolk sac, gastric mucosa	Clemedson et al., 1960
$PO_3{}^{18}F^{2-}$	Na^+	Bone, lumen of small intestine	Bone	Ericsson and Hammarström, 1965
$^{32}PO_3F^{2-}$	Na^+	Bone, liver, wall of large intestine, spleen	Bone	Ericsson and Hammarström, 1965
$^{32}PO_4H^{2-}$	Na^+	(Not studied)	Yolk sac, bone	Leder and Paschen, 1965
$^{35}SCN^-$	K^+	(Same as $^{14}CN^-$)	(Same as $^{14}CN^-$)	Clemedson et al., 1960
$^{48}V_2O_5$	—	Bone, mammary gland, liver, kidney	Yolk sac, bone	Söremark and Ullberg, 1962
$^{75}SeO_3{}^{2-}$	Na^+	Liver, kidney, spleen, myocardium	Yolk sac, liver, brain, lung	Jacobsson and Hansson, 1965

minutes after $Na_2{}^{14}CO_3$ injection, bone was the only fetal tissue visible; there was a fairly uniform fetal distribution at 30 minutes which was equal to the concentration in most maternal tissues. Maternal bone, liver, and pancreas were higher than corresponding fetal tissues (Fig. 8).

The distribution patterns of radioactivity were identical for $^{14}CN^-$ and $^{35}SCN^-$ in pregnant mice (Clemedson et al., 1960). This was attributed to rapid conversion of $^{14}CN^-$ to $S^{14}CN^-$ after injection. The highest activity was in the stomach of both mother and fetus, a fact which agrees with earlier work (Logothetopoulus and Myant, 1956) indicating active secretion of thiocyanate by gastric mucosa.

Vanadium pentoxide dissolved in saline and administered intravenously to pregnant mice accumulated primarily in maternal and fetal bone (Söremark and Ullberg, 1962). A relatively high concentration was visible in the placenta. The visceral yolk sac epithelium had the highest concentration of the soft tissues; some activity was observed 1 minute after injection. Even though significant amounts of ^{48}V were found in maternal liver, no accumulation could be detected in fetal liver or any of the other soft tissues. Vanadium oxides are used as catalysts in a wide variety of industrial applications. The studies failed to suggest a mechanism for the respiratory symptoms which are seen with human exposure.

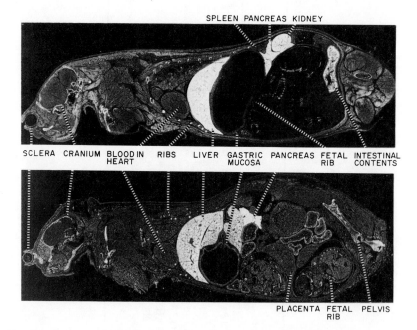

Fig. 8. Prints of autoradiograms of sections from pregnant NMRI mice injected intravenously with $Na_2{}^{14}CO_3$ a few days prior to term. The top print is from a mouse frozen 3 minutes after injection; the bottom print is from a mouse frozen 30 minutes after injection. Note the high concentration (white areas) in fetal bones.

Uteri of pregnant rats were removed 12 minutes after the mother was injected with ^{32}P-labeled orthophosphate (Leder and Paschen, 1965). In early gestation (before day 12), the highest radioactivity was in the anti-mesometrial decidua; after day 12, the highest radioactivity shifted to the yolk sac and the mesometrial decidua. This change in intrauterine location coincides with the change in fetal attachment to the uterine wall. Fetal liver and bone were the only tissues to accumulate radioactivity.

The distribution of ^{32}P and ^{18}F given as double-labeled sodium mono-fluorophosphate was studied in pregnant mice a few days before term (Ericsson and Hammarström, 1965). Sodium monofluorophosphate is absorbed from the intestine, and the fluoride is extensively removed in the body (Ericsson et al., 1961). Thirty minutes after injection of the $Na_2{}^{32}PO_3{}^{18}F$, both isotopes were found in mineralized parts of the fetal skeleton and in some small spots in the placenta. The maternal bone concentration was very high for both ^{18}F and ^{32}P. Quantitative studies on the placental transfer of $^{32}PO_3F^{2-}$, $^{32}PO_4H^{2-}$, $PO_3{}^{18}F^{2-}$, and $^{18}F^-$ showed placental concentrations of ^{18}F and ^{32}P from Na_2PO_3F to be significantly lower than from NaF and orthophosphate. However, by 4 hours, ^{32}P from both sources was approximately the same and ^{18}F from both sources was the same. The total fetal concentrations of the isotopes from all four sources were about the same at 1 hour and in all cases lower than placental concentrations. At 4 hours, ^{32}P from orthophosphate was highest in the fetus followed in decreasing amounts by $^{32}PO_3F^{2-}$, $^{18}F^-$, and $PO_3{}^{18}F^{2-}$. At this time, only ^{18}F and ^{32}P from Na_2PO_3F were lower in fetus than placenta.

Sodium selenite was studied in pregnant mice by Jacobsson and Hansson (1965). At 4 and 24 hours after injection selenium activity was high in the yolk sac. Fetal liver, brain, and lung showed some accumulation after 24 hours but it was considerably lower than the corresponding maternal tissues. Selenium concentrations were determined in maternal and fetal tissues of 26 ewes fed a muscular dystrophy-producing hay for 2 years (Hidiroglou et al., 1969). The pattern of distribution was the same for mother and fetus but maternal concentrations were always higher than the corresponding fetal tissues. As with the pregnant mice, kidney, liver, spleen, and adrenal gland had the highest accumulation of selenium. The authors found the gestational age to have little effect on the selenium concentration in maternal or fetal tissues.

C. Distribution of Organic Molecules

1. DRUGS ACTING ON THE CENTRAL NERVOUS SYSTEM

Drugs whose primary action is on the central nervous system and whose distribution patterns have been studied by whole-body autoradiog-

TABLE V Maternal and Fetal Distribution of Central Nervous System Drugs in Pregnant Animals in Last Trimester of Gestation—Tissues Are Those with Increased Concentration after Allowing Time for Equilibration

Drug	Species	Principal maternal tissues	Principal fetal tissues[a]	Reference
Barbiturates				
14C-Barbital	Mouse	Uniform except excretory organs high	Yolk sac (fetus = mother)	Lal et al., 1964
14C-Phenobarbital	Mouse	Uniform except higher in liver, bile, myocardium, intestine	Yolk sac, bile, intestine, myocardium, liver	Cassano et al., 1967a; Waddell, 1971b
14C- and 35S-Thiopental	Mouse, rat	Liver, fat, lung	Yolk sac, liver, brain, lung	Cassano et al., 1967a; Schechter and Roth, 1967
Other sedatives				
3H- and 14C-Meprobamate	Mouse	Uniform except excretory organs high	Yolk sac, urinary bladder	Ewaldsson, 1963; Van der Kleijn, 1969b
14C-Carisoprodol	Mouse	Liver, intestine, kidney	Yolk sac (fetus = mother)	Van der Kleijn, 1969b
14C-Tybamate	Mouse	Liver, kidney, myocardium	Yolk sac (fetus = mother)	Van der Kleijn, 1969b
14C-Glutethimide	Mouse	Liver, fat, myocardium, mammary gland	Liver, myocardium, gastric mucosa, renal medulla	Koransky and Ullberg, 1964
14C-Thalidomide	Mouse	Uniform except excretory organs high	Yolk sac, gastric mucosa and lumen, kidney	Koransky and Ullberg, 1964; Waddell, 1972a
14C-Ethanol	Monkey	Not studied	Liver, pancreas, kidney, lung, thymus, brain, bone marrow	Idänpään-Heikkilä et al., 1971b; Ho et al., 1972
Anticonvulsants				
14C-Diphenylhydantoin	Mouse	Adrenal cortex, liver, myocardium, intestine	Yolk sac, myocardium, liver, adrenal, intestine	Waddell and Mirkin, 1972
Anti-Parkinson agents				
14C-Tofenacine	Mouse	Lung, intestine, liver, placenta, brain	Yolk sac, lung, intestine, liver	Hespe and Prins, 1969

Drug	Species			Reference
Antitussives				
^{3}H-Noscapine	Mouse	Stomach, liver, kidney, bronchi (otherwise low and uniform)	Yolk sac, liver, lung, brain, skin	Idänpään-Heikkilä, 1967
Phenothiazines				
^{35}S-Chlorpromazine	Mouse	Lung, liver, brain, intestine, urinary bladder	Yolk sac, lung, liver, intestine, urinary bladder	Cassano *et al.*, 1967b; Sjöstrand *et al.*, 1965; Cassano, 1968; Idänpään-Heikkilä *et al.*, 1968
^{35}S-Promethazine	Mouse	Lung, liver, brain, intestine, urinary bladder	Yolk sac, eye	Hansson and Schmiterlöw, 1961b; Schmiterlöw, 1965
Other tertiary amines				
^{14}C-Imipramine	Mouse	Lung, intestine, urinary and gallbladder, brain	Yolk sac, intestine, liver, lung, brain	Cassano and Hansson, 1966
^{14}C-Anitriptyline	Mouse	Lung, liver, brain, intestine, salivary gland	Yolk sac, brain, lung, liver, intestine, urinary bladder	Cassano *et al.*, 1965; Hansson and Cassano, 1966; Cassano, 1968
^{3}H-Oxypertine	Mouse	Adrenal medulla, liver, kidney, intestinal contents	Yolk sac, lung, liver, intestinal contents, intervertebral discs	Airaksinen and Idänpään-Heikkilä, 1967
^{14}C-FG5111 (butyrophenone derivative)	Mouse	Gallbladder, salivary gland, gastrointestinal tract, liver	Yolk sac	Einer-Jensen and Hansson, 1965
^{14}C-Diazepam	Mouse	Fat, liver, brain, myocardium, intestine	Yolk sac, liver, fat, heart, gastrointestinal tract	Van der Kleijn, 1969a
	Mouse	(Information not given)	Liver, brain, spinal cord	Idänpään-Heikkilä *et al.*, 1971c
	Hamster	(Not studied)	Fetal concentration relatively uniform; spinal cord slightly higher	Idänpään-Heikkilä *et al.*, 1971c
	Monkey	(Not studied)	Liver, intestine, fat, spinal cord, cerebellum, peripheral nerves, retina	Idänpään-Heikkilä *et al.*, 1971c
^{14}C-Chlordiazepoxide	Mouse	Liver, myocardium, intestine, urinary bladder, brain	Yolk sac, liver, brain, heart, intestine, urinary bladder	Cassano *et al.*, 1967b; Placidi and Cassano, 1968; Cassano and Hansson, 1969

TABLE V (*continued*)

Drug	Species	Principal maternal tissues	Principal fetal tissues[a]	Reference
[14]C-Chloroquine	Mouse	Eye	Eye	Ullberg et al., 1970; Lindquist and Ullberg, 1972
[14]C-Chlorcyclizine	Mouse	Kidney, liver, intestinal contents, CNS, salivary gland, myocardium	Yolk sac, liver, intestinal contents, CNS, myocardium	Waddell, 1973b
[14]C-CRD-401 (benzo-thiazepine derivative)	Mouse	Intestine, liver, kidney, Harder's gland, lung, myocardium	Yolk sac, liver, intestine, lung	Sakuma et al., 1971
Quaternary phenothiazines				
[35]S-Aprobit	Mouse	Liver, intestine, salivary gland, brown fat	None	Hansson and Schmiterlöw, 1961b; Schmiterlöw, 1965
[35]S-Secergan	Mouse	Liver, intestine, gastric mucosa, pancreas, kidney	None	Allgén et al., 1960
Psychedelics				
[14]C-LSD	Mouse	Hypophysis, kidney, liver, lung, brain, intestine	Yolk sac, lung, liver, intestine, brain, myocardium	Idänpään-Heikkilä and Schoolar, 1969
[14]C-Psilocin	Rat	Liver, intestine, salivary gland, brain	Yolk sac, liver	Kalberer, 1966a,b
[14]C-Mescaline	Monkey	(Not studied)	Liver, brain, kidney, lung	Taska and Schoolar, 1972
Other quaternary ammonium compounds				
[14]C-Cetipin	Mouse	Liver, intestine, kidney, salivary gland, gastric mucosa	None	Hansson and Schmiterlöw, 1961a

[a] Comparisons of maternal and fetal concentrations, i.e., =, >, or <, in parentheses signifies a relatively uniform distribution in the fetal tissues other than those specifically named.

raphy in pregnant animals in late gestation are listed in Table V. A few compounds such as the quaternary phenothiazines are included here even though their primary action may not be on the central nervous system; their distributions were studied in order to compare them with the analogous tertiary compounds. ^{14}C-Barbital was studied by Lal *et al.* (1964) in cats and mice. Although the gestational age was not stated, the animals appear to be in mid or late gestation. At 30 minutes after injection the concentrations in fetal tissues and placenta were less than those in maternal tissues although the same tissues of the mother and fetus had increased amounts of the compound. Fetal brain was equal to other fetal tissues suggesting a less restrictive blood–brain barrier to barbital in the fetus. At 4 hours after injection the distribution was more uniform and the fetal and placental concentrations were approximately the same as maternal liver and kidney, which were higher than all other tissues of the mother. The other long-acting barbiturate, phenobarbital, which was studied in pregnant mice near term (Waddell, 1971b), clearly shows the similarity in distribution in the fetus and in the mother (Figs. 9 and 10). Fetal bile could be discerned with a high concentration of radioactivity, obviously suggesting that the fetal liver was functioning to an extent that would allow accumulation of metabolites in the fetal bile. This same pattern was seen in the mother. Phenobarbital distributed fairly uniformly in both mother and fetus; increased affinity was observed in maternal liver, bile, adrenal cortex, corpora lutea, myocardium, and intestine and in the fetal bile, intestine, and myocardium. At 3 and 24 hours following injection the fetal concentration was approximately equal to the maternal except for the tissues with increased affinity, listed above, in the mother.

The distribution of thiopental was studied in both mice (Cassano *et al.*,

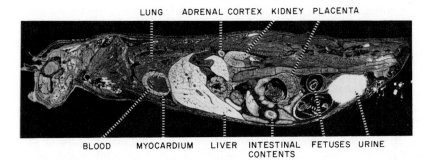

FIG. 9. A print of an autoradiogram of a 20-μm section from a C57BL mouse that received ^{14}C-phenobarbital intravenously on day 12.5 of gestation and was frozen 3 hours later.

EYE   BRAIN   STOMACH KIDNEY CORPORA LUTEA   FETAL LIVER

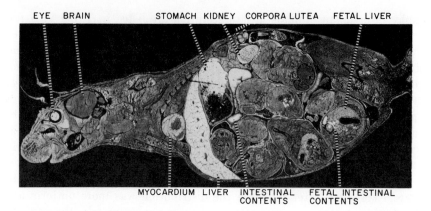

MYOCARDIUM LIVER INTESTINAL   FETAL INTESTINAL
                  CONTENTS   CONTENTS

FIG. 10. A print of an autoradiogram of a 20-μm section from a C57BL mouse injected intravenously with ^{14}C-phenobarbital on day 17.5 of gestation and frozen 24 hours later. Note the high concentration (white areas) in the fetal intestinal contents which was identified on the section as bile.

1967a) and rats (Schechter and Roth, 1967). Rats at 21 days of gestation were injected intravenously and frozen 0.5 to 30 minutes after injection. Not until 20 minutes after injection was the fetal concentration approximately equivalent to that in the mother although at 5 minutes radioactivity was clearly visible in the fetus. Fetal and maternal tissues were extracted with methylene chloride and essentially all of the radioactivity present was found to be unchanged thiopental. Cassano *et al.* (1967a) also compared the distribution of thiopental and phenobarbital in pregnant mice; thiopental in this case was labeled with ^{35}S. Although some radioactivity was present in the fetus 2 minutes after administration to the mother, thiopental did not reach its greatest fetal concentration until 10 minutes after injection. However, fetal brain continued to show a gradual increase after this time interval; and then a decrease by 4 hours after injection was recorded. Phenobarbital took an even longer time for equilibrium in the fetus. Even after 1 hour the fetal concentration was lower than that in the mother; fetal liver and brain were the tissues to show affinity at that time. Both compounds distributed rather uniformly in the fetus with liver showing a greater uptake than any other tissue. Direct fluorometric determinations of thiopental in fetal tissues revealed the liver to have the highest concentration of thiopental (Finster *et al.*, 1972a). However, at no time during the autoradiographic studies were the fetal organ concentrations higher than the maternal.

The high concentration of thiopental in the liver of the fetus was attributed to uptake by this organ as blood flowed from the placenta into the fetus. It was suggested as a protective mechanism by the fetal liver since most of the blood passes through this tissue first. Other compounds shown to have this high accumulation in fetal liver were ^{82}Br-halothane (Geddes et al., 1972), lidocaine (Finster et al., 1972b), and ^{14}C-cyclamate (Pitkin et al., 1970). However, this probably is not the full explanation since fetal liver in vitro has more than twice the affinity for ^{82}Br-halothane than maternal liver.

Van der Kleijn (1969b) compared the distribution of ^{14}C-labeled meprobamate, carisoprodol, and tybamate in pregnant mice at 19 days of gestation. Only two time intervals were studied after administration of the drugs, namely, 2 minutes and 30 minutes. None of the drugs appeared in the fetus or its membranes at 2 minutes after injection. Uniform and approximately equal concentrations were found in fetal and maternal tissues 30 minutes after injection for each of the compounds. Tritiated meprobamate was used for whole-body autoradiography in mice by Ewaldsson (1963). The rather uniform distribution in the fetus was higher than that in the mother except for maternal kidney and intestine 1 hour after intravenous injection. Marked radioactivity was said to be present in the fetal urinary bladder 1 hour after administration of the drug to the mother. Maximum fetal concentration was found 4 hours after injection; by 24 hours no detectable activity remained.

^{14}C-Thalidomide and ^{14}C-glutethimide were reported by Koransky and Ullberg (1964) to have similar distribution patterns in mice at 19 days of gestation. Four hours after oral administration of thalidomide in water, a remarkably uniform distribution pattern was observed throughout both mother and fetus except for sites of excretion. At 1 hour after intravenous injection of the thalidomide to 18-day-pregnant mice, the highest activity was found in maternal kidney and urinary bladder, and in fetal kidney (Waddell, 1972a). Fetal liver and intestine had much lower concentrations than the corresponding maternal tissues; again a high uptake was observed in fetal yolk sac. The distribution pattern of glutethimide given orally in water was not as uniform as that of thalidomide; glutethimide had a lower and more uniform concentration in the fetus than in the mother at 2 hours after administration. No other time intervals were reported.

^{14}C-Ethanol was given to Cynomologus iris monkeys in the last 30 days of pregnancy; fetuses removed 0.25, 1.5, or 12 hours later were processed for autoradiography (Idänpään-Heikkilä et al., 1971b; Ho et al., 1972). The possibility that the radioactivity seen in rapidly growing fetal tissues (see Table V) may have been in part due to acetate from metabolized ethanol must be considered. The volatility of ethanol should have allowed its escape from the sections.

[14]C-Diphenylhydantoin in pregnant mice illustrates the similarity in distribution of compounds in maternal and fetal tissues when studied a few days prior to term (Waddell and Mirkin, 1972).The specific distribution in the adrenal gland of both the mother and fetus is impressive and illustrates that with maturity of the fetus, the characteristics responsible for accumulation of the drug appear prior to delivery in several tissues. At $6\frac{1}{2}$ and 20 minutes following injection there was activity visible in the fetus but it was lower than maternal; equilibrium was reached between maternal and fetal tissues after 1 hour. Quantitative analyses of selected maternal tissues, fetus, and placenta revealed most of the radioactivity to be unchanged diphenylhydantoin (DPH), while its major metabolite, p-hydroxyphenylphenylhydantoin (HPPH), accounted for less than 5% of the radioactivity. Harbison and Becker (1971) found pretreatment with phenobarbital to lower and SKF 525A to elevate the concentration of DPH in the mouse fetus.

Sprague–Dawley rats in late gestation were given DPH and then maternal and fetal tissues were removed and analyzed by a chemical technique (Mirkin, 1971b). The highest concentration in all tissues examined occurred 1 hour after intravenous injection; the concentration in fetal tissues was approximately twice that of the corresponding maternal tissues. If the DPH were administered intraperitoneally, then the peak concentration in liver was reached at 4 hours and the concentration in maternal liver was approximately 14 times that in the fetal liver. One does not know whether the differences in concentration between mother and fetus are due to the kinetics of distribution or differences in binding affinities. For example, the amount of ^{14}C-DPH in maternal monkey liver was 2X that in fetal liver at 150 days of gestation (Gabler and Hubbard, 1972); this is the reverse of the situation found in rats following intravenous administration. The situation is further complicated because in goats the maternal plasma proteins bind twice as much DPH as fetal plasma proteins; furthermore, this protein binding accounts for the maternal–fetal plasma ratio (Shoeman et al., 1972).

Human fetuses [8.5 to 10.5 crown–rump (CR) length] taken at therapeutic abortion after the mothers had received DPH were analyzed by a chemical method for DPH (Mirkin, 1971b). Fetal livers taken 30 minutes after the administration of the DPH had greater amounts of the drug than maternal blood; adrenal, kidney, cerebral cortex, brain stem, and placenta were approximately equal to blood. The concentration of DPH was high in the adrenal, heart, and kidney of a fetus taken 25 hours after administration of the drug. The concentration of DPH in fetal plasma was the same as that in the maternal plasma of women who had received DPH throughout pregnancy. The implication has been made of an association between administration of DPH to pregnant women and cleft palate in the offspring (Mirkin, 1971a). Several cases of cleft palate have been seen in the offspring of women receiving DPH during pregnancy.

The anti-Parkinson agent, orphenadrine, is metabolized in the rat to N-demethyl orphenadrine (tofenacine). The metabolic product, ^{3}H-tofenacine, was studied by autoradiography in pregnant mice at 15, 17, and 19 days of gestation (Hespe and Prins, 1969). No correlation could be established between gestational age and concentration of radioactivity in placenta, fetal membranes, or fetus. The 19-day-old fetus showed a similar distribution pattern to that of its mother; however, the selective uptake in the fetal tissues was less pronounced in the 15- and 17-day-old fetuses. Although some activity appeared in fetal as well as maternal brain, nothing distinctive which would suggest a mechanism of action was seen. At both 1 and 4 hours after administration, the fetal concentration was still lower than that in maternal tissues.

The antitussive principle, noscapine, which is derived from opium, was labeled with tritium and studied in pregnant mice in late gestation (Idänpään-Heikkilä, 1967). At 20 minutes after intravenous injection to the mother the concentration in the fetus was at least as high as that in the mother except for maternal liver, stomach, and bronchi. The distribution pattern of mother and fetus was similar; however, by 6 hours after administration no radioactivity was discernible in the fetus.

The phenothiazines, chlorpromazine and promethazine, have a very similar structure and it is not surprising that their distributions have been found to be very similar. Four papers on the distribution of ^{35}S-chlorpromazine in mice in late gestation (Sjöstrand et al., 1965; Cassano et al., 1967b; Idänpään-Heikkilä et al., 1968; Cassano, 1968) showed the concentration to be lower in the fetuses than in maternal tissues. As early as 5 minutes after intravenous injection, radioactivity was observed in the fetus. Radioactivity was higher in the fetuses after intramuscular injection but the distribution patterns were the same after intravenous and intramuscular injection. Chromatography of maternal tissue extracts revealed that after 5–20 minutes most of the radioactivity was unchanged chlorpromazine but by 1 hour more than 50% had been metabolized. Pretreatment of the mice with cold aprobit decreased the concentration of radioactivity from chlorpromazine in fetal tissues and there were no specific tissue accumulations. However, radioactivity in the placenta and fetal membranes was not affected by aprobit. The mechanism by which aprobit pretreatment altered the maternal–fetal transfer of chlorpromazine is not clear. Aprobit itself does not penetrate the placenta; none is found in the fetus or fetal membranes after administration to the mother (Hansson and Schmiterlöw, 1961a). In the mouse, after chlorpromazine, the adrenal cortex had the highest radioactivity in the animal

at 5 minutes; a very low concentration was observed in the adrenal medulla. This difference in the adrenal remained large for 1 hour and then
decreased so that by 16 hours after injection little difference could be
demonstrated between the medulla and cortex (Vapaatalo et al., 1968).
Pretreatment with aprobit did not alter the distribution of chlorpromazine in the areas of the adrenal, but it did decrease the total radioactivity
accumulated there. The authors also observed in pregnant mice in both
groups (with and without aprobit pretreatment) at 2 and 16 hours a distinctly more radioactive zone at the border between the medulla and
cortex.

Hansson and Schmiterlöw (1961b) studied the distribution of ^{35}S-pro-
methazine a tertiary amine, which, not surprisingly, does reach the fetus
and is concentrated in what appears to be the fetal retina. Otherwise
the fetal concentration is uniform and lower than that in the mother.

The antihistamine, chlorcyclizine, which has been shown to produce
anomalies in the offspring of pregnant rats and mice was studied in pregnant mice in mid and late gestation (Waddell, 1973b). In mice which
were given the ^{14}C-labeled compound at 12.5 days of gestation and frozen
either at 3, 9, or 24 hours after injection, the concentration in the fetuses
was lower at all time intervals than that in maternal tissues; however,
the concentration was always high in the fetal yolk sac epithelium and
basophilic cells in the decidua basalis. Although the predominant anom-
aly seen from administration of this compound at this time in gestation
is cleft palate, no specific localizations could be seen in these fetal tissues.
At 17.5 days of gestation the fetal concentration was still less than the
maternal but selective affinity now was the same as in the mother. Increased uptake was present in the fetal yolk sac at 3 and 9 hours after
administration (Fig. 11).

Another amine, ^{14}C-CRD-401, which has had some use as a coronary
vasodilator, localized in the liver, intestine, and lung of the fetuses of
19-day-pregnant mice after either intravenous or oral administration.
There was an extensive and persistent accumulation in the yolk sac epithelium after oral administration to the mothers (Sakuma et al., 1971).

The same general distribution was seen for two very similar compounds, imipramine and amitriptyline, which are used clinically as antidepressants, when studied in pregnant mice in late gestation (Cassano
and Hansson, 1966; Cassano, 1968; Cassano et al., 1965; Hansson and
Cassano, 1967). After intramuscular injection more radioactivity was observed in fetal tissues. For both imipramine and amitriptyline, activity
was retained longer in the fetus than in the mother. Functioning enzymes
in the liver for metabolism of the drugs with subsequent secretion into
the intestine of the fetus most likely accounts for this high concentration.

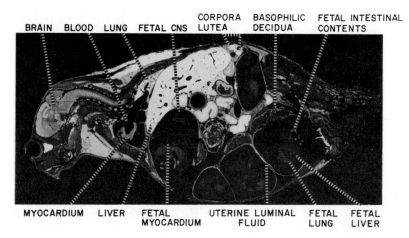

CORPORA   BASOPHILIC   FETAL INTESTINAL
BRAIN   BLOOD   LUNG   FETAL CNS   LUTEA   DECIDUA   CONTENTS

MYOCARDIUM   LIVER   FETAL   UTERINE LUMINAL   FETAL   FETAL
                     MYOCARDIUM   FLUID   LUNG   LIVER

FIG. 11. A print of an autoradiogram of a 20-μm section from an A/JAX mouse that received ¹⁴C-chlorocylizine subcutaneously on day 17.5 of gestation and was frozen 3 hours later. Increased uptake can be seen in fetal myocardium, lung, intestinal contents, and liver.

Another tranquilizer with a somewhat different structure, oxypertine, was studied in pregnant mice (Airaksinen and Idänpään-Heikkilä, 1967). One hour after administration, the fetal yolk sac had an activity as high as most maternal tissues while the fetus had a low and uniform distribution. However, by 3 hours the concentration in the fetal membranes had decreased and selective affinities were found. The concentration in the fetus was slightly lower than that in the mother.

A butyrophenone derivative with tranquilizing properties, ¹⁴C-γ-(4-methylpiperidino)-p-fluorobutyrophenone hydrochloride (FG5111), was studied in pregnant mice which were frozen 1 and 4 hours after administration of the drug to the mother (Einer-Jensen and Hansson, 1965). A low and uniform distribution was observed in the fetus. The yolk sac was the only fetal tissue with a specific localization.

There have been several reports (Cassano and Hansson, 1969; Cassano et al., 1967b; Placidi and Cassano, 1968; Van der Kleijn, 1969a; Idänpään-Heikkilä et al., 1971c) on the distribution of the two popular antianxiety agents, diazepam (Valium) and chlordiazepoxide (Librium). A similar pattern of distribution in mice, hamsters, and monkeys for the ¹⁴C-labeled drugs was found in both mother and fetus in late gestation. The maximal fetal concentration was found in mice and hamsters at about 2 hours; most of the radioactivity had disappeared from the fetus after 15 hours but some could still be observed in the mother. Tissue analysis revealed a rapid metabolic conversion of the drugs in the body.

Fetal fat and myocardium were the only tissues that had an increased concentration which could not be attributed to metabolic conversion.

The situation was different in monkeys. Diazepam was rapidly transferred to the fetus and remained high in certain fetal tissues. After 24 hours there was still strong activity in fetal cerebellum, spinal cord, and peripheral nerve which may explain the temporary hypoactivity and hypotonicity which has been reported to occur in human infants whose mothers received diazepam during labor. This also emphasizes the importance of species variability in drug distribution. Also in contrast to rodents, most of the radioactivity in the monkeys at the end of 24 hours represented unchanged diazepam. Autoradiographic studies on the distribution of diazepam in 2-day-old rhesus monkeys showed similar distributions in mice and monkeys (Van der Kleijn, 1969c; Van der Kleijn and Wijffels, 1971). Owing to the large size of the newborn monkey brain detailed autoradiography was possible. Rapid accumulation occurred in the gray cortical structure of the cerebrum, cerebellum, brain stem, and spinal cord and in myelinated structures in the brain stem and peripheral nerves. At later time intervals radioactivity was found in the fiber tracts of the same areas. Tissue analyses showed greater than 90% of the activity in brain, heart, and lung to be unchanged diazepam.

Pregnant women at 12–16 weeks of gestation were given ^{14}C-diazepam intramuscularly prior to hysterotomy (Idänpään-Heikkilä et al., 1971a) and the fetuses removed 1, 2, or 6 hours later. The peak concentration in all fetal tissues was at 1 hour after administration; the only tissue studied with a higher concentration than fetal blood at this time was the gastrointestinal tract. A delayed penetration of the brain was apparent but at 6 hours the concentration in the fetal brain was higher than blood. In a 31-week-old human fetus the concentration of N-demethyldiazepam was higher than that of diazepam in liver, heart, lung, brain, kidney, and placenta (Sereni, 1973).

A study of the distribution of methadone in pregnant and nonpregnant rats revealed some unexpected differences (Peters et al., 1972). The concentration of the drug in the liver of the pregnant rat was only half that in the liver of the nonpregnant rat. There was an increase in the weight of the liver of the pregnant rat, and it appeared to be metabolizing methadone more slowly. Although most fetal tissues had lower concentrations of the drug than the maternal, fetal brain had 3X the concentration of the maternal brain. This indicates that there is no barrier for the penetration of the drug to the fetus and that for some unknown reason fetal brain has a higher affinity than maternal brain.

The distribution patterns of several amines as well as barbiturates and central nervous system drugs have been summarized by Cassano (1968),

Cassano and Hansson (1969), and Cassano *et al.* (1967b). Recently, Ullberg *et al.* (1970) pointed out the extremely high affinity of several amines such as chlorpromazine and chloroquine for the fetal eye of pigmented mice. This remarkable affinity was characterized by a continued presence of these amines in the uveal tract 1 year after birth (Lindquist and Ullberg, 1972). Albino mice did not show this persistent localization; it was shown that the amines were localizing with the melanin in the tissue, and that it may somehow be related to the toxicity of these compounds in pigmented tissues.

Quaternary ammonium compounds which have been studied are the antihistamine, aprobit (Hansson and Schmiterlöw, 1961b; Schmiterlöw, 1965) and the antispasmodic agents, secergan (Allgén *et al.*, 1960) and cetiprin (Hansson and Schmiterlöw, 1961a). Several investigators have shown that tertiary amines readily penetrate the brain and placenta. The effect of cold aprobit on the distribution of its corresponding tertiary amine, chlorpromazine, has been discussed. No detectable radioactivity in the fetus, fetal membranes or maternal brain was found 1 hour after administration of the labeled quaternary ammonium compounds.

Three psychedelic agents have been studied in pregnant animals in late gestation. Idänpään-Heikkilä and Schoolar (1969) reported that LSD localized in virtually the same tissues of the mouse fetus in late gestation as in the mother. Greatest activity was found in fetal tissues 30 minutes after injection and significant amounts remained for at least 2 hours. Quantitative determinations revealed that 0.5% of the dose appeared in the fetus and about 70% of this was unchanged LSD 5 minutes after administration. However, during the first trimester of pregnancy 2.5% of the maternal dose appears in the fetus in 5 minutes. Thus, when the fetus is most sensitive to teratogenic agents it received more LSD than did the fetus in late gestation. A radioactive zone in the middle part of the adrenal cortex exhibits the highest maternal concentration. Whether this is related to the high cortical secretion of 17-ketosteroids and 17-hydroxycorticoids caused by LSD is unknown.

Psilocin (Kalberer, 1966a,b) has a rather uniform distribution in the rat fetus 30 minutes after administration, with perhaps a slightly higher concentration in the fetal liver. This study must be interpreted with caution since the animal was sectioned at room temperature (3–4 minutes required).

Two reports on the distribution of ^{14}C-mescaline (Taska and Schoolar, 1972; Shah *et al.*, 1973) in monkeys and mice revealed a high concentration of drug in fetal brain. The rapid accumulation in the brain of mice is similar to that found for methadone (Peters *et al.*, 1972); this could be due either to a less extensive blood–brain barrier in the fetus or to an increased affinity by some constituent of brain. Essentially all the radioactivity was unchanged mescaline. A wide variety of substances have been seen by autoradiography to appear in fetal brain in a higher concentration than in fetal blood in early and mid gestation; therefore, it is more likely that binding substances are present in the brain which account for this accumulation instead of differences in the blood–brain barrier. ^{14}C-Mescaline had a distribution pattern very similar to that of morphine and other bases in mice at 12.5 days of gestation (Fig. 12). At 3 hours after injection there was an accumulation of radioactivity in the uterine lumen. Slightly increased amounts of isotope were present in decidua basalis and in the CNS of the fetus (W. J. Waddell, unpublished).

Table VI summarizes central nervous system drugs which were studied in pregnant mice in early or mid gestation. High concentrations of radioactivity were found in maternal liver, intestinal contents, Harder's gland, fat, corpora lutea, and adrenal cortex after administration of ^{14}C-Δ^9-tetrahydrocannabinol (THC) to mice at 12 days of gestation (Kennedy and Waddell, 1972). The concentration was low in maternal brain and in the fetuses at all time intervals after intravenous or subcutaneous injection; although the fetal CNS had the highest concentration of all fetal tissues. Intravenous administration produced high radioactivity in maternal lung and spleen which was probably due either to trapping of the radiocolloid in the capillaries or phagocytic action of cells in these tissues. Another clue to the mechanism of action of this drug may be its accumulation in corpora lutea and adrenal cortex. Interference with steroid hormone metabolism may be common to a variety of drugs. Harbison and Mantilla-Plata (1972) excised and counted whole mouse fetuses and ma-

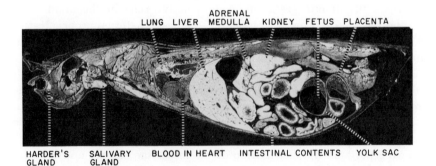

Fig. 12. A print of an autoradiogram of a 20-μm section from an A/JAX mouse injected intravenously with ^{14}C-mescaline on day 12.5 of gestation and frozen 20 minutes later.

TABLE VI Maternal and Fetal Distribution of CNS Drugs in Pregnant Mice in First 2 Weeks of Gestation

Drug	Days of gestation	Principal maternal tissues	Principal fetal tissues[a]	Reference
[14]C-Phenobarbital	12.5	Fairly uniform, excretory organs slightly higher	Yolk sac, CNS (fetus = mother)	W. J. Waddell, unpublished
[14]C-Pentobarbital	12.5	Fairly uniform, brain low, intestine and urine high	Yolk sac, CNS (fetus > mother)	Waddell, 1972a
[14]C-Thalidomide	12.5	Fairly uniform, excretory organs and eye higher	Yolk sac, CNS (fetus = mother)	W. J. Waddell, unpublished
[14]C-Morphine	12.5	Gallbladder, intestine, salivary gland, kidney, liver	Yolk sac, CNS (fetus < mother)	Waddell, 1972a
[14]C-LSD	1st week	Hypophysis, kidney, liver, lung, intestine	(High)	Idänpään-Heikkilä and Schoolar, 1969
[14]C-Mescaline	12.5	Adrenal medulla, salivary gland, gallbladder, intestine, kidney, liver	Yolk sac, CNS (fetus < mother)	W. J. Waddell, unpublished
[14]C-Δ⁹-THC	12.5	Liver, intestinal contents, Harder's gland, fat	Yolk sac, CNS (fetus < mother)	Kennedy and Waddell, 1972

[a] Comparisons of maternal and fetal concentrations, i.e. =, >, or <, in parentheses signifies a relatively uniform distribution in the fetal tissues other than those specifically named.

ternal tissues after intraperitoneal administration of ^{14}C-Δ^9-THC. Low concentrations were found in the fetus and in maternal brain.

^{14}C-Morphine localized in maternal salivary gland, liver, kidney, and intestinal contents of A/JAX mice at 12.5 days of gestation; the fetal CNS was the only tissue of the fetus itself that had a distinct accumulation (Waddell, 1972a). The fetal yolk sac, the uterine lumen, and parts of the decidua basalis have very high amounts of radioactivity (Fig. 13). Pretreatment of pregnant rats with cold dihydromorphine (DHM) to induce tolerance before administration of radiolabeled DHM increased the concentration of DHM in fetal blood (Yeh and Woods, 1970). Maternal and fetal brain also contained more labeled DHM in pretreated animals at early time intervals after injection of the isotope. It is not clear which of several possibilities accounts for this observation.

The presence or absence of a compound in the fetus and its effect on growth and differentiation of the fetus may not be related. Female rats treated with morphine and then withdrawn 5 days before mating produced offspring whose growth was retarded at 3–4 weeks of age. Since the offspring were not exposed to morphine *in utero* or postnatally, the presence of the drug apparently was not necessary for the effect (Friedler and Cochin, 1972). Another experiment illustrated the residual effects of morphine in 12-day-old rats whose mothers had received the morphine on the last day of pregnancy (Jóhannesson *et al.*, 1972). The analgesic response to a test dose of morphine at 12 days of age was different from that of controls. Although the concentration of morphine after the initial dose was less in fetal blood than that in maternal blood, the concentration of the drug in the fetal brain was almost four times that in maternal brain. This infusion of morphine did not alter the DNA or RNA ratio or the overall nucleic acid and protein composition of maternal or fetal brain or their isolated nuclei.

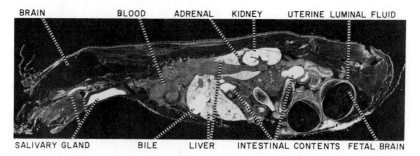

Fig. 13. A print of an autoradiogram of a 20-μm section from an A/JAX mouse that received ^{14}C-morphine intravenously on day 12.5 of gestation and was frozen 1 hour later.

^{14}C-Pentobarbital is an example of a drug that is found in higher concentration in the fetus than it is in maternal tissues (Fig. 14). However, the only time interval studied was 3 hours after injection, and this apparently high concentration may be an artifact because of the rapid elimination from the mother through metabolism and excretion during this 3-hour period. The concentration was quite uniform throughout most maternal tissues; however, the tremendous amount of activity seen in intestinal contents is consistent with extensive maternal elimination of the drug (Waddell, 1972a).

The only fetal tissue to accumulate radioactivity consistently in early and mid gestation was the yolk sac. There was a fairly consistent uptake of all types of drugs in the central nervous system of the fetus. This nonspecific affinity is peculiar to the brain and its reversal with postnatal maturation has been shown, at least for tetracycline (Sereni, 1973). Another generalization is that acidic drugs appeared in higher concentration in the fetus, and basic drugs appeared in lower concentration in the fetus. It is tempting to suggest that fetal tissues are more alkaline than maternal tissues and that this may, in part, account for this distribution pattern.

2. LOCAL ANESTHETIC AGENTS

Three local anesthetic agents labeled with ^{14}C have been studied by whole-body autoradiography. Sprague–Dawley rats in late gestation were used in the study for ^{14}C-lidocaine (Katz et al., 1968) and for ^{14}C-prilocaine (Katz, 1969). Mepivacaine labeled with ^{14}C was studied in 19-day-

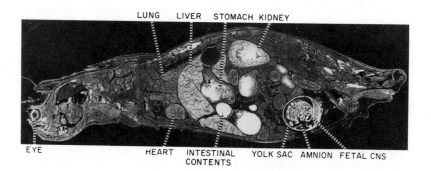

LUNG   LIVER   STOMACH   KIDNEY

EYE   HEART   INTESTINAL   YOLK SAC   AMNION   FETAL CNS
                      CONTENTS

FIG. 14. A print of an autoradiogram of a 20-μm section from an A/JAX mouse injected intravenously with ^{14}C-pentobarbital on day 12.5 of gestation and frozen 3 hours later. Note that there is a higher concentration (white areas) in the fetal tissues than in the maternal tissues.

pregnant mice (Kristerson *et al.*, 1965). The maximum survival time for any of the animals which received the local anesthetics was 1 hour. The maternal distributions correlate well with organs of excretion or metabolism of the compounds (see Table VII) and although a small amount of radioactivity was seen in the fetuses after lidocaine or prilocaine, no specific fetal tissues could be discerned. No radioactivity could be seen in the fetus on the autoradiograms of the animals that received mepivacaine; however, the authors state that a uniform but low distribution was observed in the fetus. Biopsies of frozen material taken from the rats which received prilocaine were analyzed for total radioactivity. The fetal concentration was approximately ten times that in the maternal blood; however, since the maternal tissue concentrations were much higher than that of maternal blood this probably is just a reflection of high tissue-to-blood concentrations in any tissues, maternal or fetal. The pH gradient between blood and tissues could account for the high tissue concentrations. The placental-to-fetal concentration ratio did not change with time or with the maternal blood concentration.

The accumulation of lidocaine in the fetal guinea pig liver (Finster *et al.*, 1972b) is in marked contrast to that described above in mice and rats. The concentration of lidocaine in fetal liver was higher than that in maternal liver at all time intervals from 1 to 25 minutes; no other fetal tissue had a concentration higher than the corresponding maternal tissue. Although this was explained by passage of placental blood first through the fetal liver it is difficult to understand why the studies with mice and rats did not show a high accumulation in fetal liver.

TABLE VII   **Maternal and Fetal Distribution of Local Anesthetic Agents in Pregnant Rats and Mice near Term**

Agent	Principal maternal tissues	Principal fetal tissues[a]	Reference
^{14}C-Lidocaine	Liver, kidney, brain, salivary gland	Yolk sac (fetus < mother)	Katz *et al.*, 1968
^{14}C-Prilocaine	Kidney, liver, lung, brain, bone marrow	Yolk sac (fetus < mother)	Katz, 1969
^{14}C-Mepivacaine	Liver, bile, gastrointestinal tract, salivary gland	(Fetus < mother)	Kristerson *et al.*, 1965

[a] Comparisons of maternal and fetal concentrations, i.e. =, >, or <, in parentheses signifies a relatively uniform distribution in the fetal tissues other than those specifically named.

3. Agents That Affect the Autonomic Nervous System or Neuromuscular Junction

The distribution of compounds which affect the autonomic nervous system or the neuromuscular junction is shown in Table VIII.

Nicotine and its metabolite, cotinine, were studied in pregnant albino mice in late gestation by whole-body autoradiography (Hansson and Schmiterlöw, 1962; Schmiterlöw et al., 1965; Tjälve et al., 1968; Bowman et al., 1964). Radioactivity after nicotine administration appeared in the fetus 15 minutes after injection and reached its peak at 30 minutes; at this time maternal concentration was only slightly higher. Placental concentration was high compared to the fetus; the accumulation was highest in the decidua basalis and remained high even after the blood concentration had fallen considerably. Metabolic studies with isolated tissues revealed that maternal liver, and to a small extent fetal liver, would convert nicotine to cotinine. Thus, the metabolites found in the fetus most likely originate in the mother. By 15 minutes after injection of the intact animals, 50% of the radioactivity was present in the fetus as unchanged nicotine and 50% was cotinine. It was for this reason that cotinine labeled with ^{3}H was studied alone. Cotinine passage into the fetus was slower than nicotine, but 0.5, 1 and 4 hours after injection, maternal and fetal concentrations were approximately equal. However, in rats (Mosier and Jansons, 1972) fetal plasma and tissues had a greater proportion of nicotine to metabolites than did maternal plasma from 5 minutes to 20 hours after injection.

Pigmented mice have an intense and rapid accumulation of radioactivity corresponding to the distribution of melanin (Waddell and Marlowe, 1973) following the administration of ^{14}C-nicotine. This striking accumulation in the eye may be seen in Fig. 15; it is identical to that reported for the other bases, chlorpromazine and chloroquine (Lindquist and Ullberg, 1972). If this accumulation accounts for some of the toxic effects of chloroquine and chlorpromazine on the eye, perhaps nicotine can be shown to have an action here. Furthermore, an intense localization which had not been described before for nicotine was noted in the walls of the bronchi in both pigmented and albino mice. There was no melanin in these bronchi, and it is possible that metabolic conversion of nicotine by cells in the bronchi explains this increased radioactivity.

The autoradiographic technique has been used to study the distribution of 2-^{14}C-dihydroxyphenylalanine (dopa) in mice in advanced pregnancy (Rosell et al., 1963; Ullberg, 1962). No details concerning fetal accumulation were stated, other than that a similar uptake to that of the mother

TABLE VIII   Distribution of Agents That Affect the Autonomic Nervous System and Neuromuscular Junction in Mice and Rats near Term

Drug	Principal maternal tissues	Principal fetal tissues[a]	Reference
Ganglionic drugs			
^{14}C-Nicotine	Kidney, adrenal medulla, liver, stomach, salivary gland, bronchi, intestine	Yolk sac, lung, trachea, larynx, adrenal, kidney, intestine	Hansson and Schmiterlöw, 1962; Schmiterlöw et al., 1965; Tjälve et al., 1968; Waddell and Marlowe, 1973
^{3}H-Cotinine	Fairly uniform; excretory organs higher	Yolk sac (tissues not identified)	Bowman et al., 1964
Adrenergic drugs			
^{14}C-Dihydroxyphenylalanine	Pancreas, intestinal mucosa, kidney, liver, adrenal medulla	Yolk sac (fetus similar to mother)	Ullberg, 1962; Rosell et al., 1963
Adrenergic blocking agents			
^{14}C-Propranolol	Brain, lung, liver, kidney, Harder's gland	(Fetus < mother)	Masuoka and Hansson, 1967
^{3}H-Terbutaline	Intestinal contents, gallbladder, urinary bladder, liver	Yolk sac	Bodin et al., 1972
Antimuscarinic agents			
^{3}H-Atropine	Salivary gland, gastric mucosa, Harder's gland, liver, lung, adrenal medulla	Yolk sac	Albanus et al., 1968
^{14}C-Anisotropine	Gallbladder, liver, salivary gland, pancreas, kidney, gastric musoca	Liver	Shindo et al., 1971
Cholinesterase inhibitors			
^{32}P-Tabun	Lung, liver, kidney, bone	Bone	Heilbronn et al., 1964
Muscle relaxants			
^{3}H-D-Tubocurarine	Kidney, lung, liver, myocardium, spleen, salivary gland, placenta	None	Cohen et al., 1968
^{3}H-Gallamine	(Same as D-tubocurarine)	(Very low in fetus)	Cohen et al., 1968
^{3}H-Decamethonium	(Same as D-tubocurarine)	Yolk sac	Cohen et al., 1968

[a] Comparisons of maternal and fetal concentrations, i.e. =, >, or <, in parentheses signifies a relatively uniform distribution in the fetal tissues other than those specifically named.

HARDER'S GLAND   BRONCHI   LIVER   SPLEEN   ISLETS IN PANCREAS

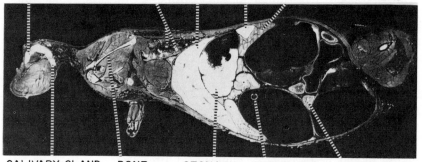

SALIVARY GLAND   BONE   STOMACH   FETAL EYE   INTESTINE

FIG. 15. A print of an autoradiogram of a 20-μm section from a C57BL/6J mouse that received ¹⁴C-nicotine intravenously on day 16.5 of gestation and was frozen 6 minutes later. An intense concentration of radioactivity (white areas) can be seen in the fetal eye.

was observed 30 minutes after injection. Activity was evident in adrenal medulla where it persisted for 4 hours when no other radioactivity remained in the body. The accumulation of exogenous L-dopa was studied in the chicken embryo with a fluorescent technique (Gripenberg and Penttilä, 1970). The L-dopa was injected into the yolk sac of 11- and 14-day-old embryos, and samples were taken at 1-day intervals for 5 days. There were two cell types in duodenum, two in the heart, and one in the stomach storing L-dopa specifically.

The distribution of ³H-norepinephrine in the human fetus in early gestation was determined by removal of tissues and counting of total radioactivity 15 minutes after injection into either the umbilical or jugular vein. The placenta had the highest concentration of radioactivity after either route of administration; the liver and lung had the next highest concentrations (Saarikoski and Castrén, 1971). Metabolic products were found in the fetus suggesting activity of the sympathetic nervous system in the early fetus. The β-receptor adrenergic blocking agent, ¹⁴C-propranolol was studied by Masuoka and Hansson (1967). Pregnant mice were frozen either 20 minutes or 4 hours after injection; although radioactivity was present in the fetuses, the concentration at both time intervals was lower in the fetal than in the maternal tissues. No specific localizations were observed in the fetus. Bodin et al. (1972) studied the distribution of ³H-terbutaline, a β-receptor stimulating agent with action predominantly on trachael muscle, by whole-body autoradiography in mice. No radioactivity was seen in near-term fetuses at 0.5, 1, and 4 hours after intravenous administration; there was a faint accumulation in the yolk sac.

Atropine and the synthetic antimuscarinic agent, anisotropine, which is a quaternary ammonium compound, were studied in pregnant mice in late gestation. Atropine (Albanus *et al.*, 1968) was found in a very low concentration in the fetus although it was high in the fetal membranes. This base would be expected to be distributed to some extent according to pH gradients in the body. Anisotropine methobromide (Shindo *et al.*, 1971) was not detectable in the fetus 1 hour after administration; 3 hours after subcutaneous injection radioactivity was seen in the fetal liver but it was low compared with that in the maternal liver.

The chemical warfare agent, Tabun, which is an organophosphorus inhibitor of cholinesterase was administered after protective doses of atropine had been given to the pregnant mice (Heilbronn *et al.*, 1964). ^{32}P-Tabun appeared in the fetus 20 minutes after injection and was mainly localized in bone. When mice were also pretreated with TMB-4, an antidote for Tabun, there was a 10–20% decrease in radioactivity reaching the tissues but no change in the pattern of distribution was observed.

The organic phosphorus cholinesterase inhibitor, demeton, which is used as an insecticide was administered to pregnant mice on the fourteenth day of gestation and its distribution studied by the wet method of autoradiography; this reveals the presence of only tightly bound drug. Placental tissue, fetal muscle, and osteogenic mesenchyme were heavily labeled within 20 minutes; the radioactivity decreased with longer time intervals (Budreau and Singh, 1973).

The three muscle relaxant drugs, D-tubocurarine, gallamine, and decamethonium, each labeled with tritium, were administered to anesthetized rats that were connected to mechanical respirators (Cohen *et al.*, 1968). The rats were in late gestation and the sacrifice time for each of the compounds was 15 minutes after injection. Very little, if any, of the isotopes reached the fetus; however, there was evidence of a small but increasing concentration of gallamine in the fetus. This may be due to the very high ionic character of the compounds. Quantitative studies revealed placental concentrations of gallamine and decamethonium at 15 and 60 minutes after injection which surpassed all tissues examined except kidney. However, ^{14}C-dimethyltubocurarine did appear in first trimester human fetuses 20 minutes after it had been administered to the mothers (Kivalo and Saarikoski, 1972). The highest concentrations were in fetal lung and liver but all the levels were much lower than maternal plasma.

4. ORGANOMERCURY COMPOUNDS

Table IX summarizes the distribution of various organic mercury compounds.

TABLE IX Maternal and Fetal Distribution of Organomercury Compounds

Compound	Species[a]	Principal maternal tissues	Principal fetal tissues[b]	Reference
^{203}Hg-Phenylmercuric acetate	Mouse (2)	Kidney, myocardium, liver, brain, thymus	Yolk sac (fetus < mother)	Berlin and Ullberg, 1963b
	Mouse (10)	Kidney, liver, myocardium, intestine	Yolk sac (fetus < mother)	Berlin and Ullberg, 1963c; Berlin and Rylander, 1964
	Mouse (18)	Kidney, liver, blood, lung, bone marrow, spleen	Yolk sac, liver (fetus < mother)	Berlin and Ullberg, 1963b; Berlin and Rylander, 1964
^{203}Hg-Phenylmercuric nitrate	Quail (15)	Kidney, liver, lung, intestine	Yolk sac, liver, gastrointestinal tract, Wolffian body, gallbladder	Bäckström, 1969
^{203}Hg-Methylmercuric dicyandiamide	Mouse (10)	Uniform except high in kidney	Yolk sac (fetus = mother)	Berlin and Ullberg, 1963c; Berlin et al., 1965
	Mouse (18)	Blood, kidney, spleen	None	Berlin and Ullberg, 1963c; Berlin et al., 1965
^{203}Hg- and ^{14}C-Methylmercuric nitrate	Quail (10)	Fairly uniform	Albumin very high; none in yolk or embryo	Bäckström, 1969
	Quail (15)	Fairly uniform	Yolk sac, bill, feather follicles, scales, intestine	Bäckström, 1969
^{203}Hg-Methoxyethyl mercuric hydroxide	Quail (4)	Kidney, pancreas, bill, liver, spleen	Yolk	Bäckström, 1969
^{203}Hg-Dimethyl mercury	Mouse (15)	Fairly uniform except kidney high	Yolk sac, eye and hair follicles (fetus = mother)	Östlund, 1969
	Mouse (19)	Bronchi, nasal, oral and esophageal mucosa, liver, kidney, hypophysis	Yolk sac, bronchi, nasal oral and esophageal mucosa, liver	Östlund, 1969
^{203}Hg-Ethyl mercuric chloride	Rat (15)	Liver, kidney, blood, placenta	Yolk sac, blood, liver (fetus < mother)	Takahashi et al., 1971
	Mouse (late)	Kidney, liver, placenta, lung, blood	Yolk sac (fetus = mother)	Ukita et al., 1969

[a] Days of gestation or incubation are included in parentheses.
[b] Comparisons of maternal and fetal concentrations, i.e. =, >, or <, in parentheses signifies a relatively uniform distribution in the fetal tissues other than those specifically named.

The organic mercury compounds are even more successful in gaining access to the fetus than the inorganic mercury compounds. Labeled phenylmercuric acetate was administered to pregnant mice at 2, 10, or 18 days of gestation. All of the mice were killed on day 18 of gestation; therefore, the time allowed for distribution varied from 16 days to 1 hour (Berlin and Ullberg, 1963b,e; Berlin and Rylander, 1964). In each case the concentration in the fetal membranes was high and some radioactivity had penetrated to the fetuses. Radioactivity in the fetal membranes was highest in the mouse with a 16-day survival time and lowest in the 1-hour survival time. The 18-day-pregnant mouse sacrificed 1 hour after the administration of the Hg compound showed an accumulation in what appeared to be fetal liver.

Bäckström (1969) studied the distribution of ^{203}Hg- or ^{14}C-labeled phenyl mercuric nitrate in hen quail and incubated eggs. In growing follicles, a very intense concentration of Hg appeared in the yolk; eggs ovulated immediately after injection had radioactivity in the periphery of yolk, and the entire yolk accumulated radioactivity in eggs ovulated later. Only a slight uptake was observed in the white of eggs. Intense radioactivity was seen in the internal yolk sac of the chick in late incubation. The excretion of Hg via the eggs during the first week was determined to be 7% after a 4-μg dose and 30% after a 16-μg dose. Chick fetuses accumulated Hg from the earliest stages of development. Compared with the mother, only small amounts of radioactivity were present in the kidneys. However, high concentrations were seen in the Wolffian body which functions as the excretory organ prior to kidney maturation. When the phenylmercuric nitrate was labeled with ^{14}C a different distribution pattern was seen after 1 hour, indicating decomposition of the phenyl mercury. The inorganic mercury portion accumulated in kidney, liver, and yolk while the organic part of the molecule was found in other tissues.

Japanese quail were given labeled methyl mercuric nitrate intravenously and the amount of radioactivity excreted in the eggs was studied. Fifty percent of the radioactivity of the injected dose was excreted by eggs laid during the first week after injection. The highest amount of mercury was in eggs laid 3 days after injection. For eggs incubated for 10 days, the highest amount of radioactivity was in albumin with little in the yolk and none in the fetus. In eggs incubated for 15 days the mercury had now transferred from the albumin to the yolk with a rather uniform distribution in the embryo. The highest concentration of all was in the yolk sac (Bäckström, 1969). Analysis of Hg in blood, liver, kidney, muscle, and brain of adult quail revealed as much as 100 times more methyl mercury retained in these tissues in the male than the female, apparently because of the extensive excretion in eggs by the female. Of all the Hg compounds studied in the quail, methyl mercury showed the greatest sex difference in distribution and the highest excretion in eggs. In contrast to phenyl mercury, methyl mercury was found to be stable; [14]C- or [203]Hg-labeling of methyl mercury gave essentially the same distribution patterns. There was an intense accumulation of radioactivity in the lens of fetal eye after administration of methyl mercury to pregnant mice; no other fetal tissues of the mouse showed a pronounced accumulation. The maternal lens in the mouse as well as the lens of the fish and quail eye also accumulated mercury, perhaps due to the high content of sulfhydryl groups. The fetal cerebellum of rats in late gestation contained the highest concentration of [203]Hg compared to other parts of the fetal and maternal brain following the administration of $CH_3{}^{203}HgCl$ (Yang et al., 1972).

Methyl mercuric dicyandiamide is a compound widely used in Sweden as a pesticide; its distribution is important in the ecology of wildlife exposed to this compound. Methyl mercuric dicyandiamide administered to pregnant mice at 10 or 18 days of gestation and sacrificed at 18 days of gestation allowed the comparison of distribution times of either 1 hour or 8 days (Berlin and Ullberg, 1963c; Berlin et al., 1965). In late gestation, after 1 hour equilibration time, no activity was detected in the fetus. Curiously, mice sacrificed 8 days after injection, in mid gestation, had a fairly uniform distribution throughout the fetus and the concentration was comparable to that in the mother. In contrast to inorganic and phenyl mercury, BAL had a pronounced effect on the fetal distribution of methyl mercuric dicyandiamide. No activity was detected in the 18-day-old fetus up to 1 hour after injection in the Hg-treated mice; however, after BAL, maternal and fetal concentrations of Hg were approximately equal. There was little effect on the 10-day-old fetus sacrificed 8 days later.

When the Swedish government prohibited the use of alkylmercurials in 1966, alkoxyalkyl mercurials were substituted. The distribution and excretion of [203]Hg-methoxyethyl mercuric hydroxide was studied in the quail (Bäckström, 1969). During the first week after injection 50% of the 16-μg dose was recovered in the eggs; the largest concentration was found on days 5, 6, and 7 after injection. Autoradiographic studies showed activity in the wall of ovarian follicles in the process of accumulating yolk as early as 10 minutes after injection; 10 days later the entire yolk had accumulated Hg. No significant concentration was found in egg white. No information was presented concerning the distribution in chick fetuses.

Dimethyl mercury was studied in pregnant mice at 19 days of gestation after allowing 5 minutes or 1 hour for equilibration (Östlund, 1969). To study the distribution of dimethyl mercury or its metabolites, the plane surface of one-half of the mouse was used to obtain the autoradiogram. Regular sagittal sections from the other half of the mouse were allowed to dry for 2 days to evaporate labeled volatile compounds; the resulting autoradiograms represented nonvolatile metabolites of dimethyl mercury. At 1 hour after intravenous administration or inhalation of mercury vapor, the two sets of autoradiograms were similar; however, no activity was detectable in fat, CNS and placenta in the autoradiograms of the nonvolatile metabolites. In the fetus marked accumulation was found in nasal, oral, and esophageal mucosa and in bronchi and liver. Mice injected on approximately day 15 of gestation and sacrificed 4 days later had a fairly high concentration in the fetus; the fetal eye had a higher concentration than the maternal eye.

The distribution of ^{203}Hg-labeled ethyl mercuric chloride was studied in pregnant mice and rats in late gestation (Ukita et al., 1969; Takahashi et al., 1971). Fetal blood and liver had the highest activity in the 15-day rat fetus after 24 hours equilibration. The other fetal tissues were fairly uniform. In mice a relatively high and fairly uniform distribution was found in the fetus 4.5 hours after intraperitoneal injection. Suckling newborn mice whose mother received the isotope showed the highest activity in liver, gastrointestinal tract, and muscle. The remaining tissues were fairly uniform.

The organic mercurial diuretic, chlormerodrin, labeled with ^{197}Hg was given to a woman 24 hours prior to hysterotomy (Sy et al., 1972). The highest concentration of radioactivity in the 25-cm CR-length fetus was in the kidney with lesser amounts in liver, lung, and heart. This probably indicates that the renal enzymes, affected by the diuretic, were present since this is the same distribution pattern seen in the adult.

5. CHEMOTHERAPEUTIC AGENTS

Table X lists the distribution studies performed using compounds which have been used in the chemotherapy of bacterial, parasitic, and neoplastic diseases.

Benzylpenicillin was the first compound to be studied by whole-body autoradiography (Ullberg, 1954a,b). Thirty minutes after injection of the compound to a pregnant mouse in late gestation, 15% as much radioactivity was found in fetal blood as was found in maternal blood. Apparently the blood–brain barrier of the fetus is not as great as that of the adult since an almost uniform concentration was found in the fetus. A low concentration was found in fetal lung in contrast to the high concentration found in the adult and newborn lung.

Dihydrostreptomycin was rather uniformly distributed throughout the fetus but with a slightly increased concentration in bone 30 minutes after

TABLE X   **Maternal and Fetal Distribution in Mice of Agents Used in Chemotherapy of Bacterial, Parasitic, and Neoplastic Diseases**

Drug	Days of gestation	Principal maternal tissues	Principal fetal tissues[a]	Reference
^{35}S-Benzylpenicillin	Late	Kidney, liver, blood, lung	Yolk sac (fetus < mother)	Ullberg, 1954a,b; Ullberg, 1959
^{3}H-Dihydrostreptomycin	Late	Kidney, lung, blood, liver, placenta, bone	Yolk sac, bone (fetus < mother)	André, 1956
^{3}H-Tetracycline	Late	Liver, kidney, spleen, brown fat, lung, bone	Yolk sac, bone (fetus < mother)	André, 1956
Demethylchlortetracycline	Late	Bone, liver, kidney, salivary gland, spleen	Yolk sac, bone	Blomquist and Hanngren, 1966
^{14}C-p-Aminosalicylic acid	Late	Intestine, kidney, liver, lung	Yolk sac, intestine, kidney, cartilage, liver, lung	Hanngren, 1959
^{14}C- and ^{35}S-Salicyl azosulfapyridine	Late	Connective tissue, liver, intestine, peritoneal, pleural, and synovial fluids	Yolk sac	Hanngren et al., 1963a,b; Svartz, 1964
^{14}C-m-Aminosalicylic acid	Late	Connective tissue, peritoneal, pleural, and synovial fluids, cartilage, intestine	Kidney, urinary bladder, eye, pleural fluid	Hanngren et al., 1963a
^{35}S-Sulfapyridine	Late	Uniform; liver slightly higher	(Fetus = mother)	Hanngren et al., 1963b; Svartz, 1964
^{14}C-Metronidazole	?	Liver, intestine, kidney, brain	(Fetus uniform)	Placidi et al., 1968
^{35}S-β,β'-Dichlorodiethyl sulphide	Late	Nasal secretion, kidney, liver; otherwise uniform	Liver, gastric mucosa (fetus < mother)	Clemedson et al., 1963a,b

[a] Comparisons of maternal and fetal concentrations, i.e. =, >, or <, in parentheses signifies a relatively uniform distribution in the fetal tissues other than those specifically named.

injection (André, 1956); tetracycline was reported in the same study to be low in the fetus 30 minutes after injection with the only specific uptake in the fetal skeleton. For both of these isotopes fetal blood contained only 15–25% of the concentration in maternal blood. The selective uptake of tetracycline by fetal skeleton was confirmed by Blomquist and Hanngren (1966) using a fluorescence technique in which whole-body sections were irradiated with ultraviolet light. They also studied the distribution of demethylchlortetracycline using this same technique. Five hours after administration of the compound to the mother, discrete localization in the fetal skeleton and fetal yolk sac was apparent. No other fetal tissues were visible.

The antitubercular agent, p-aminosalicylic acid, localized in the walls of the neural tube in early gestation, but in late gestation there was no activity in the CNS (Hanngren, 1959). The author comments that as long as the tissue of the neural tube has an epithelial character, it has the same activity as the surface epithelium.

The distribution of salicylazosulfapyridine and its two metabolic products, m-aminosalicylic acid and sulfapyridine, were compared in pregnant mice in what appears to be late gestation (Hanngren et al., 1963a,b; Svartz, 1964). The parent compound penetrated very slowly into the fetus; even after 1 hour virtually no radioactivity was seen. However, much radioactivity was found in fetal yolk sac, endometrium, and vaginal secretions. The m-aminosalicylic acid residue reached the fetus to approach an equilibrium concentration with maternal tissues at 1 hour after administration. Not surprisingly, maternal and fetal concentrations were similar to those of p-aminosalicylic acid. The other half of the drug, sulfapyridine, penetrated very rapidly into the fetus; by 20 minutes after administration to the mother, the fetal concentration was essentially the same as the maternal. In contrast, the parent compound was still much lower in the fetus 4 hours after administration of the drug to the mother.

Salicyclic acid labeled with ^{14}C was rapidly transferred to fetal mice of both the A/JAX and CBA strains; equilibrium between the mother and fetuses was achieved by 30 minutes (Eriksson and Larsson, 1971). Since the A/JAX strain is more sensitive to the teratogenic action of salicylic acid, this susceptibility cannot be accounted for by a difference in concentration of the compound in the fetus. Pretreatment with pentobarbital or cold salicylate did not significantly affect the concentration of radioactivity in maternal blood or fetus.

Although autoradiograms were not shown for the distribution pattern of the antitrichomonal and amebicidal agent, metronidazole, it was reported that the compound rapidly passed the placental barrier and was quite uniformly distributed in all organs of the fetus, in pregnant mice apparently near term (Placidi et al., 1968).

The alkylating agent, β,β'-dichlorodiethyl sulfide appeared in the fetus as early as 5 minutes after intravenous administration of the compound to pregnant mice in what appeared to be late gestation. The distribution pattern was similar in mother and fetus. No radioactivity was specifically discernible in the fetus 1 hour after administration, or as a matter of fact, in most maternal tissues; the compound must be so rapidly metabolized and eliminated that only sites of excretion such as kidney and intestinal contents show radioactivity at this time interval (Clemedson et al., 1963a,b).

The antimetabolites, azathioprine and azauridine, are transferred fairly rapidly to human (Saarikoski and Seppälä, 1973) and rat (Gutová et al., 1971) fetuses. Only limited tissues of the fetus were analyzed for azathioprine and no specific fetal tissues were isolated for azauridine; consequently tissues or areas with specific affinities remain unknown.

6. HORMONAL AGENTS

Table XI summarizes the maternal and fetal tissues in which hormonal agents are localized.

Appelgren (1967) studied the distribution in pregnant mice of three of the steroids which are intermediates in the synthesis of steroid hormones. Cholesterol, labeled in either the 4 or 26 position and given intramuscularly to pregnant mice in late gestation, did not appear to any appreciable extent in the fetus as late as 24 hours after injection. In some animals an accumulation in yolk sac epithelium was observed; however, in autoradiograms of mice killed at 24 hours no activity was detectable. Uptake in corpora lutea was dependent on the stage of gestation but appeared to be highest in the animals in the first trimester of pregnancy. Those corpora lutea in nonpregnant animals that failed to accumulate the cholesterol were found to be more eosinophilic than the highly labeled ones. No effects of the estrous cycle were seen in the labeling of ovaries with cholesterol. Thin-layer chromatography of the endocrinologically active tissues revealed that 4 hours after injection virtually all of the radioactivity was still present as unchanged cholesterol and cholesterol esters. Most of the cholesterol in fetal rhesus monkeys at term appears to reach there from the maternal blood (Pitkin et al., 1972).

4-^{14}C-Pregnenolone, however, was rapidly converted to other compounds; only 30% of the radioactivity was unchanged pregnenolone in most tissues 5 minutes after administration to pregnant animals (Appel-

TABLE XI Maternal and Fetal Distribution of Hormonal Agents

Compound	Species[a]	Principal maternal tissues	Principal fetal tissues[b]	Reference
^{14}C-Cholesterol	Mouse (late)	Adrenal cortex, liver, ovary, intestine, lung	None	Appelgren, 1967
^{14}C-Pregnenolone	Mouse (late)	Adrenal cortex, liver, ovary intestine, bronchi	Yolk sac	Appelgren, 1967
^{14}C-Progesterone	Mouse (7.5)	Liver, kidney, stomach and intestinal contents, bronchi, urine, bile	(Fetus < mother)	W. J. Waddell, unpublished
	Mouse (12.5)	Liver, stomach and intestinal contents, bile, bronchi, urine, kidney	Yolk sac, CNS (fetus < mother)	Waddell, 1972a
	Mouse (15)	Adrenal cortex, corpora lutea, liver, kidney, urinary bladder, small intestine	Yolk sac, adrenal, kidney, small intestine	Freudenthal et al., 1972
	Mouse (17.5)	Liver, bile, stomach and intestinal contents, urine	Yolk sac (fetus < mother)	W. J. Waddell, unpublished; Appelgren, 1967
	Human (CR 20–22 cm)	Not studied	Adrenal cortex, pituitary, testes, liver, kidney, intestine, eye, thyroid, thymus	Bengtsson et al., 1964
^{14}C-Norethindrone	Mouse (15)	Adrenal cortex, corpora lutea, liver, kidney, urinary bladder, small intestine	Yolk sac, adrenal, kidney, small intestine	Freudenthal et al., 1972
^{14}C-Ethynodiol diacetate	Mouse (15)	Adrenal cortex, corpora lutea, liver, kidney, urinary bladder, small intestine	Yolk sac, adrenal	Freudenthal et al., 1972
^{3}H-Pregnanediol	Mouse (late)	Gallbladder, intestinal contents, liver	Very low in fetus	Yoshikawa et al., 1971

Compound	Species (stage)	Tissue distribution	Yolk sac	Reference
^{14}C-Deoxycorticosterone	Mouse (12.5)	Liver, bile, intestinal contents, kidney, urinary bladder	Yolk sac, CNS (fetus < mother)	Waddell, 1972b
^{14}C-Corticosterone	Mouse (12.5)	Liver, bile, intestinal contents, kidney, urinary bladder	Yolk sac, CNS (fetus < mother)	Waddell, 1972b
^{14}C-Hydrocortisone	Mouse (12.5)	Liver, bile, intestinal contents, kidney, urinary bladder	Yolk sac, CNS (fetus < mother)	Waddell, 1972b
	Mouse (late)	Liver, intestine, kidney, urinary bladder, bronchial mucosa	Yolk sac, adrenal cortex, gastric mucosa, cerebrospinal fluid	Hanngren et al., 1964
^{14}C-Cortisone	Mouse (10.5 and 12.5)	Bile, liver, intestinal contents, kidney	Yolk sac (fetus < mother)	Waddell, 1971a
	Mouse (late)	Liver, intestine, kidney, urinary bladder, bronchial mucosa	Yolk sac, adrenal cortex, gastric mucosa, cerebrospinal fluid	Hanngren et al., 1964
^{14}C-Testosterone	Mouse (late)	Liver, kidney, adrenal cortex, corpora lutea (ductus deferens in male)	Yolk sac, liver, intestine, adrenal	Appelgren, 1969
^{14}C-Estradiol	Mouse (12.5)	Bile, liver, intestinal contents, adrenal cortex	Yolk sac (fetus > mother)	W. J. Waddell, unpublished
^{3}H- and ^{14}C-Estradiol	Mouse (late)	Adrenal cortex, liver, gastric mucosa, intestine, bile	Yolk sac (fetus > mother)	W. J. Waddell, unpublished; Ullberg and Bengtsson, 1963
^{14}C-Estrone	Mouse (late)	Adrenal cortex, liver, gastric mucosa, intestine, bile	Yolk sac (fetus > mother)	Ullberg and Bengtsson, 1963
^{14}C-Diethylstilbestrol	Mouse (late)	Adrenal cortex, liver, intestine, bronchi, salivary gland	Yolk sac, liver, intestine, gallbladder, adrenal cortex	Bengtsson and Ullberg, 1963; Ullberg, 1965

TABLE XI (*continued*)

Compound	Species[a]	Principal maternal tissues	Principal fetal tissues[b]	Reference
[14]C-Polydiethylstibestrol	Mouse (late)	Liver, spleen, lymph nodes, bone marrow, lung, adrenal cortex	Yolk sac	Bengtsson *et al.*, 1963
[32]P-Polydiethylstibestrol	Mouse (late)	Liver, spleen, bone marrow, lung, intestine	None	Bengtsson, 1963
[14]C-F6060	Mouse (late)	Corpora lutea, liver, kidney	Yolk sac	Hanngren *et al.*, 1965a,b
[14]C-F6066	Mouse (late)	Liver, kidney, corpora lutea	Yolk sac	Hanngren *et al.*, 1965a,b
[14]C-Alloxan	Mouse (late)	Fairly uniform, except pancreatic islets and bone high	Yolk sac (fetus = mother)	Hammarström and Ullberg, 1966
[14]C-Thiourea	Mouse (late)	Thyroid	Thyroid	Ullberg and Hammarström, 1969

[a] Days of gestation are found in parentheses.

[b] Comparisons of maternal and fetal concentrations, i.e. =, >, or <, in parentheses signifies a relatively uniform distribution in the fetal tissues other than those specifically named.

gren, 1967). Nevertheless, 1 hour after administration very little radioactivity had appeared in the fetus but the yolk sac epithelium was highly labeled. A rather uniform distribution in ovaries of nonpregnant animals was found while in the pregnant mouse the corpora lutea were specifically labeled; the concentration was one of the highest in the entire animal. Since pregnenolone rapidly accumulates in adrenals, ovaries, and testes while the uptake of cholesterol is delayed, this suggests that pregnenolone is more efficiently converted to hormones than is cholesterol. The chromatographic studies which found pregnenolone to be rapidly metabolized substantiated this. Appelgren demonstrated, histochemically in whole-body sections of pregnant mice, the presence of "secondary alcohol dehydrogenase" activity in Harder's gland, brown fat, bronchi, and liver; Δ^5-3β-hydroxysteroid dehydrogenase activity, with pregnenolone as substrate, was seen in adrenal cortex, corpora lutea, and placenta.

[14]C-Progesterone distribution was studied in pregnant mice of various gestational ages (Appelgren, 1967; Waddell, 1972a). In the 7.5-, 12.5-, and 17.5-day-old fetus only a very low and fairly uniform concentration was detected. A slightly increased uptake was detected in fetal CNS in mid-gestation. Evidence for the secretion of progesterone or its metabolites by the yolk sac is presented in Figs. 16 and 17. At 7.5 days of gestation, before the yolk sac is fully functional, there is no radioactivity in the uterine lumen 3 hours after injection. At 12.5 days of gestation, when yolk sacs are larger, the uterine lumen is filled with radioactivity 3 hours after injection (Waddell, 1972a). Chromatographic studies revealed progesterone to be rapidly metabolized (Appelgren, 1967). In contrast to pregnenolone, the nonpregnant animals accumulated activity in the corpora lutea, and no increased affinity was observed in the animals in late gestation. Previable human male fetuses were perfused with ^{14}C-labeled progesterone and processed for autoradiography (Bengtsson et al., 1964). The fetuses were 20–22 cm in length (corresponding to approximately 6-months gestational age). One fetus was perfused for 28 minutes by the

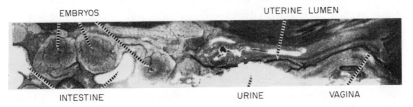

EMBRYOS   UTERINE LUMEN

INTESTINE   URINE   VAGINA

FIG. 16. A detail of a print of an autoradiogram of a 20-μm section from an A/JAX mouse that received ^{14}C-progesterone subcutaneously on day 7.5 of gestation and was frozen 3 hours later. Note the absence of radioactivity in the uterine lumen and in the area of the embryos.

SITE OF INJECTION BRONCHI ADRENAL KIDNEY UTERINE LUMEN

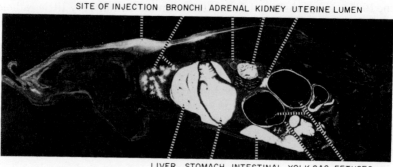

LIVER STOMACH INTESTINAL YOLK SAC FETUSES
CONTENTS

Fig. 17. A print of an autoradiogram of a 20-μm section from an A/JAX mouse that received ¹⁴C-progesterone subcutaneously on day 12.5 of gestation and was frozen 3 hours later. At this stage of gestation, a high concentration (white area) is noted in the uterine lumen and yolk sac.

umbilical vein and the other was injected intramuscularly 53 minutes before freezing. The overall distribution pattern was essentially the same for both routes of administration although the blood level was lower following intramuscular injection. This suggests that the uptake by the fetal tissues is specific and indicates either an affinity mechanism or metabolism. Since the subcellular distribution of progesterone indicates that the molecule merely associates with membranes, an affinity mechanism for membranes in general may account for this distribution pattern (Smith and Brush, 1971). Maeyama et al. (1969) studied the distribution of radioactivity in fetal liver after administration of 4-¹⁴C-progesterone to previable human male fetuses. At 13 weeks of gestation and 8 minutes after injection, 49% of the radioactivity was 20α-dihydroprogesterone and 34% was unchanged progesterone. Only about 5% was progesterone in the 17- and 22-week-old fetuses sacrificed at 12 and 18 minutes; 30 and 35%, respectively, was 20α-dihydroprogesterone. Other metabolites found were 17α- and 16α-hydroxyprogesterone and pregnanediol but each represented only 2% of the total radioactivity. No difference could be detected in these metabolites at different gestational ages.

Pregnanediol, the reduced metabolic product of progesterone, did not localize to any appreciable extent in mouse fetuses 0.5, 2, or 24 hours after administration to the mother (Yoshikawa et al., 1971) although a uniform but very low uptake was observed at the 30-minute sacrifice time. Furthermore, no radioactivity was seen in the yolk sac in these autoradiograms.

The distributions of the progestational agents, 4-¹⁴C-norethindrone and 4-¹⁴C-ethynodiol diacetate were compared with that of 4-¹⁴C-progesterone in 15-day-pregnant mice (Freudenthal *et al.*, 1972). Each of these steroids localized in sites of steroid hormone metabolism and excretion; no remarkable difference was noted among the three compounds. Although the authors found progesterone to be localized in specific fetal tissues, this was not apparent in the published autoradiograms.

The autoradiographic studies of ^{3}H-cortisone by Nasjleti *et al.* (1967) were done in mice at 12.5 days of gestation, but the fetuses were fixed in solutions which would obviously remove or translocate the radioactivity; consequently, the autoradiograms are of limited value. There is a greater binding of cortisone to fetal tissues of the A/JAX strain than there is to tissues of the C57BL strain, which is less susceptible to the teratogenic action of cortisone (Reminga and Avery, 1972). Hanngren *et al.* (1964) found the same distribution pattern for cortisone and cortisol 20 minutes after injection of the isotopes to mice in late gestation. Penetration of both hormones into the fetus was poor; however, a specific accumulation was noted in the fetal adrenal cortex, gastric mucosa, and cerebrospinal fluid. The fetal concentrations were lower than maternal except for the adrenal cortex. A high uptake in maternal adrenal cortex was found 5 minutes after injection; however, by 20 minutes this decreased so that little activity remained. At 20 minutes the concentration in the adrenal medulla was higher. Also, studies by Waddell (1971a) in mice found high accumulations of cortisone throughout the cortex and low amounts in the medulla at 8 minutes, 9, and 24 hours; at intervening time intervals only the zona glomerulosa and medulla had high concentrations. At 12.5 days of gestation no increased concentration of radioactivity could be seen in the palatal buds of mice *in utero*. This lack of an increased concentration of the compound at the site of teratogenic action raises certain questions about the mechanism of action of teratogenic compounds (Waddell, 1971a). The remarkable accumulation and apparent secretion of cortisone by the yolk sac epithelium was pointed out in this study. Whether or not the yolk sac is an organ for the nonspecific secretion of compounds into the uterine lumen awaits further experiments.

Hydrocortisone, deoxycorticosterone, and corticosterone all have essentially the same distribution pattern as that of cortisone (Waddell, 1972b). Since deoxycorticosterone is not teratogenic, the mechanism of teratogenic action of these compounds remains unknown. The increased concentration of deoxycorticosterone in liver and decreased concentration in yolk sac relative to that for cortisone, hydrocortisone, or the natural hormone of the mouse, corticosterone, may, however, be a suggestion of the relative fetal and maternal metabolic rates for these steroid hormones. Human fetal urine at 16 to 19 weeks of gestation contained a greater fraction of conjugated hydrocortisone than fetal plasma and amniotic fluid suggesting that fetal urine voiding is one pathway by which corticosteroids are added to the amniotic fluids (Abramovich and Wade, 1969). Removal of tissues from rats for counting after administration of 4-^{14}C-corticosterone revealed a significantly higher concentration of radioactivity in the fetal hypothalamus than in the rest of the brain (Zarrow et al., 1970). Fetal liver contained only a slightly higher concentration of corticosterone than fetal plasma while the 2-day-old liver had about eight times the plasma concentration and the maternal liver 50 times the plasma concentration. This could be due to either increased hepatic binding or metabolism with maturation.

The only androgenic agent which has been studied is 4-^{14}C-testosterone (Appelgren, 1969). Mice in late gestation showed essentially the same distribution patterns after intramuscular or intravenous administration at 0.5, 1, and 2 hours.

Both estradiol and estrone were stated to have the same, relatively uniform, distribution patterns in fetuses 1 hour after injection of the mother in late gestation (Ullberg and Bengtsson, 1963). Activity in fetal membranes and fetuses was always high while the placental concentration was low. Fetal blood concentration was comparable to maternal liver at 1 hour, and at 4 hours fetal serous fluids showed a concentration higher than fetal blood. In general, the fetal concentration was higher than maternal; the only exception was liver. A lower uptake of the estrogens in the adrenal cortex of pregnant animals may be due to an excess of endogenous estrogens compared to nonpregnant females. Of all mice studied the males had the highest uptake in the adrenal cortex. The elegant studies by Stumpf (1968) which have identified the hypothalamic receptors for estradiol in female rats suggest that sex differences may exist for estradiol binding.

The synthetic estrogenic agent, diethylstilbestrol, was studied at 20 minutes and 4 hours after administration to pregnant mice in late gestation (Bengtsson and Ullberg, 1963; Ullberg, 1965). The greatest difference between the distribution of this compound and the natural estrogens was seen in the fetus. Fetal concentrations of diethylstilbestrol remained lower than maternal. Fetal excretory organs and adrenal cortex showed a distinct accumulation. Specific affinity for both types of estrogens was observed in the same target tissues, viz., adrenal cortex, ovary, testis, and hypophysis. As with the natural estrogens, diethylstilbestrol was found to be lowest in the adrenal cortex of the pregnant animals. Herbst et al. (1971) have found an increased incidence of adenocarcinoma of the vagina in 15- to 20-year-old girls whose mothers received diethylstilbestrol starting in the first trimester and continuing throughout pregnancy. This type of cancer is rare in women under 50 years of age. It thus appears that a latent effect exists in female offspring.

A macromolecular synthetic estrogen, polydiethylstilbestrol phosphate, was studied when labeled either with [14]C (Bengtsson et al., 1963) or with [32]P (Bengtsson, 1963). Although no radioactivity was seen in fetuses or fetal membranes of mice in late gestation 4 hours after administration of the ^{32}P-labeled compound to the mother, the visceral yolk sac epithelium had a high concentration when the ^{14}C compound was substituted. Also, the target tissues for estrogens failed to show an uptake of the ^{32}P compound while the ^{14}C compound showed a persistent accumulation in these organs. This was interpreted to mean the ^{14}C activity in the adrenal cortex, ovary, testis, etc., represents the monomolecular diethylstilbestrol or its metabolites after hydrolytic removal of the phosphate.

An intense and almost specific localization in the corpora lutea of female mice of the nonsteroid, antigestagen F6060 and its acetylated derivative, F6066, suggested that the antigestagenic properties might be due to interference with the metabolism of progesterone (Hanngren et al., 1965a,b). The radioactivity seemed to be confined to the corpora lutea of the mother and the visceral yolk sac epithelium of the fetus for at least 24 hours after administration. However, the fact that other compounds localize in the corpora lutea and in the yolk sac epithelium obscures this as a mechanism of action for this compound. The compound was tried as a chemical abortifacient clinically in Sweden in the mid-1960's.

Although alloxan selectively localized in the pancreatic islets of adult mice, there was no accumulation in the pancreatic islets of the fetuses of mice in late gestation 4 hours after the administration of alloxan to the mother. The accumulation of this compound in the islets, whose β cells it destroys, presumably suggests a correlation between localization and action. The lack of accumulation in the pancreatic islets of the fetuses suggests that the fetal pancreas is not yet functioning in the production of insulin, even in late gestation (Hammarström and Ullberg, 1966). There was a high uptake in the visceral yolk sac while fetal concentration was uniform and approximately equal to maternal.

The remarkably specific localization of thiourea in both the maternal and fetal thyroid 4 hours after the injection of ^{14}C-thiourea in the pregnant mouse in late gestation may be related to fetal hypothyroidism seen after medication with thiourea during pregnancy (Ullberg and Hammarström, 1969). The thyroid glands of fetal rabbits and dogs in late gestation accumulate 2-^{14}C-thiouracil to very high concentrations (Quinones et al., 1972); total thyroid concentrations 16 times those of fetal blood were seen within a few hours after administration of the compound to the mother. Since this is the same distribution as that found in the adult, the explanation for any hypothyroid function in these infants is obvious.

Radioactivity appeared in 16- to 20-week-old human fetuses when 9-^{3}H-prostaglandin $F_{2\alpha}$ was given intravenously to mothers prior to therapeutic abortion (Beazley et al., 1972). A consistently high level of radioactivity was found in fetal liver, but in all the other tissues studied levels were similar to those found in maternal tissues.

Peptide hormones do not appear to cross from mother to fetus and vice versa to any significant extent. Parathyroid hormone labeled with ^{125}I was administered intravenously to either the mother or fetus (via the chorionic vitelline vein) in rats in late gestation; no transfer could be demonstrated in either direction across the placenta. The highest concentration of radioactivity was in the fetal liver and some activity was seen in the gastrointestinal tract and kidney (Garel and Dumont, 1972).

Since most small molecules do not encounter any great difficulty crossing the placenta it is not surprising that melatonin which is a modified amino acid gains ready access to the fetus from the mother. Unchanged acetyl-^{3}H-melatonin was demonstrated in whole fetuses and certain selected fetal tissues 30 minutes after administration of the labeled hormone to pregnant rats on day 18 of gestation (Klein, 1972).

7. VITAMINS

Table XII summarizes the distribution of vitamins in maternal and fetal tissues of pregnant animals.

Thiamine (Hammarström et al., 1966) and a long-acting derivative of thiamine, ^{35}S-o-butyrylthiamine disulfide (Takahashi et al., 1969) in pregnant mice in late gestation had essentially the same distribution patterns 24 hours after administration of the compounds to the mother. The high metabolic activity of the fat and other tissues in which the compounds were localized may be related to the affinity for the compounds. A comparison of the distribution of ^{35}S-thiamine and ^{14}C-glucose showed several similarities indicating the role of thiamine in glucose metabolism. Glucose was taken up more rapidly than thiamine and to a greater extent. Thiamine gradually accumulated in fetuses and reached equilibrium with the mother 4 days after injection, while glucose was approaching equilibrium as early as 20 minutes after injection. An extension of the whole-body autoradiographic technique was employed by Tubaro and Bulgini (1971) to study thiamine distribution in guinea pig fetuses. Nonradioactive thiamine was given to guinea pigs via the umbilical artery and whole-body sections were taken. These sections were then inoculated with thiamine-dependent Escherichia coli and after incubation, thiamine distribution was visualized with triphenyltetrazolium.

Nicotinamide was studied in pregnant mice at 12.5 and 17.5 days of

BROWN FAT   BLOOD   ADRENAL CORTEX   KIDNEY   INTESTINE

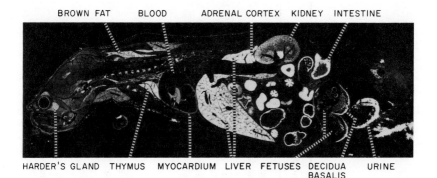

HARDER'S GLAND   THYMUS   MYOCARDIUM   LIVER   FETUSES   DECIDUA   URINE
                                                         BASALIS

FIG. 18. A print of an autoradiogram of a 20-μm section from an A/JAX mouse injected intravenously with ¹⁴C-nicotinamide on day 12.5 of gestation and frozen 1 hour later.

gestation (Waddell, 1973a). This vitamin has been reported to prevent the teratogenic action of nicotinic acid antagonists and carbonic anhydrase inhibitors (Landauer and Wakasugi, 1967). Figures 18 and 19 show its distribution which was apparently in the tissues with high metabolic activity. At 12.5 days of gestation the concentration in the fetus was fairly uniform with a slightly increased affinity observed in the CNS. Maternal and fetal concentrations were approximately equal in the 12.5- and 17.5-day-old fetuses. However, specific uptake was observed in late gestation. Maternal adrenal cortex showed one of the highest accumulations in the entire animal at both gestational ages. However, it seems that the uptake in corpora lutea was related to the gestational age of the mother. In the 17.5-day-pregnant mouse, corpora lutea exhibited the

HARDER'S GLAND   BROWN FAT   KIDNEY   CORPORA LUTEA   DECIDUA BASALIS

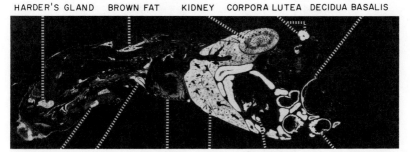

LYMPH NODE   THYMUS   MYOCARDIUM   LIVER   FETAL BROWN FAT   INTESTINE

FIG. 19. A print of an autoradiogram of a 20-μm section from an A/JAX mouse that received ¹⁴C-nicotinamide intravenously on day 17.5 of gestation and was frozen 1 hour later. The concentration in the corpora lutea was the highest in the entire animal. Also note the high uptake in fetal brown fat.

TABLE XII Maternal and Fetal Distribution of Vitamins

Vitamin	Species[a]	Principal maternal tissues	Principal fetal tissues[b]	Reference
[35]S-Thiamine	Mouse (19)	Liver, kidney, myocardium, brown fat, Harder's gland	Brown fat, myocardium, liver, gastric mucosa, kidney, bone	Hammarström et al., 1966
[35]S-o-Butyrylthiamine	Guinea pig (?)	Not studied	Liver, brown and perirenal fat, myocardium	Tubaro and Bulgini, 1971
[14]C-Nicotinamide	Mouse (late)	Liver, kidney, myocardium, brown fat, gastric mucosa, brain	Yolk sac, brown fat, liver, myocardium, G.I. mucosa, bone	Takahashi et al., 1969
	Mouse (12.5)	Wall of intestine, adrenal cortex, liver, kidney, myocardium	Yolk sac, CNS (fetus = mother)	Waddell, 1973a
	Mouse (17.5)	Wall of intestine, adrenal cortex, eye, liver, kidney, myocardium	Yolk sac, adrenal cortex, eye, intestine, liver, myocardium, brown fat	Waddell, 1973a
[14]C-Ascorbic acid	Mouse (17–19)	Liver, kidney, intestine, salivary gland, thymus, brain, adrenal	Yolk sac, adrenal, retina, spinal cord, brain	Hammarström, 1966
[14]C-Dehydroascorbic acid	Mouse (17–19)	Brain, salivary gland, thymus, adrenal, liver, pancreatic islets	Yolk sac, brain, adrenal, retina, spinal cord	Hammarström, 1966

^{14}C-α-Tocopherol	Mouse (late)	Liver, bone marrow, spleen, ovary, intestine, lung	Yolk sac	Ullberg, 1965
^{57}Co-, ^{58}Co-, ^{60}Co-Cyanocobalamin	Mouse (3)	Brown fat, liver, adrenal, placenta, hypophysis, brain stem	(Fetus = mother)	Ullberg et al., 1967; Flodh, 1968b
	Mouse (9)	Placenta, kidney, adrenal, gastric mucosa	Yolk sac (fetus > mother)	Ullberg et al., 1967; Flodh, 1968b
	Mouse (15)	Placenta, ovary, brown fat, liver	Yolk sac, gastric mucosa, kidney, brown fat, choroid plexa, pituitary, intestine	Ullberg et al., 1967; Flodh, 1968b
	Mouse (18–19)	Placenta, liver, thyroid, choroid plexa, gastric mucosa	Yolk sac, kidney, adrenal, gastric mucosa, choroid plexa, brown fat, pituitary, intestine	Ullberg, 1965; Ullberg et al., 1967; Flodh, 1968b
^{14}C-Retinol	Mouse (late)	Retina, lung, liver, gastric mucosa, intestine	Slightly in liver	Ullberg, 1965

[a] Days of gestation are found in parentheses.

[b] Comparisons of maternal and fetal concentrations, i.e. =, >, or <, in parentheses signifies a relatively uniform distribution in the fetal tissues other than those specifically named.

highest concentration in the body; somewhat less uptake was found in the 12.5-day-pregnant mouse. In the nonpregnant animal the concentration in the corpora lutea was no higher than that in several other maternal tissues. Basophilic areas in the decidua basalis had high amounts of radioactivity at all stages of gestation studied. These are the same areas that were seen to accumulate other bases such as chlorcyclizine, nicotine, and morphine. This localization may be pH dependent.

Ascorbic acid and dehydroascorbic acid were each studied in pregnant mice in late gestation at 2 minutes, 4 hours, 24 hours, and 3 days after administration of the compound to pregnant mice (Hammarström, 1966). By 3 days after injection of ascorbic acid, the concentration in fetal brain, retina, spinal cord, and adrenal was higher than that in the corresponding maternal tissues. Even though these same fetal tissues showed an increased affinity for the ^{14}C-dehydroascorbic acid, the fetal concentration never exceeded that of the mother. Since uptake of activity in fetal CNS was delayed after the injection of dehydroascorbic acid it was thought that it must be reduced to ascorbic acid before or during transfer to the fetus. Initially there were great differences in the maternal distribution of the two compounds. Ascorbic acid accumulated more rapidly in adrenal cortex, kidney, and intestinal mucosa than did dehydroascorbic acid. The central nervous system, liver, and pancreatic islets accumulated the dehydroascorbic acid more quickly. Chromatographic studies revealed that regardless of which of the forms was injected most of the radioactivity was due to ascorbic acid. Less than 3% of the activity was dehydroascorbic acid; at all time intervals and in all tissues examined the ratio of the activity of these two isotopes remained constant.

In spite of the fact that in small rodents vitamin E deficiency causes fetal death and resorption, Ullberg (1965) found no activity in the fetus 4 hours after vitamin E administration to a pregnant mouse. Transfer of ^{3}H-α-tocopherol to the fetal lamb was determined quantitatively by Hidiroglou et al. (1969). Pregnant ewes in the last month of gestation who had been fed a muscular dystrophy-producing hay were treated orally with the radiolabeled vitamin E. Highest maternal and fetal concentrations were found in adrenal, liver, spleen, and gastrointestinal tract. Up to 5 days after dosing, maternal concentrations were always higher than the corresponding fetal tissues but this gradually changed so that by 13 days after dosing, maternal and fetal concentrations were approximately the same. Comparison of radioactivity in the fetal tissues to that in the newborn lambs showed higher concentrations in the lambs. This increase was obviously due to the high α-tocopherol content in milk.

Vitamin B$_{12}$ was given to pregnant mice at all stages of gestation; with one exception, the mice were killed 2 days before delivery (Flodh,

1968b; Ullberg, 1965; Ullberg et al., 1967). The additional pregnant animal was injected on day 9 of gestation and sacrificed 1 day later. A unique placental transfer of the B_{12} was found. As early as 15 minutes after injection approximately 55% of the injected dose was localized in the placenta and no activity was detected in the fetus. The placental concentration reached a peak of about 70% of the injected dose at 1 hour, and thereafter its concentration fell while the fetal concentration started to increase. Between 4 to 5 hours after injection both placenta and fetus each contained about 40% of the injected dose and by 24 hours almost 80% of the activity was concentrated in the fetus. However, this fetal uptake was dose dependent. After small doses, 40 to 100 times the concentration in maternal tissue was found in the fetuses; at extremely high doses this ratio decreased to less than two. In late gestation, activity was first observed in fetal intestine with none in the maternal intestine. At later time intervals this uptake gradually disappeared and by 4 hours accumulation was in fetal blood, kidney, adrenal cortex, gastric mucosa, and choroid plexus. From 4 hours to 4 days after injection every fetal tissue had a significantly higher concentration than the corresponding maternal tissue. The highly selective localization in the pituitary (high in pars intermedia and pars distalis but none in pars nervosa) was found in both fetus and mother. With time, increased concentration was observed in maternal CNS and brown fat; this was also true for the fetus. In the mouse injected on the third day of gestation and sacrificed 16 days later, maternal and fetal concentrations were approximately equal. For the one animal sacrificed in early gestation localization was highest in the placenta and fetus. Lower fetal and placental concentrations were observed if the female mouse was injected 12 days before mating and then sacrificed on day 19 of gestation. The author interprets this to indicate that most fetal B_{12} is derived from maternally ingested B_{12} during pregnancy and not from maternal tissue stores.

Various vitamin B_{12} analogues were administered to pregnant mice before giving the radiolabeled B_{12} (Flodh, 1968b); both placental passage in female mice and intestinal absorption in male mice were determined. The greatest inhibitory effect was found for methyl-B_{12}, coenzyme-B_{12}, and cold B_{12} in both transfer processes. Factor B had the least effect. Chromatographic studies showed that the radioactivity in all tissues was intact vitamin B_{12} even in those tissues where there was a delayed accumulation. Most endocrine and reproductive organs exhibited a high uptake of the radioactive B_{12}. Several tissues where rapid cell growth occurs exhibited a high localization; these included testicular tubuli, ovarian follicles, gastrointestinal mucosa, fetuses and tumors. One notable exception was the lack of activity in the bone marrow.

The unusual technique of Tubaro and Bulgini (1971) was again used to study the distribution of vitamin B_{12} in a newborn guinea pig. Highest concentrations were present in brown fat, liver, myocardium, and perirenal fat.

Vitamin A was not found in fetal retina even though a high accumulation was noted in this maternal tissue (Ullberg, 1965). Fetal liver did show a slight accumulation of vitamin A. The localization of vitamin A was detected in tissue sections by fluorescent microscopy in pregnant rats on the tenth, eleventh, and twelfth day of gestation; the vitamin A had been administered orally on days 7, 8, and 9 of gestation (Geelen, 1972). Fluorescence was seen in decidua capsularis, decidua basalis, Reichert's membrane, parietal yolk sac epithelium, giant cells, and uterine musculature; none was seen in the visceral yolk sac epithelium or embryo.

8. MISCELLANEOUS COMPOUNDS

A summary of the distribution of these compounds is listed in Table XIII.

The two chlorinated hydrocarbon insecticidal agents, DDT and dieldrin, appeared in the fetus of mice in late gestation; the mice were sacrificed as early as 1 hour and as late as 16 days after intramuscular administration of the compound (Bäckström et al., 1965). It is not clear how the treatment schedule was arranged for the mice killed many days after administration. Apparently, the pregnant mice were injected with the compound 16 days prior to term and killed at term. For compounds that are retained in maternal tissues to such a remarkable extent as DDT and dieldrin, it is not surprising that the distribution pattern after 16 days is typical for that for fetuses in late gestation. There is simply a redistribution continually occurring in the pregnant animals. No appreciable uptake was observed in either mother or fetus until six hours after injection. At this time and all later time intervals studied, the same maternal and fetal tissues showed a high affinity for the isotopes. Fetal concentrations were always lower than the maternal. The slow absorption after injection and distribution into maternal and fetal tissue may be due to the poor solubility of this nonpolar material in blood; the presence of α-globulins in the fetal circulation has been shown to enhance the transfer of dieldrin into the fetus, presumably from binding of dieldrin to this protein (Eliason and Posner, 1971). Newborn mice allowed to suck for 2 days from their mothers who received the isotopes 3 days prior to delivery showed a higher concentration than the fetuses, indicating a high excretion of DDT and dieldrin in the milk and/or a lower rate of elimination in the newborn than in the fetal–maternal unit. There was a fivefold greater concentration of DDT in the livers of 10-hour-old rats that had sucked than there was in the livers of neonatal rats before sucking (Woolley and Talens, 1971). Tissue analysis of fetal brain, liver, and fat at different stages of gestation confirmed the transfer of DDT to the fetus after it was administered to the mother (Schmidt and Dedek, 1972).

The teratogenic herbicides, 2,4-dichlorophenoxyacetic acid (2,4-D) and 2,4,5-trichlorophenoxyacetic acid (2,4,5-T), each show a selective uptake in the yolk sac epithelium of pregnant mice (Lindquist and Ullberg, 1971). The uptake and retention by the yolk sac epithelium of 2,4,5-T was more rapid and persistent than 2,4-D. Since both compounds clearly cross into the fetus and since quantitative determinations of the compounds in fetal blood were not done in this study, it is impossible to know whether they reached the yolk sac via maternal or fetal blood. A structurally similar environmental pollutant, 2,3,5-triiodobenzoic acid, was also found to reach the fetus (McDowell et al., 1971).

The hydroxylated derivative of tryptophan, 5-hydroxytryptophan, and the decarboxylated active autocoid, 5-hydroxytryptamine, have both been studied in pregnant mice (Ritzén et al., 1965). The 5-hydroxytryptophan rapidly reached the fetus; 20 minutes after injection, the fetal concentration was appreciable. Most of the radioactivity disappeared after 1 day. Decarboxylation to 5-hydroxytryptamine almost totally prevented accumulation of radioactivity in the fetus; at either 1 hour or 4 days after administration, no radioactivity was seen in the fetus. Radioactivity, however, was still present in the adrenal medulla, spleen, and blood of the mother after 4 days. Since the amine as well as the 5-hydroxytryptophan accumulated in the adrenal medulla this accumulation is probably due to storage instead of decarboxylating enzymes. High-resolution autoradiography was used by Gershon and Ross (1966) to study the sites of 5-hydroxytryptamine storage after administration of ^{3}H-5-hydroxytryptophan. The amine was taken up rapidly and retained for long periods of time by adrenal medullary chromaffin cells, gastric enterochromaffin cells, blood platelets, thyroid parafollicular cells, β cells of pancreatic islets, mast cells, and septal cells of the lung.

The alkyl-substituted theobromine, SK-7, which is 1-hexyl-3,7-dimethylxanthine, was studied by whole-body autoradiography in pregnant mice which were sacrificed 5 minutes, 20 minutes, 1 hour, and 4 hours after injection. The concentration was low in the fetuses at each of these time intervals although the yolk sac epithelium contained a high concentration (Sjöstrand and Schmiterlöw, 1968). A slightly increased affinity was observed in the fetal eye 3 days after administration of the ^{14}C-labeled isotope to the mother.

TABLE XIII Maternal and Fetal Distribution of Various Compounds in Pregnant Mice and Rats in Late Gestation

Compound	Principal maternal tissues	Principal fetal tissues	Reference
^{14}C-DDT	Fat, liver, intestine, kidney, mammary gland, brain, ovary	Yolk sac, fat, liver, intestine	Bäckström et al., 1965
^{14}C-Dieldrin	Fat, liver, intestine, bone marrow, mammary gland, ovary	Yolk sac, fat, liver, intestine	Bäckström et al., 1965
^{14}C-2,4,5-T	Relatively uniform	Yolk sac (fetus similar to mother)	Lindquist and Ullberg, 1971
^{14}C-2,4,D	Relatively uniform	Yolk sac (fetus similar to mother)	Lindquist and Ullberg, 1971
^{14}C-5-Hydroxytryptophan	Pancreas, adrenal medulla, thyroid, bone marrow, spleen, lung, intestine	Yolk sac, adrenal medulla, intestine, skin	Ritzén et al., 1965
^{14}C-5-Hydroxytryptamine	Adrenal medulla, spleen, lung, bone marrow, thyroid, islets of Langerhans	Yolk sac	Ritzén et al., 1965
^{14}C-SK-7	Liver, blood, intestine, kidney, lung, eye, bone marrow	Yolk sac, eye	Sjöstrand and Schmiterlöw, 1968
^{14}C-Cyclamate	Kidney, gastrointestinal tract	Yolk sac (fetus > mother)	Schechter and Roth, 1971
^{35}S-Cysteamine	Pituitary gland, salivary gland, liver, spleen, intestine, retina, bone marrow	Liver, skeleton, intestine, retina, bone marrow, kidney, myocardium	Nelson and Ullberg, 1960
^{35}S-Glutathione	Liver, renal cortex, pancreas, salivary gland, gastrointestinal mucosa	Bone, liver, eye, brain	Takahashi and Sato, 1968

^{14}C-Glutamine	Pancreas, intestine, salivary gland, bone marrow, spleen, thymus, lymph nodes	Yolk sac (fetus similar to mother)	Cassano and Hansson, 1965
^{14}C-Ethionine	Liver, pancreas	Yolk sac (fetus > mother)	Hansson and Garzo, 1961
^{75}Se-Selenomethionine	Pancreas, intestine, salivary gland, liver, kidney, mammary gland, gastric mucosa, bone marrow	Yolk sac, pancreas, gastrointestinal tract	Hansson and Jacobsson, 1966
^{14}C-p-Fluorophenylalanine	Pancreas, gastrointestinal mucosa, salivary gland, liver, bone marrow	(Fetus similar to mother)	Garzo et al., 1962
^{125}I-4-Iodophenylalanine	Pancreas, renal pelvis, (epididymis in males)	Yolk sac, optic lens	Ullberg and Blomquist, 1968
^{125}I-3,4-Diiodophenyl-alanine	Pancreas, renal parenchyma	Yolk sac, optic lens	Ullberg and Blomquist, 1968
^{125}I-3-Hydroxy-4-iodo-phenylalanine	Walls of large blood vessels, renal parenchyma	Optic lens	Ullberg and Blomquist, 1968
^{14}C-Urea	Aorta, cartilage, bone, vibrissae, vibrissal sinuses	Cortex of bone, vibrissae, vibrissal sinuses	Waddell, 1968
^{14}C-DMO	Periphery of lens of eye, retina, salivary gland	Eye, bone (fetus > mother)	Waddell, 1971b
^{14}C-Nitrilotriacetic acid	Bone, kidney, urinary bladder, liver, nasal mucosa, spleen	Bone	Tjälve, 1972
^{14}C-3-Methylcholanthrene	Lung, intestinal contents, gallbladder, liver, kidney	Intestinal contents, liver, kidney	Takahashi and Yasuhira, 1973
^{14}C-Bilirubin	Liver, kidney, lung, intestine	(Fetus similar but less than mother)	Lüders, 1971

The distribution of ^{14}C-cyclamate in 21-day-pregnant rats was observed 5 minutes or 7 hours after intravenous administration (Schechter and Roth, 1971). The 7-hour interval was selected because this is the estimated biological half-life of the compound. At the earlier interval very high accumulations were observed in the placenta and yolk sac but no activity was detectable in the fetus. However, at the later time the only activity visible in the mother was found in kidney and gastrointestinal tract; high fetal concentrations were apparent. The authors proposed that the fetus may store the cyclamate by removing it from the maternal circulation. This mechanism may exist for many compounds. The degree depends on such factors as the affinity of fetal tissues for the drug, the rates of transfer of the drug between mother and fetus, and the rate of elimination of the drug from the mother.

^{14}C-Cyclamate was given to five women in early pregnancy at the time of therapeutic abortion and sterilization by abdominal hysterectomy (Pitkin et al., 1970). This unusual but valuable experimental design undoubtedly will be done with more drugs in the future. The uterus and its contents were studied by liquid scintillation counting and autoradiography; extracts of the tissues were subjected to thin-layer chromatography to establish the chemical identity of the radioactivity. The fetal crown–rump lengths ranged from 4.7 to 10.8 cm. Fetal liver, spleen, intestine, pancreas, and kidney had greater amounts of radioactivity than did blood in all or almost all fetuses. Lung, skin, placenta, and chorioamnion frequently had greater amounts than did fetal blood. Radioactivity in the sinusoids of the liver was clearly seen in the autoradiograms.

Pitkin et al. (1971) studied the distribution of ^{14}C-saccharin in rhesus monkeys at 140–160 days of gestation. Considerable amounts of radioactivity were transferred to the fetus and were slowly eliminated from the fetus. It was distributed to all fetal tissues studied except brain; no tissue had consistently higher levels than fetal blood although there was extensive excretion by the fetal kidney.

In an effort to add information to the possible action of agents which protect against the effects of ionizing radiation, female mice in advanced pregnancy were injected intravenously with ^{35}S-cysteamine and sacrificed 0.33, 1, 4, and 24 hours later (Nelson and Ullberg, 1960). At no time did the fetal uptake equal that of the mother. The highest activity was found in the fetal liver at the earliest time interval; after 4 hours fetal skeleton dominated other tissues. These authors found that the fetal uptake of amino acids exceeded that of the maternal in contrast to the distribution of cysteamine. Another major difference was the lack of cysteamine accumulation in the pancreas; the accumulation of amino acids was higher in pancreas than in any other tissue. ^{35}S-Glutathione accumulated in fetal bone, liver, eye, and brain of mice when studied by whole-body autoradiography (Takahashi and Sato, 1968). The amino acid, ^{14}C-glutamine, was studied in pregnant mice in late gestation, 1, 4, and 24 hours after intravenous administration. Maternal tissues which are known to have a high rate of protein synthesis rapidly accumulated the radioactivity. Essentially the same distribution pattern was observed in the fetus (Cassano and Hansson, 1965).

The amino acid analogues, ethionine, selenomethionine, and methionine have been studied in rodents by autoradiography. In mice, there was accumulation of ^{14}C-ethionine and ^{75}Se-selenomethionine in fetal tissues, particularly pancreas, liver, and yolk sac (Hansson and Garzo, 1961; Hansson and Jacobson, 1966). These authors were able to demonstrate that the ethionine accumulated in these tissues but was not incorporated into the tissue proteins, whereas there was rapid incorporation of the methionine into the protein fraction. Proffit and Edwards (1962) injected pregnant rats on days 12–15 of gestation and sacrificed them 4 hours later. ^{3}H-Methionine localized in fetal liver and developing epithelial structures; ^{3}H-ethionine had a relatively uniform distribution in fetal tissues.

Other amino acid analogues, p-fluorophenylalanine, 4-iodophenylalanine, 3,4-diiodophenylalanine, and 3-hydroxy-4-iodophenylalanine were studied in pregnant mice in late gestation (Garzo et al., 1962; Ullberg and Blomquist, 1968). A remarkable accumulation was seen in the lens of the eye of the fetus which was not seen in the mother's lens. The fetal yolk sac was the only other site of prominent accumulation.

^{14}C-Urea was used as an indicator of total tissue water (Waddell, 1968) in pregnant mice in late gestation. By including a wide range of time intervals between intravenous injection of the compound and the freezing time of the animal, it was possible to visualize the kinetics of distribution and elimination affecting the relative maternal and fetal concentrations. At early sacrifice times, the fetal concentration was very low relative to that in maternal tissues. At later time intervals, the fetal concentration was very high relative to maternal concentration. This can readily be explained by a slow rate of exchange of the drug between mother and fetus and a rapid rate of renal elimination of the compound from the mother. A higher concentration of urea was found in certain collagen-rich structures than could be accounted for by their water content. This apparent binding of urea to collagen may not be great enough to invalidate the use of urea as an indicator of total body water but it prevents its use for this purpose in collagen-rich structures. Since fetal urea is higher than maternal and it is excreted by the fetus across the placenta, the distribution of the ^{14}C-urea at later time intervals may be closer to that which is actually present (Gresham et al., 1971, 1972).

The demethylated metabolite of the antiepileptic trimethadone, ^{14}C-5,5-dimethyl-2,4-oxazolidinedione (^{14}C-DMO) was studied in pregnant mice in late gestation by autoradiography (Waddell, 1971b). DMO has been widely used as an indicator of intracellular pH (Waddell and Bates, 1969) and its distribution by autoradiography was anticipated to indicate tissue gradients of pH which could not be discerned by the usual techniques of tissue removal and homogenization. Although the study by autoradiography was not as successful as had been hoped, some sites of higher pH could be inferred. Fetal tissues had a higher concentration of the compound than maternal, suggesting that fetal tissues may be more alkaline than maternal. (See summary for Section III,C,1.) It was also of interest that other tissues capable of a high rate of anaerobic glycolysis such as retina and tumor tissue appeared to have higher pH values.

Iophenoxic acid is the most persistent drug that has been employed clinically. When administered as a cholecystographic agent, it will usually interfere with protein-bound iodine determination for the lifetime of that individual. Although it is extensively bound to plasma albumin the free portion crosses the placenta and equilibrium ultimately occurs between maternal and fetal fluids (Miller et al., 1972). By 7 days after administration to pregnant guinea pigs maternal and fetal plasma have the same concentration of the compound. The fetal yolk sac of guinea pigs shows the highest affinity of any fetal tissue. The remarkable persistence of this drug and its transfer to the fetus are a unique example of the transfer of a drug to the offspring. The plasma protein-bound iodine level in children born to mothers who received the drug is about the same as that in the mother for at least several years after birth.

Nitrilotriacetic acid has been used in recent years as a replacement for phosphates in detergents. The compound has a high affinity for the fetal skeleton; it accumulates there rapidly and persists for days at least (Tjälve, 1972). Perhaps this affinity for bone is related to its chelating properties.

The carcinogenic hydrocarbon, 3-methylcholanthrene, is transferred to fetal mice from the mother in amounts sufficient to induce tumors in the offspring (Tomatis et al., 1971; Takahashi and Yasuhira, 1973). Less than 1% of the unchanged drug administered to the mothers could be recovered from the fetuses. However, fetal livers near term were metabolizing the drug and secreting it via the bile into the fetal intestine. Very little radioactivity could be detected in the fetal tissues which developed tumors. The possible localization of 3-methylcholanthrene or an active metabolite in only a few cells of the tissue where the tumor arises could certainly have been overlooked in these studies.

^{14}C-Bilirubin has essentially the same distribution pattern in fetal rats as in maternal tissues; the material does not readily penetrate into the fetal brain (Lüders, 1971). The distribution in the fetus and placenta of the Gunn rat was no different from that in the normal rat.

D. Concluding Remarks

Comparisons of maternal and fetal distributions allow certain inferences (see Tables XIV and XV). Similarities or lack of similarities may suggest certain mechanisms. In summary, it may be said that the localization of drugs in the fetus appears to be accounted for by one or more of the following mechanisms.

1. Ready transfer to the fetus and distribution in water compartments of mother and fetus. Examples are Br^-, I^-, urea, thiocyanate, benzylpenicillin, dihydrostreptomycin, etc. (see Tables XIV and XV).

2. Ready transfer to the fetus and localization in calcifying tissues due to specific affinities between the substance and the calcifying tissue. Examples are Na^+, Ca^{2+}, F^-, Fe^{2+}, and most of the rare earths.

3. Transfer into the fetus and apparent concentration in tissues which are in fact metabolizing the drug. Examples are those which are found in fetal liver in late gestation. Concentration in the yolk sac may be due to this mechanism; studies have not been done to clarify this question. Localization of drugs in the fetal adrenal in late gestation may also be due to this mechanism.

4. Active absorption and/or secretion by the fetal yolk sac may account for the localization of an extremely wide variety of substances. The rodent yolk sac appears to concentrate more substances than any other fetal tissue. In late gestation, the fetal kidney concentrates substances by active secretion.

5. Specific affinities for binding sites for endogenous substances such as hormones. The localization of DPH, phenobarbital, chlorcyclizine, and others in sites of steroid hormone metabolism and action may be due to structural similarities with steroids. The rare earths may be another example.

6. Gradients of pH between certain tissues, areas, or cells may account for localization of acids and bases. The accumulation of bases such as morphine, cotinine, nicotine, imipramine, etc., in areas which stain basophilic may be an example. The concentration of acids such as barbiturates and DMO in the whole fetus may be due to an alkalinity of these tissues.

TABLE XIV   Ions Which Localize in Same Tissues of Mother and Fetus

Ion	Conjugate ion	Species	Days of gestation or incubation	Sacrifice time	Reference
$^{14}CO_3^{2-}$	Na^+	Mouse	17–19	30 min	Waddell et al., 1969
$^{14}CN^-$	K^+	Mouse	19	1 hr	Clemedson et al., 1960
$^{18}F^-$	Na^+	Mouse	19–20	30 and 60 min	Ericsson and Ullberg, 1958; Appelgren et al., 1961; Ericsson and Hammarström, 1964
$PO_3^{18}F^{2-a}$	Na^+	Mouse	Late	30 min	Ericsson and Hammarström, 1965
$^{22}Na^{+a}$	?	Mouse	18–19	4 and 24 hr	Huggert et al., 1961
$^{32}PO_3F^{2-a}$	Na^+	Mouse	Late	30 min	Ericsson and Hammarström, 1965
$^{35}SCN^-$	K^+	Mouse	19	1 hr	Clemedson et al., 1960
$^{45}Ca^{2+a}$	Cl^-	Mouse	19	30 min	Appelgren et al., 1961; Ericsson and Hammarström, 1964
$^{48}V_2O_5{}^a$	—	Mouse	18–19	48 hr	Söremark and Ullberg, 1962
$^{59}Fe^{3+}$	Citrate	Mouse	?	5 and 20 min, 4 hr	Ullberg et al., 1961
$^{60}Co^{2+a}$	Cl^-	Mouse	?	4 days	Flodh, 1968a
$^{65}Zn^{2+a}$	Na^+	Mouse	?	4 and 8 hr	Bergman and Söremark, 1968
$^{75}SeO_3{}^{2-}$	NH_4^+	Mouse	Late	24 hr	Jacobsson and Hansson, 1965
$^{82}Br^{-a}$	Cl^-	Mouse	19	60 min	Söremark, 1960; Söremark and Ullberg, 1960
$^{86}Rb^{+a}$	Cl^-	Mouse	16–18	5 days	Olsson et al., 1969
$^{91}Y^{3+a}$	Cl^-	Mouse	Late	4 hr	Appelgren et al., 1966
$^{95}Nb^{5+}$	Oxalate	Mouse	Late	?	Bäckström et al., 1967
$^{95}Zr^{4+} + {}^{95}Nb^{5+}$	Oxalate	Mouse	Late	24 hr	Bäckström et al., 1967
$^{125}I^-, {}^{131}I^-$	Na^+	Mouse	19	1 and 24 hr	Ullberg and Ewaldsson, 1964; Ullberg et al., 1964
$^{137}Cs^{+a}$	Cl^-	Mouse	15	4 days	Nelson et al., 1961
$^{144}Ce^{3+a}$	Cl^-	Mouse	19	24 hr	Ewaldsson and Magnusson, 1964a
$^{147}Pm^{3+a}$	Cl^-	Mouse	19	24 hr	Ewaldsson and Magnusson, 1964a
$^{160}Tb^{3+a}$	Cl^-	Mouse	19	24 hr	Ewaldsson and Magnusson, 1964b
$^{166}Ho^{3+a}$	Cl^-	Mouse	19	24 hr	Ewaldsson and Magnusson, 1964b
$^{203}Hg^{2+a}$	Cl^-	Mouse	14	4 days	Berlin and Ullberg, 1963a
$^{203}Hg^{2+}$	NO_3^-	Quail	?	?	Bäckström, 1969
$^{241}Am^{3+a}$	NO_3^-	Mouse	18	24 hr	Hammarström and Nilsson, 1970

[a] Not apparent in some fetal tissues when fetal concentration is low.

7. Active metabolism and its requirement for cofactors may account for the accumulation of ascorbic acid, vitamin B_{12}, nicotinamide, etc., in brown fat, kidney, liver, myocardium, adrenal, and intestine in both maternal and fetal tissues.

8. The kinetics of distribution, metabolism, and elimination from the mother together with the rate of transfer to and from the fetus can simulate all degrees of apparent transfer to the fetus even if there is free permeability of the placenta, e.g., urea. For example, the apparent lack of transfer of the fluoride ion to the fetus after acute administration to the mother is most likely due to rapid sequestering of the ion by maternal tissues; consequently, the concentration in the blood is not high enough, long enough to allow appreciable diffusion to the fetus.

The wide variety of substances whose distributions have been characterized in fetal tissues of experimental animals, particularly the mouse, make the generalizations fairly clear. In the future, emphasis should be mostly in two directions. One should be the elucidation, at the cellular, subcellular, and molecular level, of the events responsible for the specific affinities seen in the adrenal, corpora lutea, liver, yolk sac, and calcifying tissues. The other direction should be to define the distribution and events responsible for this distribution in human fetuses. The species differences in distribution and metabolism of drugs and in placentation and differentiation compel the use of human material if one is to characterize the processes and abnormalities of human fetal growth.

IV. Metabolism of Drugs in the Fetus

Several recent reviews have appeared concerning drug metabolism in the fetus and newborn. For further details and other aspects of the effects of drugs on the developing and immature animal, one might see Done (1964, 1966), Dutton (1966b), Schmid and Lester (1966), Yaffe and Back (1966), Arias (1970), Fleischner and Arias (1970), Rane and Sjöqvist (1972), and Rane et al. (1973a,b).

A. Appearance of Enzyme Activity before Birth

Although metabolites of many drugs administered to pregnant animals may be found in the tissues of the fetuses of that animal, no implication can be made from such in vivo studies of the site of metabolism of the drug. In vitro incubations of isolated tissues are the only source of information on the maturation of drug-metabolizing enzymes in the develop-

TABLE XV   Compounds Which Localize in Same Tissues of Mother and Fetus

Compound	Species	Days of gestation or incubation	Sacrifice time	Reference
14C-Phenobarbital	Mouse	17	3 and 24 hr	Waddell, 1971b
35S-Thiopental	Mouse	17–18	1 hr	Cassano et al., 1967a
3H-Meprobamate[a]	Mouse	Late	1 hr	Ewaldsson, 1963
14C-Glutethimide	Mouse	19	2 hr	Koransky and Ullberg, 1964
14C-Thalidomide	Mouse	18–19	1 and 4 hr	Koransky and Ullberg, 1964; Waddell, 1972a
14C-Diphenylhydantoin	Mouse	17	1, 3, and 9 hr	Waddell and Mirkin, 1972
3H-Tofenacine	Mouse	19	1 and 4 hr	Hespe and Prins, 1969
3H-Noscapine	Mouse	Late	20 min	Idänpään-Heikkilä, 1967
35S-Chlorpromazine	Mouse	17–18	1 hr	Idänpään-Heikkilä et al., 1968; Sjöstrand et al., 1965
14C-Imipramine	Mouse	19	1 hr	Cassano and Hansson, 1966
14C-Amitriptyline	Mouse	Late	1, 4, and 24 hr	Cassano et al., 1965
3H-Oxypertine	Mouse	Late	3 hr	Airaksinen and Idänpään-Heikkilä, 1967
14C-Diazepam	Mouse	19	0.5 and 4 hr	Van der Kleijn, 1969a
14C-Chlordiazepoxide	Mouse	Late	4 and 12 hr	Placidi and Cassano, 1968
14C-Chlorcyclizine	Mouse	17	3 and 9 hr	Waddell, 1972a
14C-CRD-401	Mouse	19	0.5–2 hr	Sakuma et al., 1971
14C-LSD	Mouse	Late	5 and 30 min	Idänpään-Heikkilä and Schoolar, 1969
14C-Psilocin[a]	Rat	Late(?)	30 min	Kalberer, 1966a,b
14C-Nicotine	Mouse	16–18	30 min	Hansson and Schmiterlöw, 1962; Tjälve et al., 1968
14C-Dopa	Mouse	Late	30 min	Rosell et al., 1963; Ullberg, 1962
14C-Anisotropine[a]	Mouse	Late	3 hr	Shindo et al., 1971
32P-Tabun[a]	Mouse	Late	0.33 and 4 hr	Heilbronn et al., 1964

Compound	Species	Age (days)	Time	Reference
203Hg-Phenylmercuric acetate[a]	Mouse	18	1 hr	Berlin and Ullberg, 1963b
203Hg-Phenylmercuric nitrate	Quail	15	?	Bäckström, 1969
203Hg-Methyl mercuric dicyandiamide	Mouse	10	8 days	Berlin and Ullberg, 1963c; Berlin et al., 1965
203Hg-Methyl mercuric nitrate	Quail	15	?	Bäckström, 1969
203Hg-Methyl mercuric nitrate	Mouse	Late	4 days	Bäckström, 1969
203Hg-Dimethyl mercury	Mouse	15	4 days	Östlund, 1969
203Hg-Dimethyl mercury	Mouse	19	1 hr	Östlund, 1969
203Hg-Ethylmercuric chloride[a]	Rat	15	24 hr	Takahashi et al., 1971
3H-Dihydrostreptomycin[a]	Mouse	Late	30 min	André, 1956
3H-Tetracycline[a]	Mouse	Late	30 min	André, 1956
Demethylchlortetracycline[a]	Mouse	Late	5 hr	Blomquist and Hanngren, 1966
14C-p-Aminosalicylic Acid	Mouse	Late	30 min	Hanngren, 1959
14C-m-Aminosalicylic acid	Mouse	Late	1 hr	Hanngren et al., 1963a
35S-β,β'-Dichlorodiethyl sulphide	Mouse	Late	5 min	Clemedson et al., 1963a,b
14C-DDT	Mouse	17–19	6 hr	Bäckström et al., 1965
14C-Dieldrin	Mouse	17–19	2 and 4 days	Bäckström et al., 1965
14C-Hydrocortisone	Mouse	Late	20 min	Hanngren et al., 1964
14C-Cortisone	Mouse	Late	20 min	Hanngren et al., 1964
14C-Testosterone	Mouse	Late	0.5, 1 and 2 hr	Appelgren, 1969
14C-Diethylstilbestrol	Mouse	Late	4 hr	Bengtsson and Ullberg, 1963; Ullberg, 1965
14C-Thiourea	Mouse	Late	4 hr	Ullberg and Hammarström, 1969
35S-Thiamine	Mouse	19	24 hr	Hammarström et al., 1966
35S-o-Butyrylthiamine disulfide	Mouse	Late	24 hr	Takahashi et al., 1969
14C-Nicotinamide	Mouse	17	1 hr	W. J. Waddell, unpublished
14C-Ascorbic acid[a]	Mouse	17–19	4 hr, 1 and 3 days	Hammarström, 1966
14C-Dehydroascorbic acid[a]	Mouse	17–19	1 and 3 days	Hammarström, 1966
58Co-, 57Co-, 60Co-Cyanobalamin	Mouse	15	4 days	Flodh, 1968b; Ullberg et al., 1967
58Co-, 57Co-, 60Co-Cyanobalamin	Mouse	18–19	4 and 24 hr	Flodh, 1968b; Ullberg et al., 1967
14C-Oxalic acid	Mouse	Late	4 hr	Hammarström, 1966
14C-5-Hydroxytryptophan	Mouse	Late	4 hr	Ritzén et al., 1965

TABLE XV (*continued*)

Compound	Species	Days of gestation or incubation	Sacrifice time	Reference
^{14}C-SK-7[a]	Mouse	Late	3 days	Sjöstrand and Schmiterlöw, 1968
^{35}S-Cysteamine	Mouse	19	0.33, 1, 4, and 24 hr	Nelson and Ullberg, 1960
^{14}C-Glutamine	Mouse	Late	1, 4, and 24 hr	Cassano and Hansson, 1965
^{57}Se-Selenomethionine	Mouse	Late	1, 2, and 48 hr	Hansson and Jacobsson, 1966
^{14}C-p-Fluorophenylalanine	Mouse	19	4 hr	Garzo et al., 1962
^{14}C-DMO	Mouse	Late	0.33 and 4 hr	Waddell, 1971b
^{14}C-Urea	Mouse	Late	0.33, 1, 3, and 9 hr	Waddell, 1968
^{14}C-Nitrilotriacetic acid[a]	Mouse	18	2 hr	Tjälve, 1972
^{14}C-Bilirubin	Rat	?	10 min	Lüders, 1971

[a] Not apparent in some fetal tissues when fetal concentration is low.

ing fetus. Nevertheless, when one is attempting to ascertain the time of appearance or disappearance of specific enzymes in the fetus, the fetal tissues must be separated in some manner from maternal tissues. The ready transfer of virtually all small molecules between mother and fetus constrains the elimination of maternal enzymes from the system. Isolation of the uterine–placental–fetal preparation from the maternal circulation still leaves the possibility open for metabolic conversion by nonfetal tissues. The significant metabolism of aminopyrine in such a preparation in dogs (Benzi *et al.*, 1968) does not prove that the metabolism occurred in fetal tissues and says even less about metabolism in the specific fetal tissues in which the metabolites were found.

1. LIVER

a. Oxidations.   Table XVI summarizes the oxidative reactions by fetal liver incubations *in vitro*.

i. Guinea pig.   The fetal guinea pig liver near term does not significantly demethylate monomethylaminoantipyrine nor hydroxylate benzo-[a]pyrene (Jondorf *et al.*, 1958; Juchau and Pedersen, 1973).

ii. Rabbit.   The liver from animals of this species has been studied with aminopyrine (Hart *et al.*, 1962; Berté and Benzi, 1967; Mascherpa, 1968), chlorcyclizine, benzo[a]pyrene, testosterone (Gillette *et al.*, 1973), hexobarbital (Hart *et al.*, 1962; Dixon and Willson, 1968), zoxazolamine (Dixon and Willson, 1968), and strychnine (Pecile *et al.*, 1969) as substrates. The first two are primarily demethylation reactions and the remainder hydroxylations. The discrepancy between the extensive metabolism of aminopyrine found by some investigators and essentially no metabolism found by others has not been explained. The hydroxylation of zoxazolamine follows a pattern distinctly different from that of other compounds; it is more extensively metabolized in earlier gestation than 3 days before term. There was minimal, if any, metabolism of the other compounds by the fetal rabbit liver without pretreatment. Pretreatment with phenobarbital enhanced the metabolism of strychnine and hexobarbital at term but pretreatments were without effect on aminopyrine and zoxazolamine.

iii. Rat.   3-Methyl-4-monomethylaminoazobenzene (Bresnick and Stevenson, 1968; Welch *et al.*, 1972), p-chloro-N-methylaniline (Fahim *et al.*, 1970), p-nitroanisole (Jori and Briatico, 1973), aniline (Gabler and Falace, 1970; Jori and Briatico, 1973), benzo[a]pyrene (Nebert and

TABLE XVI   Drug Oxidations by Fetal Liver in *Vitro*

Substrate	Pretreatment	Species	Fraction	Days before term	Extent of metabolism (% of adult)[a]	Reference
Demethylations						
Aminopyrine	None or phenobarbital	Rabbit	Whole homogenate	Term–10	0	Hart et al., 1962
	None	Rabbit	9000 g Supernatant	18	0	Berté and Benzi, 1967
	None	Rabbit	Not stated	7	40	Mascherpa, 1968
	None	Opossum	9000 g Supernatant	6 (to pouch)	60	Wilson, 1967
	None	Human	105,000 g Pellet	100–125	0	Yaffe et al., 1970
	None	Human	Whole homogenate	110–210	0	Juchau and Pedersen, 1973
Monomethylamino-antipyrine	None	Guinea pig	9000 g Supernatant	2	0	Jondorf et al., 1958
3-Methyl-4-mono-methylaminoazo-benzene	None or 3-methyl-cholanthrene	Rat	9000 g Supernatant	2–4	25	Bresnick and Stevenson, 1968
	None	Rat	9000 g Supernatant	3–8	2	Welch et al., 1972
	3-Methylcholan-threne	Rat	9000 g Supernatant	3–8	4	Welch et al., 1972
Chlorcyclizine	None	Rabbit	Not stated	10	2	Gillette et al., 1973
Desmethylimipramine	None	Human	105,000 g Pellet	119–182	0–50	Rane et al., 1973b
Ethylmorphine	None	Human	105,000 g Pellet	133–182	35	Rane and Ackermann, 1972
Meperidine	None	Human	12,000 g Supernatant	113–211	0	Pelkonen et al., 1969
N-Methylaniline	None or cigarette smoke	Human	12,000 g Supernatant	70–210	(5–50)[b]	Pelkonen et al., 1971b, 1972; Pelkonen, 1973
p-Chloro-N-methyl-aniline	None or pheno-barbital	Rat	Not stated	2	75	Fahim et al., 1970

N-Monomethyl-p-nitroaniline	None or phenobarbital	Mouse	8400 g Supernatant	2	0	Pomp et al., 1969
p-Nitroanisole	None	Human	8400 g Supernatant	14–183	0	Pomp et al., 1969
	None	Swine	9000 g Supernatant	7–14	0–10	Short and Davis, 1970; Short et al., 1972
	None or phenobarbital	Mouse	8400 g Supernatant	2	0	Pomp et al., 1969
	None	Rat	9000 g Supernatant	7	3	Jori and Briatico, 1973
	Eucalyptol	Rat	9000 g Supernatant	7	5	Jori and Briatico, 1973
	None	Human	8400 g Supernatant	14–183	0	Pomp et al., 1969
Hydroxylations						
L-Amphetamine	None	Swine	9000 g Supernatant	14	6	Short and Davis, 1970
				7	0	
				0	0	
Aniline	None	Opossum	9000 g Supernatant	0 (to pouch)	0	Wilson, 1967
	None or diphenyl-hydantoin	Rat	105,000 g Pellet	2	0	Gabler and Falace, 1970
	None or eucalyptol	Rat	9000 g Supernatant	7	7	Jori and Briatico, 1973
	None	Human	105,000 g Pellet	133–182	40	Rane and Ackermann, 1972
	None	Human	Whole homogenate	110–210	(6)[b]	Juchau and Pedersen, 1973
Benzo[a]pyrene	None	Rabbit	Not stated	10	1	Gillette et al., 1973
	None	Rat	10,000 g Supernatant	1–7	3	Puolakka et al., 1971
	None	Rat	9000 g Supernatant	3–8	0	Welch et al., 1972; Conney et al., 1973
	3-Methylcholanthrene	Rat	9000 g Supernatant	3–8	10	Welch et al., 1972
	3-Methylcholanthrene	Rat	105,000 g Pellet	3–8	15	Welch et al., 1972
	Phenobarbital	Rat	105,000 g Pellet	3–8	4	Welch et al., 1972
	Benzo[a]pyrene	Rat	Not stated	2	4	Conney et al., 1973
	None	Rat	Whole homogenate	1–3	0	Nebert and Gelboin, 1969

TABLE XVI (continued)

Substrate	Pretreatment	Species	Fraction	Days before term	Extent of metabolism (% of adult)[a]	Reference
	3-Methylcholanthrene	Rat	Whole homogenate	1–3	10	Nebert and Gelboin, 1969
	None	Hamster	Whole homogenate	1	1	Nebert and Gelboin, 1969
	3-Methylcholanthrene or phenobarbital	Hamster	Whole homogenate	1	10	Nebert and Gelboin, 1969
	None	Guinea pig	Whole homogenate	10–20	2	Juchau and Pedersen, 1973
	None	Monkey	Whole homogenate	38–113	1	Juchau et al., 1972; Juchau and Pedersen, 1973
	None	Human	105,000 g Pellet	100–125	0	Yaffe et al., 1970
	None or cigarette smoke	Human	12,000 g Supernatant	70–210	(5–10)[b]	Pelkonen et al., 1971b; 1972; Pelkonen, 1973
	None or cigarette smoke	Human	Whole homogenate	110–210	(3)[b]	Juchau et al., 1972; Juchau and Pedersen, 1973
Hexobarbital	None or phenobarbital	Rabbit	Whole homogenate	4–10	0	Hart et al., 1962
	None	Rabbit	Whole homogenate	Term	0	Hart et al., 1962
	Phenobarbital	Rabbit	Whole homogenate	Term	15	Hart et al., 1962
	None, chlordane or phenobarbital	Rabbit	9000 g Supernatant	3–10	0	Dixon and Willson, 1968
	None	Human	12,000 g Supernatant	113–211	Low in some expt.	Pelkonen et al., 1969
	None	Swine	9000 g Supernatant	7–14	1	Short and Davis, 1970

Substrate	Pretreatment	Species	Preparation	Age	Activity	Reference
4-Methylcoumarin	None	Rat	Whole homogenate	1–7	30	Feuer and Liscio, 1970
	4-Methylcoumarin or phenobarbital	Rat	Whole homogenate	5	30	Feuer and Liscio, 1970
	phenobarbital			1	65	
Strychnine	None	Rabbit	11,000 g Supernatant	Term	0	Pecile et al., 1969
	Phenobarbital	Rabbit	11,000 g Supernatant	Term	20	Pecile et al., 1969
	None	Rat	11,000 g Supernatant	Term	0	Pecile et al., 1969
	Phenobarbital	Rat	11,000 g Supernatant	Term	15	Pecile et al., 1969
Testosterone	None	Rabbit	Not stated	10	0	Gillette et al., 1973
	None	Human	105,000 g Pellet	100–125	High	Yaffe et al., 1970
Zoxazolamine	None, chlordane, or phenobarbital	Rabbit	9000 g Supernatant	11	33	Dixon and Willson, 1968
				3	25	
Demethylation and hydroxylation						
Chlorpromazine	None	Human	12,000 g Supernatant	85–211	Low	Pelkonen et al., 1969, 1971a; Pelkonen, 1973
Diazepam	None	Rat	10,000 g Supernatant	1–7	0	Puolakka et al., 1971
	None	Human	10,000 g Supernatant	170–200	(10)[b]	Idänpään-Heikkilä et al., 1971a
Laurate	None	Human	105,000 g Pellet	100–125	High	Yaffe et al., 1970
Keto oxidation						
Nicotine	None	Mouse	Tissue slices	3	Small	Tjälve et al., 1968
	None	Mouse	Tissue slices	1–4	5	Stålhandske et al., 1969
Other oxidations						
Acetaldehyde	None	Human	Whole liver perfused	160–200	(20)[b]	Pikkarainen, 1971
Ethanol	None	Human	Whole liver perfused	160–200	0	Pikkarainen, 1971

[a] Calculated for nonpretreated fetuses and mothers or pretreated fetuses compared with pretreated mothers. In some instances the activity in pretreated fetal liver was higher than that in nonpretreated maternal liver.
[b] Compared to adult rat liver.

Gelboin, 1969; Puolakka et al., 1971; Welch et al., 1972; Conney et al., 1973), 4-methylcoumarin (Feuer and Liscio, 1970), strychnine (Pecile et al., 1969), and diazepam (Puolakka et al., 1971) have been used as substrates for fetal rat liver preparations. The first three compounds are metabolized primarily by demethylation, the second three compounds by hydroxylation, and the last one by both. Here again unexplained discrepancies are seen; 3-methyl-4-monomethylaminoazobenzene was metabolized at 25% of the adult value in one report and only one-tenth of that rate in another report. Another surprise is the extensive metabolism of p-chloro-N-methylaniline. The only other compound which was metabolized at a significant rate was 4-methylcoumarin. Although phenobarbital and some polycyclic hydrocarbons were ineffective in stimulating the activity for benzo[a]pyrene and 3-methyl-4-monomethylaminoazobenzene, 3-methylcholanthrene, benzo[a]pyrene, and other polycyclic hydrocarbons effected modest increases in metabolism of these two substrates. These increases are referred to as modest when comparing the pretreated fetal liver with the pretreated maternal liver; however, pretreated fetal liver activity may be 2.5 times nonpretreated maternal liver activity (e.g., Conney et al., 1973). However, phenobarbital or 4-methylcoumarin pretreatment was effective in enhancing the metabolism of 4-methylcoumarin 1 day before term. Phenobarbital was effective in enhancing strychnine metabolism and eucalyptol in p-nitroanisole metabolism. Partial hepatectomy of the pregnant rat prior to phenobarbital pretreatment did not increase the effect of the inducer on fetal liver, indicating that this effect was near maximal.

There are two studies with rat liver explants (Nebert and Gelboin, 1969; Bürki et al., 1971). Benz[a]anthracene and 3-methylcholanthrene were effective in inducing severalfold the hydroxylation of benzo[a]pyrene. The lag phase for induction with methylcholanthrene was not observed if the explants had been preincubated for 40 hours. One of the dihydroxy derivatives of methylcholanthrene was a more potent inducer than the parent molecule.

iv. Mouse. Three of the compounds whose metabolism has been studied in the fetal mouse liver are listed in Table XVI. None of these, p-nitroanisole, N-monomethyl-p-nitroaniline, or nicotine, were found to be metabolized to any significant extent. Furthermore, pretreatment with phenobarbital had no effect. However, careful genetic studies with individual fetuses demonstrate that the hydroxylation of benzo[a]pyrene by fetal tissues can be induced with 3-methylcholanthrene if the proper genetic predisposition is present (Nebert, 1973). Dramatic stimulation of the hydroxylase was seen in tissues from fetuses that contain the single autosomal dominant trait. Fetuses from the same uterus which did not contain this trait were indistinguishable from controls. Therefore it is clear that not only is the inducibility of the enzyme restricted to certain mouse strains but the individual fetus must contain the inherited dominant trait. The genetic ability to hydroxylate benzo[a]pyrene following 3-methylcholanthrene induction in adult mouse liver correlated very well with the stimulation of the hydroxylase activity by benz[a]anthracene in cultures of fetal cells from the same strain of mice. Six strains, C57BL/6N, C3H/HeN, BALB/cANN, CBA/HN, AL/N, and N:GP(SW), were inducible and four strains, DBA/2N, NZW/BLN, NZB/BLN, and AKR/N, were nonresponsive. Another interesting observation by Nebert was that strains which metabolized aromatic hydrocarbons were more susceptible to the toxic effect of the compound. He suggested that highly reactive metabolites are responsible for the toxicity and that perhaps the teratogenic action of compounds might be correlated with their metabolism in that fetus (Nebert and Gelboin, 1969; Nebert, 1973). On the other hand, an increased ability to metabolize drugs could be a protective mechanism for the fetus if the administered drug is the active form; this was the suggestion by Zimmerman and Bowen (1972) for the faster metabolism of triamcinolone by CBA mice than by A/JAX or C3H mice.

v. Hamster and Chick.   The hydroxylation of benzo[a]pyrene is the only metabolism which has been studied in the hamster fetal liver. The low basal rate was stimulated about tenfold by pretreatment with 3-methylcholanthrene or phenobarbital. Treatment with benz[a]anthracene of primary and secondary fetal cells derived from the hamster increased benzo[a]pyrene hydroxylase activity about fifteenfold. Similarly treated cell cultures from the chick increased only two- to threefold (Nebert and Gelboin, 1969).

vi. Swine.   Although the metabolism of *p*-nitroanisole, *l*-amphetamine, and hexobarbital was low, it is interesting to note that the metabolism of *l*-amphetamine was greater 2 weeks before term than it was 1 week before term (Short and Davis, 1970; Short *et al.*, 1972).

vii. Opossum.   This marsupial should be a convenient experimental model for fetal studies because of the extended developmental stage in the mother's pouch. The only study of drug metabolism in this species reported that neither aminopyrine nor aniline were metabolized by these animals at the time they migrated to the maternal pouch (Wilson, 1967).

viii. Monkey.   The only substrate that has been studied in the monkey (*Macaca nemestrina*) is benzo[a]pyrene; slight activity for hydroxylation was found in mid and late gestation (Juchau *et al.*, 1972; Juchau and Pedersen, 1973).

ix. Human. The recent availability of human abortion material has prompted numerous studies of drug-metabolizing activity in the human fetus. A total of 16 different substrates which are metabolized oxidatively have been reported, all since 1969 (see Table XVI). Several important observations may be made from these reports. The first is that, in contrast to experimental animals, the human fetus has a high activity for oxidizing drugs even in early gestation. The second important observation, which must be kept in mind, is that there is a very wide variability among individual fetuses. Furthermore, it has been recognized that the properties of this enzyme system are different from those of the adult system; these differences will be discussed more fully in Section IV,C. In some reports only absolute fetal values are given which makes interpretation relative to the adult value difficult; in some cases adult rodent tissue was studied to obtain comparative values. Another fact which must be kept in mind when comparing rates among tissues is that fetal tissues frequently contain less protein per gram tissue weight than adult tissues. Values reported per gram tissue weight of fetal tissue may be deceptively low. The appearance of this oxidative metabolism was not gradual and linear during gestation. The activity appeared abruptly at 8 weeks of gestation and developed rapidly during the next 4 weeks to levels which remained essentially constant throughout the remainder of gestation (Pelkonen, 1973). This correlates well with the ultrastructural development of human liver at this stage of gestation reported by Zamboni (1965).

The compounds that were reported to be most actively metabolized were testosterone and laurate (Yaffe *et al.*, 1970), acetaldehyde (Pikkarainen, 1971), aniline and ethylmorphine (Rane and Ackermann, 1972), and desmethylimipramine (Rane *et al.*, 1973b). The disappearance of acetaldehyde is not entirely due to oxidation since some of it is converted to ethanol. A number of others were metabolized somewhat less actively and some were reported not to be metabolized at all. Possible explanations for not finding activity could be the use of the wrong fraction of the homogenate as pointed out by Rane *et al.* (1973b), the use of incorrect incubation conditions, or the instability of the fetal enzymes as demonstrated by Juchau *et al.* 1972). These factors obviously cannot be the entire story because individual fetuses from the same report can have wide variability (Pomp *et al.*, 1969; Pelkonen *et al.*, 1969, 1971b; Yaffe *et al.*, 1970; Rane *et al.*, 1973b); perhaps genetic differences or exposure to certain agents are also important. The only possible inducing agent which has been specifically examined for drug metabolism in the human fetus was cigarette smoke; this clearly enhanced the oxidative metabolism of benzo[a]pyrene in placental homogenates but had no effect on the placental metabolism of N-methylaniline or on the fetal hepatic metabolism of either of these substrates (Juchau et al., 1972; Pelkonen et al., 1972). However, prednisolone increased phosphoenolpyruvate carboxykinase activity tenfold in a 12.5-week-old fetus (Kirby and Hahn, 1973); the possible effect of other agents should certainly be investigated.

Pelkonen et al. (1971b) found that hexobarbital, barbital, chlorpromazine, N-methylaniline, and p-nitrobenzoic acid each would inhibit the metabolism of benzo[a]pyrene and N-methylaniline in fetal liver homogenates. This possibility for the explanation of decreased fetal metabolism in an experiment should always be kept in mind. Much earlier Fouts and Adamson (1959) discovered the presence of unidentified inhibitors in homogenates of developing fetal liver.

b. *Reductions and Hydrolyses.*   A few reductive and hydrolytic reactions by fetal liver have been studied and the results are summarized in Table XVII.

i. *Rabbit.*   Very low activity for the reduction of p-nitrobenzoic acid and the hydrolysis of acetylsalicylic acid was present in fetal rabbit liver (Hart et al., 1962; Eyring et al., 1973).

ii. *Mouse.*   Although the actual extent of the metabolism was not determined, the presence of large amounts of covalently bound metabolites of nitrofurazone were found in fetal liver. Nitrofurazone is reduced by xanthine oxidase rather than cytochrome P-450, and the metabolites are highly reactive. These results therefore suggest that significant activity for the reduction of nitrofurazone is present in fetal mouse liver (Gillette et al., 1973).

iii. *Swine.*   This species had the highest activity for reduction and hydrolysis; neoprontosil reduction was 30–45% of the adult and procaine hydrolysis was 15–30% of the adult (Short and Davis, 1970; Short et al., 1972). However, p-nitrobenzoic acid was not reduced (Short et al., 1972).

iv. *Opossum.*   Wilson (1967) reported only minimal activity for the reduction of p-nitrobenzoic acid in opossum liver at the time of migration to the pouch.

v. *Monkey.*   Although in late gestation the fetal monkey liver reduced p-nitrobenzoic acid to only about 5% of that of the adult rat liver, in

TABLE XVII　Drug Reductions and Hydrolyses by Fetal Liver in *Vitro*

Substrate	Pretreatment	Species	Fraction	Days before term	Extent of metabolism (% of adult)	Reference
Reductions						
Acetaldehyde	None	Human	Whole liver perfused	160–200	One-third dose reduced to ETOH	Pikkarainen, 1971
p-Nitrobenzoic acid	None or phenobarbital	Rabbit	Whole homogenate	Term–10	1	Hart et al., 1962
	None	Opossum	9000 g Supernatant	0 (to pouch)	Low	Wilson, 1967
	None	Human	12,000 g Supernatant	85–215	Low	Pelkonen et al., 1969, 1971a; Pelkonen, 1973
	None	Human	9000 g Supernatant	145–225	3[a]	Juchau, 1971; Juchau and Pedersen, 1973
	None	Monkey	9000 g Supernatant	10	5[a]	Juchau, 1971
	None	Swine	9000 g Supernatant	7	0	Short et al., 1972
Neoprontosil	None	Swine	9000 g Supernatant	7–14	30–45	Short and Davis, 1970; Short et al., 1972
	None	Human	Whole homogenate	120–215	7[a]	Juchau and Pedersen, 1973
Hydrolyses						
Acetylsalicylic acid	None	Rabbit	9000 g Supernatant	7–14	4	Eyring et al., 1973
Procaine	None	Swine	9000 g Supernatant	7–14	15–30	Short and Davis, 1970; Short et al., 1972

[a] Compared to adult rat liver.

early gestation the reduction was four times as efficient and the addition of riboflavin 5-phosphate increased the activity to that of the adult rat (Juchau, 1971).

vi. Human. The ability to reduce *p*-nitrobenzoic acid or neoprontosil by liver supernatants appeared in human fetuses as early as 7 to 8 weeks of gestation (Juchau, 1971; Juchau and Pedersen, 1973; Pelkonen, 1973). The activity for *p*-nitrobenzoic acid increased somewhat by 10 weeks of age and remained fairly constant to 21 weeks of age. However, this activity was still only about 3% of that in adult rat liver; furthermore, the reports which included boiled controls reveal that almost the same activity occurred nonenzymatically. Enzymatic activity could be increased considerably by the addition of riboflavin 5-phosphate.

Acetaldehyde is metabolized by perfused human fetal liver at about one-fifth the rate of adult rat liver. About one-third of this acetaldehyde eliminated by the human fetal liver is reduced to ethanol, presumably by alcohol dehydrogenase. The reaction from acetaldehyde to ethanol with human liver alcohol dehydrogenase is much higher than the reverse reaction which may account for this reduction of acetaldehyde to ethanol without detectable oxidation of ethanol; alcohol dehydrogenase activity of the human fetal liver is about 5–10% of the adult activity (Pikkarainen, 1971; Pikkarainen and Räihä, 1967; Blair and Vallee, 1966).

Studies for esterase activity using α-naphthyl acetate and propionate as substrates revealed activity in human liver from fetuses between 40 and 160 mm CR length. Several isoenzymes were demonstrated by starch gel electrophoresis (Taylor, 1972).

c. Conjugations. The conjugation of various substances with glucuronic acid by fetal liver *in vitro* is summarized in Table XVIII. The importance of the ability of the fetus to conjugate and eliminate bilirubin soon after birth has stimulated interest in this metabolic reaction for many years. There is a great deal of species and substrate variability in the activity of glucuronyltransferase before birth, although it appears clear from the studies listed in the table that the activity of this enzyme in the fetal liver has not reached the activity present in the mature liver. There appears to be an increase in the fetus, at least in the rat, in the ability to convert heme to bilirubin. The activity in rat fetal liver 1 week prior to term of heme oxygenase, the enzyme which catalyzes this conversion, has twice the activity of that in adult liver. This activity increases further immediately after birth and does not decrease to the adult value until the time of weaning (Thaler *et al.*, 1972).

TABLE XVIII   **Glucuronide Conjugation by Fetal Liver *In Vitro***

Substrate	Pretreatment	Species	Fraction[a]	Days before term	Extent of metabolism (% of adult)	Reference
o-Aminophenol	None	Guinea pig	80,000 g Pellet	7	10	Brown and Zuelzer, 1958
	None	Guinea pig	Slices	19–33	0	Dutton, 1959, 1963
				5–19	5	
				1–5	10	
	None	Guinea pig	Whole homogenate	19–33	10	Dutton, 1959, 1963
				5–19	20	
				1–5	40	
	None or anthranilic acid	Rat	105,000 g Pellet	Near term	25	Schmid et al., 1959
	None	Rat	Whole homogenate	2	90	Stevens, 1962
	None	Rat	Slices	3	75	Gartner and Arias, 1963
	None	Mouse	Whole homogenate	4–5	1	Dutton, 1966a
				2–3	20	
	None	Chick	Slices or whole homogenate	7–10	25	Dutton, 1963
	None	Human	Slices	150–180	1	Dutton, 1959
	None	Human	Slices	126	(13)[b]	Gartner and Arias, 1963

Substrate	Inducer	Species	Preparation			Reference
p-Nitrophenol	None	Rat	Whole homogenate	2	180	Dutton, 1966a
	None	Rat	Sonicated whole homogenate	5–7	25	Henderson, 1971
Phenolphthalein	None	Human	12,000 g Supernatant[c]	1–3	100	Pelkonen et al., 1969
	None	Guinea pig	80,000 g Pellet	113–211	0	Brown and Zuelzer, 1958
	None	Guinea pig	9000 g Supernatant[d]	12	0	Jondorf et al., 1958
	None	Rat	Whole homogenate	2	0	Dutton, 1966a
	None	Mouse	Whole homogenate	5–6	10	Dutton, 1966b
				3–4	20	
				2	40	
					60	
	None	Swine	105,000 g Pellet	7–14	15	Short and Davis, 1970; Short et al., 1972
Oxazepam	None	Guinea pig	9000 g Supernatant	13–15	40	Berté et al., 1968
	None	Rat	9000 g Supernatant	1	35	Berté et al., 1968
	None	Rat	9000 g Supernatant	3	10	Manzo et al., 1969
	Oxazepam or phenobarbital	Rat	9000 g Supernatant	3	25	Manzo et al., 1969
Bilirubin	None	Guinea pig	80,000 g Pellet	12	0	Brown and Zuelzer, 1958
	None	Rabbit	Slices	1	15	Flint et al., 1964
	None	Rat	Whole homogenate	5–10	0	Grodsky et al., 1958
	None	Rat	Slices	3	10	Flint et al., 1964

[a] No UDPGA was added to tissue slices; whole homogenates, supernatants, and microsomal fractions were fortified with UDPGA unless otherwise stated.

[b] Value relative to adult rat.

[c] Incubation system not stated.

[d] Incubation system contained UDP-glucose instead of UDPGA.

i. Guinea pig. Although the fetal guinea pig liver *in vitro* did not conjugate bilirubin nor phenolphthalein, it conjugated oxazepam almost half as well as the adult (Brown and Zuelzer, 1958; Jondorf *et al.*, 1958; Berté *et al.*, 1968). An indication that this is not simply a substrate variability is seen in the conjugation of *o*-aminophenol which is conjugated at percentages of 0–40% of the adult rate depending on the fraction and age (Brown and Zuelzer, 1958; Dutton, 1959, 1963).

ii. Rabbit. The only compound which has been studied in rabbit liver was bilirubin which is conjugated by slices at 15% of the adult rate (Flint *et al.*, 1964).

iii. Rat. The variability for conjugation among liver fractions is most apparent in the rat. The conjugation of *o*-aminophenol and *p*-nitrophenol varied from low values to rates equal to or greater than that of the adult (Schmid *et al.*, 1959; Stevens, 1962; Gartner and Arias, 1963; Dutton, 1966a; Henderson, 1971). The conjugation of phenolphthalein, bilirubin, and oxazepam were low although oxazepam was conjugated as much as 35% of the adult rate in some experiments (Dutton, 1966a; Grodsky *et al.*, 1958; Flint *et al.*, 1964; Berté *et al.*, 1968, Manzo *et al.*, 1969). Pretreatment with phenobarbital or oxazepam was shown to have an effect on enhancing the ability to conjugate oxazepam (Manzo *et al.*, 1969).

iv. Mouse. Although both *o*-aminophenol and phenolphthalein were conjugated to varying rates with age, the conjugation of phenolphthalein was much more extensive (Dutton, 1966a,b).

v. Chick. The only substrate which was studied with the chick was o-aminophenol which was conjugated about one-fourth as efficiently as the adult (Dutton, 1963).

vi. Swine. Conjugation of phenolphthalein by the microsomal fraction of this fetal liver was only about 15% of the adult (Short and Davis, 1970; Short *et al.*, 1972).

vii. Human. Little if any ability of the fetal human liver to conjugate *o*-aminophenol or *p*-nitrophenol was found between about 3 and 7 months of gestation (Dutton, 1959; Gartner and Arias, 1963; Pelkonen *et al.*, 1969).

The *in vitro* studies summarized in Table XVIII offer some information on the maturation of glucuronyltransferase. However, other processes are involved in the elimination of substances by the liver *in vivo* (Plaa, 1968). Furthermore, the study of isolated liver or liver subfractions *in vitro* may give deceptively low activities compared with the *in vivo* situation because of the inadequate supply of other cofactors for the reaction. This is especially true when the full sequence of events in the transfer of substances from blood to bile is not yet known. Consequently, more informative studies are those performed in the intact animal. There are a few reports done by this more difficult approach.

Lester *et al.* (1970) and Jackson *et al.* (1971) surgically prepared dogs and monkeys so that radio-labeled bilirubin and bile acids could be administered to dog and monkey fetuses *in utero*. Samples of fetal blood and bile could be taken without disturbing the intact, lightly anesthetized preparation. Comparison of maternal and fetal blood, bile, and intestinal contents gave information on the ability of the fetal liver to conjugate and/or secrete these substances into fetal bile, as well as information on the placental transfer of these substances. The near-term fetal dog extensively conjugated ^{3}H-bilirubin with glucuronic acid and secreted it into fetal bile. In contrast, no ^{3}H-bilirubin glucuronide appeared in the bile of near-term fetal monkeys after administration of ^{3}H-bilirubin. Most of the ^{3}H-bilirubin administered to the fetal monkeys was transferred to the mother and appeared in the maternal bile. Similar experiments in near-term guinea pigs (Schenker *et al.*, 1964) who were injected with ^{14}C-bilirubin revealed only small amounts of radioactivity in fetal bile.

Similarly, most of the ^{14}C-cholate administered to fetal dogs was recovered from the fetal gallbladder and intestine in the form of the taurine conjugate, ^{14}C-taurocholate. The rate of secretion of ^{14}C-cholate into the bile of the fetus was almost as great as the rate of secretion by the adult liver. The slightly lower rate of secretion by fetal liver could easily be accounted for with the bypass of fetal liver by portal blood through the ductus venosus. Surprisingly, the near-term fetal monkey secreted most of the administered ^{14}C-cholate as ^{14}C-taurocholate in fetal bile. Cholate in the maternal bile exists as both taurine and glycine conjugates. It appears then that whereas the near-term fetal dog is able to extensively conjugate bilirubin and cholate and secrete the conjugates into its bile, the near-term fetal monkey is only able to conjugate and secrete cholate. These studies emphasize two important points: that conjugation and biliary secretion in the near-term fetus can be as efficient as in the adult but that there are marked substrate and species differences.

In a later experiment by these same investigators (Smallwood *et al.*, 1972) 85 to 95% of the taurocholate administered to fetal dogs was excreted by the fetal liver during the 24-hour study period. Only 5% of the dose was transferred across the placenta. They concluded that bile salt is excreted by the fetal liver with remarkable efficiency but the presence or absence of an enterohepatic circulation was not determined.

Henderson (1971) sonicated rat liver homogenates in an attempt to exclude any interference by differences in transport at the microsomal membrane. One day before term these preparations had as much activity for conjugating nitrophenol as did some of the preparations from adult rats. One should not assume that this difference is due merely to sonication since other variables exist between this and other studies; a direct comparison between sonicated and nonsonicated fetal tissue was not made.

2. ADRENAL

a. *Oxidations.* The first report on the ability of the human fetal adrenal to metabolize benzo[a]pyrene showed only 3% of the adult rat liver rate (Pelkonen *et al.,* 1971b). These were determined in whole homogenates of adrenals from fetuses of about 15 to 20 weeks of gestation. Later experiments detected much higher activities for benzo[a]pyrene hydroxylation (Juchau *et al.,* 1972; Juchau and Pedersen, 1973). The fetal human adrenal rate per gram protein per hour was 47% of that from the adult male rat liver; similarly the monkey fetal adrenal at 12 to 20 weeks of gestation was 46% of that in the maternal monkey liver. The guinea pig fetal adrenal activity was only 20% of the maternal adrenal and only about 10% of that in the maternal guinea pig liver. The hydroxylation of benzo[a]pyrene in the human adrenal increased steadily between the eighth and twentieth week of gestation. Although the reports are conflicting there is evidence to indicate that cigarette smoking markedly stimulated the activity for benzo[a]pyrene hydroxylation in the human fetal adrenal.

Demethylation of *N*-methylaniline by the human fetal adrenal at 15–20 weeks of gestation varied between 2 and 10% of the rate in adult rat liver (Pelkonen *et al.,* 1971b). No demethylation of aminopyrine was detected in whole homogenates of human fetal adrenals of 9–17 weeks of gestation (Juchau and Pedersen, 1973); however the same tissue hydroxylated aniline at about 10% of the rate in adult rat liver.

b. *Reductions.* The human fetal adrenal has a greater ability to reduce *p*-nitrobenzoic acid than liver from the same specimens. This activity increased sharply, in contrast to liver, at about 15 weeks of gestation to rise to levels about one-fourth that of adult rat liver. This reductive ability of the human fetal adrenal makes this tissue an important fetal site for this reaction. Although neoprontosil was also reduced it was not as extensive. High levels of activity for reduction of p-nitrobenzoic acid were also found in the fetal monkey adrenal (Juchau, 1971; Juchau and Pedersen, 1973).

3. OTHER FETAL TISSUES

a. Oxidations. The hydroxylation of benzo[a]pyrene has been studied in a wide variety of fetal tissues. Although the earlier study by Pelkonen *et al.* (1971b) found no activity in early to mid gestation in human lung, kidney, and intestine, Juchau and Pedersen (1973) more recently reported low but significant activity in each of these tissues as well as in the spleen and pancreas. This activity in the pancreas was greater than that in the liver and second only to that in the adrenal. Perhaps the discrepancies in these two reports can be accounted for by the fact that there is a marked variability among individual fetuses (Juchau *et al.*, 1972). None of these reports found significant activity with this substrate in brain, heart, testicle, ovary, thymus, skin, or stomach. Minimal hydroxylation of this substrate was found in 9- to 20-week-old fetal monkey kidney, lung, spleen, brain, and pancreas; as in the human, pancreas was second only to the adrenal in activity. No activity was detected with heart, thymus, and skin (Juchau *et al.*, 1972; Juchau and Pedersen, 1973). The marked species variability was seen by Juchau and Pedersen (1973); guinea pig kidney hydroxylated benzo[a]pyrene more than two times as extensively as fetal guinea pig adrenal and more than ten times that of the fetal guinea pig liver. Administration of 3-methylcholanthrene to pregnant hamsters and rats a few days prior to birth stimulated benzo[a]pyrene hydroxylase activity in fetal lung, small intestine, and kidney (Nebert and Gelboin, 1969); however, cigarette smoking by the human had no apparent stimulatory effect on the kidney and lung (Juchau *et al.*, 1972).

No hydroxylation of hexobarbital was detected in 9- to 16-week-old human fetal kidney and intestine but some hydroxylation of aniline was detected in 9- to 17-week-old human fetal kidney, lung, and brain (Pelkonen *et al.*, 1969, 1971a; Juchau and Pedersen, 1973).

No N-demethylation of aminopyrine was detected in 9- to 17-week-old human fetal kidney, lung, or brain (Juchau and Pedersen, 1973); however, some of this activity was found in 25-day-old rabbit fetal kidney, lung, and brain although no activity was present in these tissues in the 14-day-old fetus (Berté and Benzi, 1967). Measurable activity for the demethylation of N-methylaniline was reported for 15- to 20-week-old human fetal kidney and intestine; insignificant activity was found with stomach, lung, brain, and testes (Pelkonen *et al.*, 1971b). In swine 1 week before term, *p*-nitroanisole was not demethylated by lung, kidney, or intestinal mucosa (Short *et al.*, 1972).

Neither diazepam was metabolized in human fetal brain and intestine nor meperidine in human fetal kidney and intestine but chlorpromazine was oxidized in kidney and intestine (Idänpään-Heikkilä *et al.*, 1971a; Pelkonen *et al.*, 1969, 1971a).

b. Reductions and Hydrolyses.   Although *p*-nitrobenzoic acid was reduced in the 12,000 *g* supernatant from human intestine from 8 to 16-week-old fetuses (Pelkonen *et al.*, 1969, 1971a), homogenates of kidney, lung, and brain from 9- to 17-week-old human fetuses did not reduce this substrate (Juchau and Pedersen, 1973). However, the addition of riboflavin 5-phosphate to whole homogenates and 9000 *g* supernatant fractions of lungs and kidneys from 7- to 18-week-old human fetuses revealed high specific activities. Heat inactivation reduced these specific activities and dialysis yielded variable results (Juchau, 1971). In sharp contrast to the absence of reduction of *p*-nitrobenzoate is the rather uniform reduction of neoprontosil by all tissues examined including kidney, lung, and brain in human fetuses of 9 to 17 weeks of gestation (Juchau and Pedersen, 1973). This is also true in the swine; 2 weeks before term, the fetal swine kidney has approximately 80% of the ability found in the adult kidney to reduce neoprontosil (Short and Davis, 1970) but it falls to 55% at 1 week before term and to 40% at birth (Short *et al.*, 1972). Azoreduction of neoprontosil was high in lung and intestinal mucosa of fetal swine 1 week before term (Short *et al.*, 1972).

Some capacity was detected for hydrolyzing procaine in fetal kidney, lung, and intestinal mucosa of swine (Short and Davis, 1970; Short *et al.*, 1972), acetylsalicyclic acid in fetal kidney, small intestine, and stomach of rabbits (Eyring *et al.*, 1973), and α-naphthyl acetate and proprionate in fetal heart and lung of humans between 8 and 20 weeks of gestation (Taylor, 1972). The specific activity for some of these tissues was as great as that in the adult (Short *et al.*, 1972). The specific activity for the hydrolysis of γ-glutamyl-β-naphthylamide by intestine from human fetuses between 13 and 24 weeks of age increased from the proximal to the distal third at every fetal age. It was approximately eight times that in the adult; this should enable the fetus to digest γ-glutamyl peptides readily (Auricchio *et al.*, 1973).

c. Conjugations.   No conjugative activity could be detected with bilirubin in the fetal rat kidney at any age (Grodsky *et al.*, 1958). Although the activity for glucuronide conjugation of *o*-aminophenol was equal to or greater than adult values in slices of guinea pig stomach after the sixth week of gestation, it was considerably less in kidney slices and none was observed in lung, spleen, or brain (Dutton, 1959). No activity was present in the 12,000 g supernatant of 8- to 16-week-old human fetal kidney and intestine for the conjugation of p-nitrophenol (Pelkonen et al., 1969, 1971a). Just prior to birth, some capability to conjugate oxazepam was found in fetal kidney, lung, brain, and muscle from rats and guinea pigs; this activity was considerably less than in the corresponding maternal tissues (Berté et al., 1968). Pretreatment of the pregnant rat with oxazepam or phenobarbital for 3 days increased the glucuronyltransferase activity for oxazepam to some extent in 18-day-old fetal kidney, but not lung and brain (Manzo et al., 1969). Although lung and intestinal mucosa of fetal swine 1 week before term did not conjugate phenolphthalein with glucuronic acid, kidney conjugated more than the adult (Short et al., 1972).

4. WHOLE FETUS

The activity for hydroxylation of benzo[a]pyrene by homogenates of whole rat fetuses between 13 and 18 days of gestation was studied by Schlede and Merker (1972). No activity could be demonstrated in these fetuses without pretreatment; pretreatment with benzo[a]pyrene induced measurable levels of benzo[a]pyrene hydroxylase. The extent of induction increased with age.

The presence of hydrolysis products of thalidomide in the embryos of rabbits given the drug may be suggestive evidence for the hydrolysis having occurred in the embryo (Fabro et al., 1967). The greater lipid solubility of thalidomide compared with its hydrolysis products may allow its rapid transfer to the fetus with retention of the polar products because of their slow transfer back to the mother. However, this explanation, no matter how plausible, should be accepted cautiously until more is known about the transport characteristics of the yolk sac placenta.

B. Rates of Appearance of Drug-Metabolizing Activity in the Postnatal Period

1. OXIDATIONS

a. In Vitro. i. Guinea pig. One of the first studies of drug-metabolizing enzymes in the perinatal period (Jondorf et al., 1958) found that the activity in the 9000 g supernatant of a homogenate of newborn liver for the oxidation of several substrates appeared during the first week of life and had reached adult levels by 8 weeks of age.

ii. Rabbit. The 9000 g supernatant of newborn liver homogenates had little activity for oxidation of barbiturate, demethylation of aminopyrine or meperidine, and other oxidative reactions (Fouts and Adamson, 1959; Pantuck *et al.*, 1968). The activities had reached adult values by 4 weeks of age; however, these studies were only done at weekly intervals and abrupt changes in activity between these time intervals could have been overlooked (Fouts and Adamson, 1959). This was the first study also in which there was indication of the presence of inhibitors in the nuclear and mitochondrial fraction of the homogenate. Fouts and Devereux (1972) later demonstrated that the rise to adult values occurred between 15 and 30 days of age for benzo[a]pyrene hydroxylase and benzphetamine demethylase activities in microsomes from rabbit liver; benzphetamine metabolism in lung microsomes was as rapid or more rapid than in liver microsomes. Benzo[a]pyrene hydroxylase activity was low in lung microsomes at all ages studied. The activity in whole homogenates for benzphetamine metabolism was similar but not exactly parallel with that in microsomes of both liver and lung. Pretreatment of the pregnant mothers or newborn animals with phenobarbital (Hart *et al.*, 1962; Pantuck *et al.*, 1968) or nursing the newborn animals from mothers that had received low, therapeutic doses of phenobarbital (Fouts and Hart, 1965) increased the activity of the supernatant for oxidizing these substrates. Chlordane administered in neonates by injection or from the milk of nursing mothers also increased the activity toward these substrates (Fouts and Hart, 1965).

iii. Rat. The neonatal rat has been studied more extensively than other species for its ability to metabolize drugs. There appears to be a fair amount of substrate variability in these animals. Virtually no activity was demonstrable in the 9000 g supernatant fraction of liver of 12-hour-old rats for metabolizing nitroanisole, hexobarbital, aminopyrine, or benzphetamine (Eling *et al.*, 1970b) and only low activity for hydroxylation of pentobarbital or N-demethylation of meperidine (Pantuck *et al.*, 1968). In contrast, Jori and Briatico (1973) reported that the p-nitroanisole demethylase activity in the liver supernatant from 1-day-old rats was approximately 15% of the adult value. Significant aniline hydroxylase activity was found in 1-day-old rat liver supernatant (Jori and Briatico, 1973) and in the hepatic microsomal fraction of the 2-day-old rat (Gabler and Falace, 1970). Significant metabolic activity for the oxidation of diazepam and benzo[a]pyrene was detected in the 10,000 g supernatant fraction from livers of 6-hour-old rats; at 3 weeks of age this activity had reached adult values for both substrates (Puolakka *et al.*, 1971). However, the demethylation of 3-methyl-4-monomethylaminoazobenzene in 9000 g supernatants of liver on the first day of life was almost half that of the adult female (Bresnick and Stevenson, 1968). On the third day of life, activity was essentially the same as the adult female and no change was seen during the second and third weeks of life.

There is also a great deal of variability in the developmental pattern of the enzymes for metabolism in the neonatal period. For example, the activity for hydroxylation of 4-methylcoumarin (as well as glucose-6-phosphatase and methionine-microsomal phospholipid methyltransferase) reached its maximum value at about 3 days after birth; this sharp peak was several times the value for the prenatal and 10-day-old rat (Feuer and Liscio, 1970). The stimulation of methylcoumarin hydroxylase by pretreatment of the rats with methylcoumarin produced a peak activity at 3 days also.

There was another increase in methylcoumarin hydroxylase activity at 4 weeks of age which Feuer and Liscio (1969) suggested might be due to the discontinued ingestion of an inhibitor in the milk of the nursing mothers. A later report from the same laboratory (Kardish and Feuer, 1972) suggested the chemical nature of this inhibitor. The hydroxylation of 4-methylcoumarin by homogenates and microsomal fractions from newborn rat liver was compared with the hydroxylation and reduction of progesterone. Since the hydroxylation of 4-methylcoumarin and progesterone were decreased in pregnant rats with a concomitant increase in the reduction of progesterone, the effect of pretreatment of the newborn rats with reduced progesterone metabolites was studied. Pretreatment of 2- to 3-week-old rats with the reduced metabolites of progesterone decreased the 16α- and 6β-hydroxylation of progesterone as well as the 3-hydroxylation of coumarin; the Δ^4-reduction of progesterone was increased. Furthermore, early weaning of rats, compared with nonweaned rats of the same age, had the reverse effect on these four enzymatic activities. In addition, treatment of weaned rats with reduced metabolites of progesterone returned these four enzymatic activities to the values of nonweaned rats. This led the authors to suggest that the presence of reduced metabolites of progesterone in the fetus received from the mother *in utero* or in the newborn via the mother's milk was responsible for the decreased hydroxylation of progesterone and 4-methylcoumarin. This however still does not explain the maximal activity for 4-methylcoumarin at 3 days of age since no such peak for the hydroxylation of progesterone was seen at this age; the peak activity for hydroxylation of progesterone occurred sharply at 4 weeks of age. However, this effect of reduced pro-

gesterone metabolites does agree with the general observation that fetal
and newborn tissues are better able to reduce compounds than they are
to hydroxylate them.

However, Henderson (1971) could find no effect of weaning on the activity for N-demethylation of aminopyrine or the glucuronidation of nitrophenol. Furthermore, neither Kato *et al.* (1964) nor Soyka (1969) were
able to demonstrate the presence of an inhibitor. Soyka and Henderson
both found a rise in activity for both female and male rats at this age
although the activity in the males rose to twice that in the females. This
difference between males and females in hepatic microsomal aminopyrine
N-demethylase was confirmed recently although the sharp rise at 3 weeks
of age was not apparent in the female (MacLeod *et al.*, 1972). In contrast, aniline *p*-hydroxylase activity increased in both sexes to reach the
same adult value at 5 weeks of age. The sharp increase which occurs
in the 9000 *g* liver supernatant for demethylation of aminopyrine at 20
days of age is well illustrated in Fig. 20 (from Henderson's paper). Catz
and Yaffe (1967) found a steep increase in nicotine and hexobarbital
metabolism between the third and fourth week of age; they point out
that this coincides with weaning and increased physical activity. Simply
because a change in enzymatic activity coincides with weaning or other
events does not establish a causal relationship between the events; each
of the events may very well be sequenced and occur independently of
the others.

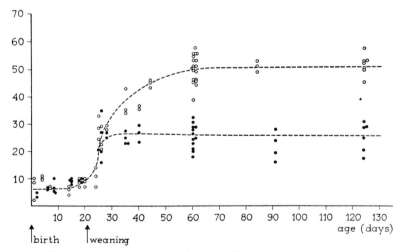

FIG. 20. Postnatal development of hepatic N-demethylation of aminopyrine in
the rat. The enzymatic activities, measured with 9000 *g* supernatants, are given as
μmoles formaldehyde produced per hour per gram dry liver. $\bigcirc$: male; $\bullet$: female.
(Reprinted by permission from Henderson, 1971. *Biochem. Pharmacol.* **20**, 1225.)

The progressive rate of change in activity of drug-metabolizing enzymes was carefully studied by Kato *et al.* (1964) in rats from 1 to 250 days of age. The results from *in vitro* incubations of the 9000 *g* supernatant fraction of liver homogenates, from incubations of liver slices, and from *in vivo* studies were consistent. The rate of metabolism of hexobarbital, pentobarbital, meprobamate, carisoprodol, and strychnine increased from a low level at birth to a maximum at 30 days of age and then declined with increasing age (Figs. 21 and 22). This change in rate with age is dramatic; the rate at 30 days of age is more than 20 times that at 1 day and approximately three times that at 250 days of age. The dramatic peak in enzyme activity at 30 days of age did not coincide with the increase in microsomal RNA and protein with age. This is different from the maximum activity found by Feuer and Liscio (1970) at 3 days for methylcoumarin hydroxylase. The developmental pattern of rat liver microsomal enzymes for drug metabolism was studied also by Basu *et al.* (1970) between the ages of 6 and 100 days. The activity of biphenyl-2-hydroxylase attained a maximum at 21 days and fell to a negligible value after 52 days. The biphenyl-4-hydroxylase activity reached a maximum at 24 days and declined to 40% of this value at

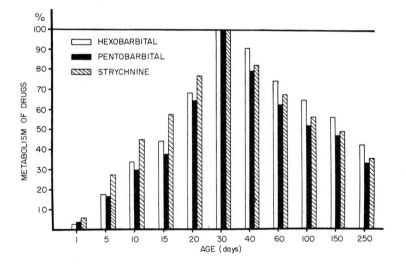

FIG. 21. Metabolism of hexobarbital, pentobarbital, and strychnine in the microsomal preparation obtained from different aged rats. The enzyme activities of 30-day-old rats are expressed as 100. The average enzyme activities (±S.E.) of 30-day-old rats are following: hexobarbital (252 ± 7.8 μg/gm per hour), pentobarbital (82 ± 5.1 μg/gm per hour), and strychnine (158 ± 7.6 μg/gm per hour). The values given represent averages obtained from at least six determinations. (Reprinted by permission from Kato *et al.* 1964. *Biochem. Pharmacol.* 13, 1037.)

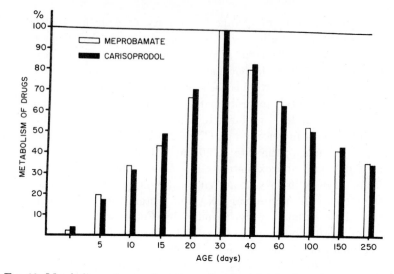

FIG. 22. Metabolism of meprobamate and carisprodol in the microsomal preparation obtained from different aged rats. The metabolic activities of 30-day-old rats are expressed as 100. The average enzyme activities (±S.E.) of 30-day-old rats are following: meprobamate (85 ± 7.3 μg/gm per hour), carisprodol (103 ± 7.5 μg/gm per hour). The values represent averages obtained from at least six determinations. (Reprinted by permission from Kato et al. 1964. Biochem. Pharmacol. 13, 1037.)

85 days. Eling et al. (1970b) studied the activity in the 9000 g liver supernatant of rats at 5 and 10 days of age. The activity for reducing nitrobenzoic acid or oxidizing hexobarbital was greater at 5 days than at 10 days. The reverse was true for nitroanisole, aminopyrine, and benzphetamine.

The effect of pretreatment with enzyme inducers has been studied in rats in the perinatal period. Pretreatment of pregnant rats with diphenylhydantoin (DPH) for 1 week prior to parturition had no effect on the activity at birth. Although pretreatment with DPH increased the activity toward most substrates at both 5 and 10 days of age the extent of the increase differed among the substrates (Eling et al., 1970b). Aniline hydroxylase and benzo[a]pyrene hydroxylase activity were unaffected by DPH treatment at either age. Pretreatment of pregnant mothers with phenobarbital for 4 days prior to delivery increased the enzyme activity in the 9000 g liver supernatant toward pentobarbital and meperidine in rats (Pantuck et al., 1968). Stimulation of the enzymes for the hydroxylation of aniline and the demethylation of p-nitroanisole was demonstrated in 1-day-old rat liver when pregnant mothers were pretreated with eucalyptol for 4 days prior to delivery. However, eucalyptol administration to the mothers after delivery did not induce these drug-metabolizing enzymes in the suckling rats (Jori and Briatico, 1973), although direct administration of eucalyptol to the suckling rats did induce these enzymes. There was a wide variation in the extent of stimulation of the enzymes. Pretreatment of neonatal, 2-week-, or 3-week-old rats with methylcholanthrene increased the activity for demethylation of 3-methyl-4-monomethylaminoazobenzene (Bresnick and Stevenson, 1968). The enzyme activity could not be induced in fetal liver after administration of the drug directly into the amniotic sac of the pregnant rat. However, administration of the methylcholanthrene into the amniotic sac of rats 2–3 days before delivery caused an elevation in the demethylase activity of these rats on the first day after birth. Conney et al. (1960) demonstrated that pretreatment of rats with a variety of drugs caused a marked increase in the activity of microsomal oxidative enzymes at about 3 weeks of age.

iv. Mouse. The activity of mouse liver supernatant for the metabolism of nitroanisole, *N*-monomethyl-*p*-nitroaniline (Pomp *et al.*, 1969), and nicotine (Stålhanske *et al.*, 1969) increased during the neonatal period to reach the adult activity at about 3 weeks of age. Formation of cotinine was maximal at 4 weeks of age; the conversion to cotinine thereafter decreased while the conversion to other metabolites increased. This peak activity is similar to that found in rats at about the time of weaning.

v. Hamster. The negligible benzo[a]pyrene hydroxylase activity in fetal hamster liver increased thirtyfold by the second day of life; this was still only one-sixth of the adult activity (Nebert and Gelboin, 1969). Administration of methylcholanthrene to the newborn hamster increased the hydroxylase activity fivefold in 24 hours.

vi. Swine. The time course of the appearance of enzymes in liver from swine after birth was studied by Short and Davis (1970) for the oxidation of hexobarbital, zoxazolamine, nitroanisole and L-amphetamine. All of these activities increased linearly from very low levels at birth to maximum or near-maximum values at about four weeks of age. The rate of demethylation of *p*-nitroanisole rose to adult values within the first week after birth in the kidney and intestinal mucosa; little if any activity for this substrate was found in lung at any age (Short *et al.*, 1972).

b. In Vivo. i. Rabbit. An increased disappearance of pentobarbital from rabbits was seen *in vivo* when the pregnant mothers were pretreated with phenobarbital for 4 days prior to delivery (Pantuck *et al.*, 1968).

ii. Rat. The extent of meprobamate metabolism in young rats at several time intervals would suggest that the activity might be higher in the newborn than at any other age. The *in vivo* metabolism of meprobamate decreased after 4.5 weeks of age; the rate of metabolism of the drug at 4.5 weeks was twice that of the adult. Furthermore, pretreatment with phenobarbital or phenaglycodol increased the activity more in the immature animal than in the adult (Kato *et al.*, 1961).

iii. Mouse. The disappearance of aminopyrine, Phenacetin, and hexobarbital from intact mice increased from birth to 3 weeks of age; this correlated with a decreased sleeping time from hexobarbital during the same time interval (Jondorf *et al.*, 1958). The sleeping times at 3 weeks of age were still longer than those in the adult.

iv. Human. The rate of disappearance of tolbutamide from the serum of full-term newborn infants was only one-sixth that of adults (Nitowsky *et al.*, 1966). After 2 days of age the rate of appearance of carboxyltolbutamide in the urine of these infants was the same as that in adults; this was interpreted to indicate maturation of the liver oxidative enzyme systems by 2 days of age. Newborn infants who had received ethanol from the mother *in utero* eliminated the compound at about half the maternal rate during the first 4–8 hours of life (Idänpään-Heikkilä *et al.*, 1972), which suggests a deficiency of alcohol dehydrogenase in the newborn human. The disappearance of nortriptyline from the plasma of the mother who had taken an overdose of the drug 1 day prior to delivery was compared with the disappearance of the drug from the plasma of her newborn infant (Sjöqvist *et al.*, 1972). The concentration of the drug in the mother's plasma was five times that in the fetal plasma and the half-lives of the drug in the mother and fetus were 17 and 56 hours, respectively.

Extremely sensitive analytic techniques using gas chromatography and gas chromatography–mass spectrometry that make possible the identification of microgram amounts of drugs and their metabolites have been applied to studies of human newborn plasma and urine (Horning *et al.*, 1969). This technique has been used to identify in newborn urine the metabolites of a large number of drugs administered to the mother prior to delivery; it is impossible, however, to know whether these metabolites were produced in maternal or newborn tissues. Three drugs that had been given to the newborn shortly after birth were studied. Hydroxylated derivatives of secobarbital, phenobarbital, and diphenylhydantoin were identified in the urine of each infant, but quantitative rates of formation were not made. The metabolites of secobarbital and phenobarbital found in newborn urine are the same as those which are predominantly found in adult urine, namely hydroxysecobarbital, secodiol, and p-hydroxyphenobarbital, respectively (Horning *et al.*, 1973). No unchanged secobarbital was found but there was unchanged phenobarbital as is common in the adult. The major metabolites of diphenylhydantoin were 5-phenyl-5-(p-hydroxyphenyl)hydantoin and 5-phenyl-5-(3,4-dihydroxy-1,5-cyclohexadien-1-yl)hydantoin; small amounts of unchanged diphenylhydantoin were present. Although caffeine was not given to newborn infants, differences in excretion patterns of newborns and mothers allowed certain inferences. Only 26% of caffeine was excreted unchanged by the mothers; the remainder was present as demethylated metabolites. In contrast, 75–83% of urinary xanthine was present as unchanged caffeine in the newborn; 19–25% of the total xanthine excreted were monomethyl- and dimethylxanthines.

Administration of diphenylhydantoin and barbiturates had no effect on the urinary steroid excretion patterns in the first 5 days in human newborns (Reynolds and Mirkin, 1973). Thus these two drugs do not stimulate 6β-steroid hydroxylase in the human newborn although they do in the adult human. The activity of this 6β-hydroxylase, however, is normally higher in the newborn than in the adult. Much more needs to be done on the interactions between drug and steroid hydroxylations; drugs have a profound effect on the steroid excretion patterns of the newborn human (Horning *et al.*, 1969) and steroids have an effect on hydroxylations *in vitro* in newborn rat liver homogenates (Kardish and Feuer, 1972).

2. REDUCTIONS AND HYDROLYSES

a. In Vitro. i. Rabbit.   Newborn rabbit liver is deficient in the ability to reduce nitrobenzoic acid. The activity increased to reach adult levels by about 4 weeks of age (Fouts and Adamson, 1959). Hart *et al.* (1962) and Fouts and Hart (1965) reported that the reduction of nitrobenzoic acid in whole liver homogenates from newborn rabbits could be increased by pretreating the pregnant or newborn rabbits with phenobarbital or chlordane. The hydrolytic conversion of acetylsalicyclic acid to salicyclic acid increased rapidly in neonatal rabbit liver, small intestine, and stomach homogenates to reach its maximum activity at 4 weeks of age; no activity was detected in the kidney (Eyring *et al.*, 1973).

ii. Rat.   The 9000 g supernatant fraction of the liver of 12-hour-old rats had no ability to metabolize nitrobenzoic acid (Eling *et al.*, 1970b).

Pretreatment of the pregnant rats with DPH for 1 week prior to parturition had no effect on this activity. Pretreatment with DPH increased the reductive activity about 50% in the rats which were sacrificed on the fifth day of life; pretreatment with DPH increased the reductive activity two and a half times that of the controls in the rats which were killed on the tenth day of life. Furthermore, the activity of nitrobenzoate reductase was greater at 5 days than at 10 days in the controls but essentially the same at these two ages after pretreatment with DPH. Basu et al. (1970) found that the peak activity of p-nitrobenzoate reductase was reached at 38 days and followed by slow decline to 60% of this value at 100 days when rat liver microsomal enzymes were studied between 6 and 100 days of age.

iii. Swine. Azoreductase activity for neoprontosil was studied in 9000 g supernatant fractions of both liver and kidney homogenates by Short and Davis (1970). The significant activity in both the fetus and newborn pig remained essentially unchanged in the kidney whereas the activity in the liver increased over a period of about 6 weeks to reach a value three times that present at birth. In a later study (Short et al., 1972) the rate of azoreduction of neoprontosil by kidney at 6 weeks of age was more than double that at birth; a peak in activity at 6 weeks of age in lung and intestinal mucosa of about twice the newborn rate declined in the adult to the same rate as that in the newborn. In contrast, the rate of reduction of p-nitrobenzoic acid in liver increased steadily from 10% of the adult value at birth to reach 72% of the adult value at 6 weeks of age.

The ability of the 9000 g supernatant fractions from swine liver and kidney homogenates to hydrolyze procaine was studied from birth to 10 weeks of age (Short and Davis, 1970). Although only minimal activity was found at birth, hepatic procaine esterase activity increased to the maximum value by 4 weeks of age. At this time there was a slight decline in the rate of hydrolysis for the remaining 6 weeks studied. Renal metabolism of procaine was minimal but increased slightly during the period studied. A peak in the rate of procaine hydrolysis was seen at 4–6 weeks of age in lung, liver, kidney, and intestinal mucosa (Short et al., 1972). For liver and kidney this peak was only slightly above the adult value and the newborn rate was about one-third of the adult value. For lung and intestinal mucosa the peak at 4 weeks was two to three times the adult value and the rate in the newborn was the same as that in the adult. More complete cell disruption was suggested for the higher metabolic rates seen in the later study.

3. CONJUGATIONS

a. In Vitro. i. Guinea pig. Liver homogenates, fortified with UDPGA, had 20% of adult activity for glucuronidation of o-aminophenol at birth (Brown and Zuelzer, 1958) and about 30% of adult activity at 2–3 days (Gartner and Arias, 1963). Adult activity was reported to be reached at 5 days (Dutton, 1959) or at 20 days (Brown and Zuelzer, 1958). The activity in liver slices was reported to be greater than that in homogenates by Gartner and Arias (1963) and lower than in homogenates by Dutton (1959). These discrepancies were attributed to strain variability (Dutton, 1966b) or a deficient UDPG-dehydrogenase or cellular transport mechanism. Pretreatment of newborn animals with benzo[a]pyrene increased glucuronyltransferase activity in the microsomal liver fraction 1–3 days after birth (Inscoe and Axelrod, 1960).

Either 0% (Jondorf et al., 1958) or only 10% (Brown, 1957; Brown and Zuelzer, 1958) of adult activity for conjugation of phenolphthalein was found in newborn guinea pig liver homogenates. Adult activity was reached by 3 weeks (Brown, 1957; Brown and Zuelzer, 1958) or 8 weeks (Jondorf et al., 1958).

No glucuronyltransferase activity for bilirubin could be demonstrated in microsomal fractions of newborn guinea pig liver (Brown and Zuelzer, 1958). Slices of liver, kidney, and small intestine of the newborn guinea pig are relatively inactive in conjugating salicylate (Schachter et al., 1958, 1959), but approximately adult activities were reached at about 3 days.

ii. Rabbit. The conjugation of o-aminophenol by rabbit liver slices or homogenates developed slowly and progressively during the first month of life to reach adult levels at about 4 or 5 weeks of age (Flint et al., 1964; Lathe and Walker, 1958a), whereas the activity for the conjugation of p-nitrophenol in rabbit liver homogenates increased from about 70% of the adult value on day 1 to 100% on day 21 (Tomlinson and Yaffe, 1966; Yaffe et al., 1968). Newborn rabbit kidney slices conjugated considerably more glucuronic acid with salicylate than did the adult kidney, and liver had about the same activity as the adult (Schachter et al., 1959). Conjugation of bilirubin with glucuronic acid by slices or homogenates of rabbit liver was very low at birth, 20–40% of adult activity at 7 days, and equal to adult activity at 10 days (Lathe and Walker, 1958a; Flint et al., 1964). In liver homogenates the activity had also reached adult levels by 10 days of age but did not peak until about 20 days of age before returning to the adult activity at 30 days of age (Flint *et al.*, 1964). The peak activity at 20 days was almost double that in the adult. This same sharp rise from very low levels at birth to activity exceeding that of the adult was described by Tomlinson and Yaffe (1966).

A careful study of cofactor requirements, inhibitors, developmental patterns, and solubilization properties clearly shows the wide differences in the properties of the enzymes for glucuronidation of bilirubin and *o*-aminophenol in the rabbit (Tomlinson and Yaffe, 1966; Yaffe *et al.*, 1968).

iii. Rat. Although Inscoe and Axelrod (1960) found low glucuronyltransferase activity with *o*-aminophenol (OAP) in the microsomal fraction of rat liver, 1–3 days after birth, others (Dutton *et al.*, 1964; Gartner and Arias, 1963; Dutton, 1966a) have reported activity in 1-day-old rat liver homogenates and slices as great as that in the adult. The peak activity in rat liver slices for OAP-glucuronide formation occurred during the first day of life (Gartner and Arias, 1963) and during the fourth day of life in liver homogenates (Dutton *et al.*, 1964; Dutton, 1966a); however, Gartner and Arias reported no OAP-conjugating ability in homogenates of either newborn or adult liver. The possibility was suggested that homogenization released an inhibitor. Homogenates of rat liver had activity for the formation of OAP-glucuronide which was equal to or greater than that in the adult at approximately 1 and 3 weeks of age (Stevens, 1962); intervening values were lower than that in the adult.

At birth glucuronyltransferase activity for *p*-nitrophenol in liver homogenates was equal to that in the adult (van Leusden *et al.*, 1962; Schröter and Eggeling, 1965; Henderson, 1971). Twice the adult activity at birth which declined steadily to adult levels at about the fifth day of life has also been reported (Dutton *et al.*, 1964; Dutton, 1966a). Henderson (1971) sonicated homogenates to minimize interference by differences in transport at the microsomal membrane and found a peak activity at 4 days of age which declined rapidly to the adult level by 10 days. The peak at 4 days was three times as high as the activity at birth or at 10 days.

The activity in liver homogenates for conjugation of phenolphthalein was about one-third of the adult value at 1 day of age and increased to reach the adult activity by 5 days (Dutton, 1966a). Newborn liver was many times more active than maternal liver in its ability to conjugate glucuronic acid with salicylic acid (Schachter *et al.*, 1959).

Newborn liver slices and homogenates conjugate bilirubin with glucuronic acid about one-half as efficiently as the adult (Flint *et al.*, 1964; Grodsky *et al.*, 1958; Thaler, 1970); this increases to reach the adult activity after a few days (Thaler, 1970) or a few weeks (Grodsky *et al.*, 1958). In contrast, Bakken (1969) found no bilirubin–glucuronic acid conjugating activity in newborn liver homogenates. A week or more was required for the activity to reach adult values.

The importance of the genetic difference in strains of rats and their ability to conjugate bilirubin and glucuronic acid is illustrated when normal rats are mated with Gunn rats which have an enzymatic defect in bilirubin conjugation. Heterozygous rats of two types with different developmental patterns for the appearance of the conjugating enzymes are seen (Thaler, 1970). The presence of bilirubin is associated with the induction of the enzyme; bilirubin stimulation of the enzyme was confirmed by Bakken (1969).

The inhibition of bilirubin conjugation in rat liver slices by serum from pregnant women and newborn infants (Lathe and Walker, 1958b) is apparently due to the presence of pregnane-3α,20β-diol in these sera (Fleischner and Arias, 1970). Infants nursing from mothers who secrete this steroid in their milk have a prolonged neonatal jaundice.

Pretreatment with chlorcyclizine, 3,4-benzpyrene, chloroquine, and pamaquine stimulates glucuronyltransferase activity in the liver of newborn and young rats for *o*-aminophenol and bilirubin (Arias *et al.*, 1963a,b; Inscoe and Axelrod, 1960). Treatment of pregnant rats with benzo[*a*]pyrene in the last 7–10 days of gestation did not increase OAP or bilirubin glucuronide formation in the newborn; however, similar treatment with chloroquine or chlorcyclizine increased glucuronide formation 1.5 to 2.5 times that observed in controls (Inscoe and Axelrod, 1960; Arias *et al.*, 1963a,b). It immediately becomes apparent, when one is aware of the wide variety of compounds that can stimulate or inhibit the transferase, how conflicting reports on the transferase activity in the newborn could arise.

iv. Mouse. The activity of liver homogenates or slices for conjugation of OAP or phenolphthalein with glucuronic acid was zero (Jondorf *et al.*, 1958; Dutton, 1959, 1963) or 20% (Dutton, 1966a) at birth. The activity increased over the next few weeks at rates which differ widely among techniques and investigators (Jondorf *et al.*, 1958; Lathe and Walker, 1958a; Dutton, 1959, 1963, 1966a). The ability to conjugate *p*-nitrophenol and phenolphthalein in liver homogenates is near the adult value at birth (Dutton, 1966a). The activity of liver homogenates to conjugate bilirubin and glucuronic acid was one-third of that in the adult on the first day of life (Catz and Yaffe, 1968) and the same as the adult on day 2 (Lathe and Walker, 1958a). Addition of UDPGA was necessary to demonstrate full activity. The activity continued to increase to about four times that of the adult on the tenth day of life and then declined slowly over a matter of weeks to the adult value (Catz and Yaffe, 1968).

Pretreatment of the pregnant mother or newborn mice with barbital or phenobarbital increased glucuronyltransferase activity with bilirubin and OAP but not with phenolphthalein (Catz and Yaffe, 1962).

v. Chick. Remarkable maturity of liver UDPGT for OAP exists in the chick embryo (Dutton, 1963, 1966b). As early as at 8 days of incubation there is significant activity for conjugation of OAP. The activity falls to low levels at the time of hatching and then rises again as the chick matures. Bilirubin has not been studied as a substrate for the transferase. In contrast to the situation in mammalian liver, UDPGA was high in early chick embryo liver.

vi. Cat and Hamster. Newborn cat liver slices conjugate bilirubin with glucuronic acid as extensively as do those of the adult, while the newborn hamster liver is only one-half as efficient as that of the adult (Flint *et al.*, 1964).

vii. Swine. The ability of the liver of swine to conjugate glucuronic acid with phenolphthalein was studied during the first ten weeks of life by Short and Davis (1970). Studies at weekly intervals indicated that the activity rose from very low values at birth rapidly over the first 3 weeks of life to reach essentially adult levels by the third week without any further significant change. There was approximately a thirtyfold increase in the activity during these first 3 weeks of life. No phenolphthalein glucuronide formation could be demonstrated in the kidney at any of these ages. More complete cell disruption increased the apparent activity in the liver of the newborn than it did at later ages (Short *et al.*, 1972); the rise to the peak activity at 4 weeks was only nine times that of the newborn. This conjugation in lung, kidney, and intestinal mucosa also peaked at 4–6 weeks of age.

viii. Human. Minimal ability of the human premature or newborn liver was found for the conjugation of glucuronic acid with bilirubin, OAP, or *p*-nitrophenol (Lathe and Walker, 1957, 1958a; van Leusden *et al.*, 1962); newborn human liver suspensions did not conjugate bilirubin even in the presence of UDPGA (Lathe and Walker, 1957).

b. In Vivo. Conjugation of glucuronic acid with bilirubin and other substrates is one of the steps in the elimination of such substances from the intact animal. In recent years it has become apparent that mechanisms other than enzymatic conjugation are rate limiting in the excretory process. As early as 1963, Vest and Rossier obtained evidence that the most likely cause of increased plasma retention of bromsulfophthalein (BSP) in the newborn human is due to a deficiency of cellular transport and/or secretion of the BSP conjugates. Schenker and Schmid (1964) also demonstrated an excretory defect for conjugated ^{14}C-bilirubin in 1-day-old guinea pigs but concluded that the rate-limiting step was the impaired ability of the liver to conjugate ^{14}C-bilirubin.

i. Rabbit, rat, and mouse. Newborn and 4-day-old rabbits have an accelerated disappearance of bilirubin from their serum after phenobarbital pretreatment. This rapid disappearance of circulating bilirubin suggests a cellular mechanism which has been stimulated by phenobarbital for the uptake of bilirubin (Catz and Yaffe, 1968). Two hepatic cytoplasmic protein fractions, Y and Z, which have a high affinity for bilirubin, BSP, and other anions, have been suggested as the substances responsible for the liver's ability to sequester bilirubin (Levi *et al.*, 1969). However, phenobarbital has been reported not to affect these carriers in rat liver (Fanska *et al.*, 1970).

Roberts and Plaa (1967) demonstrated an enhanced disappearance of bilirubin from plasma and an enhanced biliary excretion in phenobarbital-treated mice. There was no change in the bilirubin concentration in the bile and the increase in bilirubin excretion was apparently due to an increase in bile volume. Increased bile flow in phenobarbital-treated animals apparently accounts for the increased excretion of chlorothiazide and probenecid in the bile of rats (Hart *et al.*, 1969).

Although the chemical identity of the ouabain excreted into the bile of young rats was not determined, the extent of this excretion was decreased in neonatal rats and accounted for the increased toxicity of the drug. The plasma concentration of ouabain, after the same dose per gram body weight, was seven times higher in 7-day-old rats than in 39-day-old rats. A much higher concentration of ouabain in the liver, but not other tissues, of the older rats suggested an inability of the liver of the newborn rat to concentrate and excrete ouabain (Klaassen, 1972).

Further clarification of the neonatal animal's defect in biliary excretion came from comparing the disposition of sulfobromophthalein, sulfobromophthalein-glutathione, and indocyanine green (Klaassen, 1973). Each of these compounds was excreted by the neonatal liver at a slower rate than that in the adult. Since the latter two are not biotransformed during their passage through the liver, a decrease in the hepatic organic acid transport mechanism would account for the decreased excretion of all three compounds. In the *in vivo* situation a deficiency of the organic anion-binding protein (Y) or in conjugation can account for decreased hepatic excretion of compounds that are conjugated; comparisons among conjugated and nonconjugated substances must be made to identify the defect as were done by Klaassen.

The activity of phenosulfotransferase using p-nitrophenol sulfate as substrate and m-aminophenol as sulfate acceptor was as high in the newborn mouse liver homogenate as in the adult (Yaffe et al., 1968). There was a rise to almost three times this activity at 28 days of age which may be related to changes in other enzyme activities that occur after weaning.

ii. Human. The effect of phenobarbital in stimulating bile flow has been used clinically in intrahepatic cholestasis (Thaler, 1969; Sharp and Mirkin, 1970; Stiehl et al., 1971). Whether this mechanism or enhanced uptake by factors such as Y and Z protein accounts for enhanced biliary secretion in the newborn treated with phenobarbital is not known. However, the recent demonstration that the conjugation of salicylate, salicylamide, and acetaminophen with glucuronic acid, glycine, and sulfate is normal in two sisters with congenital, unconjugated hyperbilirubinemia responsive to phenobarbital treatment, suggests that a deficiency of hepatic anion-binding protein is an important factor in the overall excretion of bilirubin (Levy and Ertel, 1971). Studies on the excretion of acetaminophen glucuronide in newborn infants after phenobarbital treatment might help clarify the question since the formation of this glucuronide is reduced in newborn infants (Vest and Streiff, 1959).

There is normally a gradual increase in glucuronide excretion by the human infant during the first week of life (Brown, 1957); however, the disappearance of bilirubin from the blood of premature infants is as slow on the fifth day of life as it was on the first (Heringová et al., 1972); full-term hypotrophic newborns and full-term newborns of diabetic mothers excreted bilirubin at the same rate as healthy full-term infants. Administration of phenobarbital to pregnant women for 2 weeks or longer prior to delivery significantly lowered the serum bilirubin levels in their offspring in the first 4 days of life compared with control groups (Maurer et al., 1968). Administration of chloroquine, however, to pregnant women from 1–8 weeks prior to delivery had no effect on the serum bilirubin concentration of the infants in the first 5 days of life (Arias et al., 1963a).

Further evidence for the specificity of the glucuronide conjugation was the presence in urine of the glucuronide conjugate of hydroxyphenylphenylhydantoin but not the glucuronide of p-hydroxyphenobarbital after newborn infants had been given the parent drugs (Horning et al., 1973). The diphenylhydantoin had been administered for 4 or 5 days and the phenobarbital for only 1 day; perhaps 1 day was not sufficient for induction. Reynolds and Mirkin (1973) found that 88 to 99% of the hydroxyphenylphenylhydantoin was conjugated in newborn urine from infants whose mothers had received diphenylhydantoin during pregnancy.

Administration of phenobarbital to a female infant at nine months of age who had a deficiency in glucuronide conjugating activity decreased her serum bilirubin concentration to one-third of the value before phenobarbital treatment (Yaffe et al., 1966). The glucuronide conjugating deficit was also apparent for salicylamide, and it also rose to normal values with phenobarbital treatment. This was one of the first clinical applications of enzyme induction of metabolizing enzymes to accomplish a therapeutic goal.

The poor ability of the newborn infant to form the glucuronide conjugate of chloramphenicol has been known for some time to account for the high blood levels of unconjugated chloramphenicol in infants receiving this drug (Weiss et al., 1960). The mechanism by which this unconjugated chloramphenicol produced the "gray baby syndrome" was unknown. Recently, however, a mechanism for this syndrome was suggested (Leitman, 1972). Chloramphenicol inhibits mitochondrial protein synthesis in human fetal liver. It was suggested that chloramphenicol may be inhibiting the increase in mitochondrial proteins and/or numbers of mitochondria that normally would be expected in such tissues of the newborn as brain, heart, and brown adipose tissue; the consequence would be inadequate, aerobic respiration in these tissues.

In recent years newborn infants with elevated serum concentrations of bilirubin have been exposed to blue light to decrease circulating bilirubin. Although this phototherapy apparently converts the bilirubin to an unknown substance or substances which are more rapidly eliminated from the infant, the long-term consequences of this therapy are unknown. The consensus is that the use of phototherapy for hyperbilirubinemia in the newborn should be accepted with caution and applied only with informed clinical judgment (Behrman and Hsia, 1970).

C. Characteristics of the Enzyme Systems for Drug Metbolism

Although the complete enzyme system for metabolism of drugs is not yet known, some of the enzymes involved have been identified. Some studies have determined the amounts or activities of these specific enzymes during prenatal and postnatal growth. Because of marked differences in these patterns of development among tissues, the papers will be summarized by species and tissues. The four enzymes present in microsomes which are involved with drug metabolism are the ones that have been commonly studied. Cytochrome P-450 is generally thought to be the enzyme that binds to the drug and oxygen to accomplish the oxidative metabolism. Cytochrome P-450 reductase and/or cytochrome c reductase then reduce the cytochrome P-450 to make it available for another substrate molecule. NADPH then reduces the reductase. There appears to be some interaction with the cytochrome b_5 system since NADH can reduce cytochrome P-450, probably through this system.

  i. *Rabbit.* A careful study of the development of the drug-metabolizing enzyme system in the lung and liver of this species by Fouts and Devereux (1972) exemplifies the complexity of the system. Each of the enzymes thought to be involved in drug metabolism was assayed at about 4 days, 2 weeks, 4 weeks, and 5 months of age. The NADPH-generating capacity of soluble fractions in lung and liver appeared to be adequate at all ages. In contrast to experiments with neonatal rat and human fetal tissues, the relative amount of activity lost in the 9000 g pellet of immature lung and liver appeared to be similar to the activity lost in the adult tissues. The concentrations of cytochromes P-450 and b_5 were about five times higher per milligram of protein in liver microsomes than lung microsomes at all ages. Although it was difficult to assay NADPH–cytochrome P-450 reductase activity in immature lung, the activity in adult lung was as great as or higher than the activity in adult liver. The NADPH–cytochrome c reductase activity was sensitive to ionic strength, and the differences between lung and liver were not great.

  There were subtle differences in the patterns of development of these enzymes between tissues and certain correlations could be made with the metabolism of different substrates. Both cytochrome P-450 and b_5 in lung showed slow, progressive increases at the four time intervals studied. Cytochrome c reductase in lung showed a marked change in activity only between 2 and 4 weeks of age. This increase in the reductase correlated with the increase in benzphetamine metabolism suggesting that another pathway besides cytochrome P-450 might be responsible for the demethylation of benzphetamine. However, there was no significant increase in benzo[a]pyrene hydroxylation in lung at these time intervals, which is consistent with benzo[a]pyrene hydroxylation being dependent on cytochrome P-450 in this tissue.

  In the liver, however, both benzphetamine and benzo[a]pyrene metabolism rose sharply between 2 and 4 weeks of age in parallel with the rise of both cytochrome P-450 and cytochrome c reductase in this tissue. It was interesting that the increase in cytochrome b_5 in the liver did not correlate with the other two enzymes or with the metabolism of the two substrates.

  ii. *Rat.* The only tissue in the rat that has been studied for the specific enzymes in drug metabolism is liver. Care must be taken with this tissue since as much activity was found in the sediment as in the supernatant of neonatal liver homogenates. The pH optimum of this system in fetal liver was a few tenths higher than that of the adult system for the oxidation of aminopyrine (Soyka, 1969). The presence of inhibitors in the newborn (Fouts and Adamson, 1959; Soyka, 1969) or from the mother (Feuer and Liscio, 1970) has been suggested.

A low content of cytochrome P-450 in the newborn increased to reach a maximum at 31 days of age; it then declined to almost the adult value by 38 days (Dallner et al., 1965; Basu et al., 1970). However, Gram et al. (1969) found very little change in cytochrome P-450 content between 1 and 12 weeks of age. They also found that the largest changes in metabolizing activity occurred immediately after birth and at about the time of weaning; furthermore, the activities of aniline hydroxylase and ethylmorphine demethylase do not correlate with each other or with changes in cytochrome P-450. Sexual maturation of male rats did not appear to coincide with changes in enzyme activity.

MacLeod et al. (1972) confirmed the poor correlation between increasing drug-metabolism activity and the increasing concentration of cytochrome P-450 in young rats. There were also sex differences. In males the pattern of maturation of both type I and type II drug oxidations most closely followed the activity of NADPH–cytochrome P-450 reductase, however, since the sampling times are more frequent than those by Fouts and Devereux (1972) the difference in this respect between rat and rabbit liver cannot be established; in females the relationship was closer to the activity of NADPH–cytochrome c reductase. After the age of 3 weeks male rats demonstrated higher activity for aminopyrine N-demethylation than did females but there was no difference between sexes for aniline p-hydroxylation. In adult rats activities of aminopyrine N-demethylase and NADPH-cytochrome P-450 reductase and the concentration of cytochrome P-450 were lower in the female. This study suggests that in the developing rat liver the amount of cytochrome P-450 itself may not be the limiting step in drug oxidation.

Diphenylhydantoin pretreatment increased NADPH–cytochrome c reductase activity, NADPH–oxidase activity and cytochrome P-450 content of microsomes without qualitative changes as determined by the ethylisocyanide-induced difference spectra after dithionate reduction at different pH values. Eling et al. (1970a) also studied the changes in the kinetic parameters and the spectral characteristics of the hepatic microsomal mixed-function oxidase in 5-, 10-, and 30-day-old rats without and after pretreatment with DPH. A complex pattern of change and lack of change of different components of this oxidase system with aniline or benzphetamine indicates that the system undergoes qualitative as well as quantitative changes between 5 and 30 days of age. The results of DPH pretreatment on enzyme kinetics on microsomal drug spectral interactions were different from those of phenobarbital or benzo[a]pyrene pretreatment. These complex changes emphasize the need for extensive studies of all the components of these enzyme systems at closely spaced time intervals during maturation.

A difference in absorption spectra for microsomal hemoprotein in fetal liver induced by two types of substrates administered to pregnant rats was discovered by Welch *et al.* (1972). Pretreatment of pregnant rats with 3-methylcholanthrene increased activity for benzo[a]pyrene metabolism in fetal liver which was paralleled by an increase in microsomal hemoprotein concentration with an absorbancy at 448 nm when CO was added to reduced microsomes or 455 nm with ethylisocyanide. Phenobarbital pretreatment did not increase the hydroxylation of benzo[a]pyrene nor have any effect on the hemoprotein concentration in fetal liver. Thus a *P*-448 specific for benzo[a]pyrene hydroxylation was induced by 3-methylcholanthrene in fetal liver whereas the *P*-450 for other drugs was not induced by phenobarbital.

Kato *et al.* (1964) studied the microsomal RNA and protein content at intervals between birth and 250 days of age in rats. Both RNA and protein rose between about the first day of life and the thirtieth day of life where they reached roughly plateau values. There was little correlation between total RNA or protein and drug metabolism which reached a sharp peak at 30 days and then declined. It is apparent that there was little correlation between the content of these two constituents and the activity of drug metabolism. However, the variation of the microsomal NADPH–oxidase activity is almost exactly the same as that of the microsomal drug-metabolizing enzymes.

Electron microscopic studies of fetal rat liver revealed poorly developed endoplasmic reticulum until the end of gestation (Dallner *et al.*, 1965). At term there is extensive synthesis of the rough-surfaced microsomal membranes with tightly packed ribosomes. The many free ribosomes and large aggregates of glycogen particles present at birth coincide with very little smooth-surfaced endoplasmic reticulum. By 3 days after birth the highly developed endoplasmic reticulum, containing both smooth- and rough-surfaced ribosomes separated by larger distances, approaches the picture seen in the adult liver. Gabler and Falace (1970) were unable to show recognizable smooth endoplasmic reticulum in electron micrographic studies of fetal rat liver near term; pretreatment with DPH had no effect on this ultrastructure. Schlede and Merker (1972) found that treatment of pregnant rats with benzo[a]pyrene caused a moderate increase and enlargement of the cisternae of the rough endoplasmic reticulum in fetal liver cells. Franke and Klinger (1966) were unable to demonstrate an effect of barbital treatment on the smooth endoplasmic reticulum of fetal rat liver cells on the fifteenth and twenty-second day of gestation. Phenobarbital and chlordane given to immature male rats caused a proliferation of smooth-surfaced endoplasmic reticulum in hepatocytes but benzo[a]pyrene and methylcholanthrene do not (Fouts and Rogers, 1965).

Free ribosomes, which are present in rat hepatocytes as early as the eleventh day of gestation, decrease progressively to reach the adult appearance by the day of birth (Chedid and Nair, 1974). Rough endoplasmic reticulum was most prominent on the thirteenth day, and these cisternae progressively filled with electron-dense material between the fifteenth and twentieth days of gestation; this electron-dense material disappeared at birth. Smooth endoplasmic reticulum (SER) first appeared on the twentieth day of gestation and increased progressively into the postnatal period. There was much variability in the amount of SER in individual hepatocytes at birth; furthermore, phenobarbital treatment of the pregnant animals did not influence the rate of appearance of SER in the fetal hepatocytes.

Some clues of more physiological factors such as hormones which either hasten or retard the differentiation of enzymes in the perinatal period have been identified by Greengard (1973). Thyroxine administered to fetal rats *in utero* increased their NADPH–cytochrome *c* reductase activity at birth. Administration of glucagon, estradiol, or glucocorticoids altered the time of differentiation of other enzymes in rat liver in the perinatal period.

A beautiful organization of the structural and enzymatic events which occur in sequential fashion in developing rat liver has been made possible by the morphometric studies of Greengard *et al.* (1972). Their determinations of the number and volumes of parenchymal, hematopoietic, and Kupffer cells in fetal rat liver from late gestation up to adulthood allow correlations with enzyme activities determined per gram of total liver. Glycogen synthetase activity reaches a peak in parenchymal cells on the twentieth day of gestation. The mean volume of the parenchymal cell reaches a peak on the twenty-second day of gestation, just before birth; this apparently is due to the accumulation in these cells of glycogen just before birth as seen by Dallner *et al.* (1966a). Just after birth the mean volume of individual parenchymal cells decreases to about one-half without a decrease in the volume fraction of the liver occupied by hepatocytes. From this age to adulthood the volume fraction continues to be more than 85% hepatocytes although there is a second rise in the mean volume of individual parenchymal cells between days 12 and 28. Thus, the sequence of events appears to be an increase in glycogen synthetase in parenchymal cells 2 days before term followed by a peak storage of glycogen in them at term. The glycogen may be used for synthesis of endoplasmic reticulum just after birth (Dallner *et al.*, 1966a,b) and be necessary for the appearance of drug-metabolizing enzymes at this time. Short and Davis (1970) found a high glycogen content in pig liver about the time of birth, immediately preceding the increase in the content of *P*-450 and the increase in activity for drug metabolism. The fascinating correlation of the appearance of enzyme activity with glycogen accumulation was also noted by Rogers *et al.* (1963) even in adult rats.

The activity of glycogen synthetase per parenchymal cell increases sharply again between 12 and 28 days of age; this is the same age that a marked increase in the activity of drug-metabolizing enzymes was noted by Feuer and Liscio (1969), Soyka (1969), and Henderson (1971) in rat liver and by Catz and Yaffe (1967) and Stålhandske *et al.* (1969) in mouse liver. Several of these investigators attributed this to weaning and increased physical activity which occurs at about this time. However, Henderson (1971), in a direct experimental test, could not demonstrate any difference in the N-demethylation of aminopyrine or the UDP-glucuronidation of *p*-nitrophenol in weaned rats and those which continued to nurse for 10 days. It thus seems that the appearance of enzyme activities is probably sequenced before and after birth and increases merely occur at birth and at weaning which may not be due to external factors.

iii. Mouse. Comparison of hypnotic and lethal effects with *in vitro* metabolism of liver homogenates in mice of different ages and strains was made by Catz and Yaffe (1967). Differences in hypnotic and lethal effects among strains revealed that the strain exhibiting the least hypnotic effect had the highest lethal effect. The authors suggested that this may be due to the rapid formation of an intermediate product more toxic than the parent substance. Since the two enantiomers of hexobarbital are metabolized at different rates in rats (Furner *et al.*, 1969), another possibility is that increased rates of metabolism of the hypnotic enantiomer among the strains of mice unmask the more lethal enantiomer. The extreme variability among strains of mice in enzyme activity and in the regulation of enzyme induction must always be considered (Nebert and Gelboin, 1969).

The teratogenic and toxic effect of cyclophosphamide on mice *in utero* or postnatally can be altered by pretreatment with phenobarbital or SKF 525A; these alterations provide interesting clues to the mechanism of that toxic effect. Phenobarbital pretreatment of pregnant mice 3 days before delivery increases the toxic effect of cyclophosphamide administered to the newborn mice. This toxic effect can be measured by a decrease in weight gain, mortality, or growth of the tail. Pretreatment with SKF 525A 1 hour before administration of cyclophosphamide to the newborn mice offered some protection to these toxic effects. Furthermore, pretreatment with SKF 525A increased the half-life of cyclosphosphamide in these mice and phenobarbital decreased the half-life (Bus et al., 1973). This is obviously consistent with the idea that the toxic effects of cyclophosphamide are due to a metabolite of the drug. An earlier observation that SKF 525A increased the teratogenicity of cyclophosphamide is also consistent with this concept; decreased metabolism and elimination from the mother presents more drug to the fetus for slow conversion to the toxic metabolite in the fetus (Gibson and Becker, 1968). Although pretreatment of pregnant mice with SKF 525A had no effect on the binding of radioactivity from cyclophosphamide to macromolecules of the embryo, pretreatment with phenobarbital decreased the binding to embryo DNA (Murthy et al., 1973). Binding to DNA of the embryo showed a positive correlation with overall frequencies of malformations produced by cyclophosphamide.

iv. Swine. The microsomal protein in the liver of pigs increased only slightly during the period from 2 weeks prior to birth up to 10 weeks after birth (Short and Davis, 1970). They stated that the activity curves were similar when the activity was calculated either as the amount of substrate metabolized per gram of liver or as the amount metabolized per miligram of microsomal protein for oxidations, conjugations, and hydrolyses. For the reduction of neoprontosil there was a somewhat altered shape to the activity curve when plotted as micromoles per miligram of protein, resulting from the fact that the rate of metabolism of this substrate was relatively high at birth whereas the microsomal protein content was relatively low. The content of cytochrome P-450 in microsomes was measured at weekly intervals from 2 weeks before birth to 10 weeks after birth. There was a very low level of the pigment prior to birth and in the newborn; it increased in content linearly over the first 3 weeks of life to reach essentially a plateau level. This increase in the content of P-450 correlates very well with the increase in the activity of the microsomes in drug conversions found by these investigators.

A later study with swine confirmed the pattern of increase in content of cytochrome P-450 in liver, except that the maximal values obtained were substantially higher; this was attributed to differences in the method of homogenization (Short et al., 1972). Microsomal cytochrome b_5 was found in fetal liver in somewhat higher concentration than in the liver of the newborn. Lung, kidney, and intestinal mucosa were also assayed for the content of these two enzymes. Only very low levels of cytochrome P-450 were found in lung and intestinal mucosa at any age and although the content in kidney increased with age it did not approach that in liver. Little cytochrome b_5 was found in lung and intestinal mucosa. Low levels in kidney increased with age; this increase paralleled an increase in microsomal protein content.

v. Human. As would be expected from the presence of drug-metabolic activity in the human fetus, the enzymes for this system have been identified in fetal tissues. Zamboni (1965) studied by electron microscopy the livers of human embryos 7–20 weeks of age. Smooth endoplasmic reticulum was absent in the seventh and ninth weeks but by the third month a considerably developed agranular reticulum of irregular vesicles was profusely distributed in the cytoplasm. The reorganization of the ergastoplasm and the development of the agranular endoplasmic reticulum at 3 months occurred concomitantly with the appearance of glycogen and iron deposits in the liver cells. This appearance at 3 months corresponds well with the increase in drug metabolism in fetuses of this age observed by Pelkonen (1973); however, he found no change in the amount of microsomal protein in the liver during this period.

The physical properties of the fetal endoplasmic reticulum from liver are different from the adult. Only 10–15% of the fetal liver microsomes were recovered in the 105,000 g pellet. Homogenization caused much of the fetal liver endoplasmic reticulum to form long, slender cisternae that sedimented with the mitochondrial fraction. Nevertheless, the 105,000 g pellet was composed of homogeneous microsomal vesicles. Most of the activity for NADPH–cytochrome c reductase and most of the cytochrome P-450 were found in the 200 g pellet; the levels of these two enzymes were comparable to those in adult liver (Ackermann and Rane, 1971; Ackermann *et al.*, 1972). Soyka (1970) had earlier demonstrated the presence of NADPH–cytochrome c reductase and cytochrome b_5 in newborn liver.

In fetal liver of 14–25 weeks of age there were highly variable amounts of cytochrome P-450 and NADPH–cytochrome c reductase. There was no obvious correlation of either of these enzymes with the length of gestation. Although NADPH–cytochrome P-450 reductase activity was not quantitated, it was present in every sample analyzed. NADH–cytochrome c reductase and cytochrome b_5 were also present in the livers from these fetuses. Thus all the components of both the NADPH- and NADH-linked electron transport systems were present in these samples although they were unable to oxidize benzo[a]pyrene and aminopyrine. The system was capable, however, of hydroxylating testosterone and laurate.

Studies of the change in the absorption spectra revealed that substrates which were metabolized gave a type I spectral change and aminopyrine gave a type II. It was suggested that endogenous substrates with high affinities were blocking the sites for oxidizable exogenous substrates (Yaffe et al., 1970).

In another study (Rane and Ackermann, 1972), ethylmorphine was metabolized by fetal liver microsomes but induced a reverse type I spectral change. This substrate gives a type I spectral change in adult rat liver microsomes whereas testosterone causes a reverse type I in human adult liver microsomes. These substrate-induced spectral changes that vary with age and species are still incompletely understood but indicate that the enzyme probably differs in some respects with age and species (Rane et al., 1971). The pH optimum for the drug-metabolizing system in fetal liver was about one-half a pH unit higher than that in the adult and curiously, the optimal temperature was 40°–45°C (Pelkonen et al., 1971a).

The human fetal adrenal appears to be much more active than the liver in drug oxidations. This correlates with a much higher concentration of the CO-binding pigment. Adrenal microsomes had a much higher content of this pigment than hepatic microsomes; mitochondria from the adrenal and liver had amounts intermediate between these extremes. None was found in kidney or lung. The absorption maximum of this pigment when treated with CO was 448 nm which is consistent with the observation that these microsomes actively hydroxylated benzo[a]pyrene (Juchau and Pedersen, 1973; Rane et al., 1973a). The P-448 enzyme is the one that is increased in microsomes from rats pretreated with 3-methylcholanthrene. The high concentrations of NADPH and benzo[a]pyrene required to saturate the enzyme system indicate that the apparent affinity for substrate and cofactors of the human fetal system is lower than the mature rat hepatic system (Juchau and Pedersen, 1973).

D. Effects of Pregnancy on Maternal Drug Metabolism

The pregnant female apparently metabolizes drugs at a slower rate than the nonpregnant female. Bresnick and Stevenson (1968) reported that the N-demethylase activity in pregnant rats was only 80% of that in the nonpregnant female. Feuer and Liscio (1969, 1970) reported the methylcoumarin hydroxylase and glucuronyltransferase activity in pregnant rat liver to be about one-half that in the nonpregnant female; variable degrees of induction were found for these two enzyme systems after pretreatment with methylcoumarin, methylcholanthrene, and phenobarbital. Gabler and Falace (1970) found that DPH disappears from nonpregnant rats much faster than from pregnant animals. This correlated with the significantly lower activity of microsomal aniline hydroxylase in pregnant as compared to nonpregnant rats. Repeated doses of DPH further reduced enzyme activity in pregnant rats while similar treatment of nonpregnant rats increased this activity.

ACKNOWLEDGMENTS

The authors are most grateful to Dr. Ed Mayberry for his comments and suggestions on the anatomic and histological portion of the manuscript, to Miss Jo Anne Barbour for her rapid and excellent preparation of the typescript, to Mrs. Martha Crampton and Mr. Roderick Roberson for their untiring and skillful preparation of illustrations, and last, but not least, to Mrs. Jo Goulson for her versatile assistance in all stages of the preparation of the manuscript. The work was supported in part by NIH Grant No. DE-02668 and Tobacco and Health Research Grant No. KY-057.

REFERENCES

Abramovich, D. R., and Wade, A. P. (1969). *J. Obstet. Gynaecol. Brit. Commonw.* **76**, 610.

Ackermann, E., and Rane, A. (1971). *Chem.-Biol. Interact.* **3**, 233.

Ackermann, E., Rane, A., and Ericsson, J. L. E. (1972). *Clin. Pharmacol. Ther.* **13**, 652.

Adams, C. E., Hay, M. F., and Lutwak-Mann, C. (1961). *J. Embryol. Exp. Morphol.* **9**, 468.

Agnew, W. F. (1972). *Teratology* **6**, 331.

Agnew, W. F., and Cheng, J. T. (1971). *Toxicol. Appl. Pharmacol.* **20**, 346.

Airaksinen, M. M., and Idänpään-Heikkilä, J. E. (1967). *Psychopharmacologia* **10**, 400.

Albanus, L., Hammarström, L., Sundwall, A., Ullberg, S., and Vangbo, B. (1968). *Acta Physiol. Scand.* **73**, 447.

Allgén, L.-G., Ekman, L., Reio, L., and Ullberg, S. (1960). *Arch. Int. Pharmacodyn. Ther.* **126**, 1.

André, T. (1956). *Acta Radiol., Suppl.* **142**, 1.

André, T., Ullberg, S., and Winqvist, G. (1960). *Acta Pharmacol. Toxicol.* **16**, 229.

Appelgren, L.-E. (1967). *Acta Physiol. Scand.* **68**, Suppl. 301, 1.

Appelgren, L.-E. (1969). *Acta Endocrinol. (Copenhagen)* **62**, 505.

Appelgren, L.-E., Ericsson, Y., and Ullberg, S. (1961). *Acta Physiol. Scand.* **53**, 339.

Appelgren, L.-E., Nelson, A., and Ullberg, S.. (1966). *Acta Radiol., Ther., Phys., Biol.* **4**, 41.

Arias, I. M. (1970). *Birth Defects, Orig. Art. Ser.* **7**, 55.

Arias, I. M., Gartner, L., Furman, M., and Wolfson, S. (1963a). *Ann. N.Y. Acad. Sci.* **111**, 274.

Arias, I. M., Gartner, L., Furman, M., and Wolfson, S. (1963b). *Proc. Soc. Exp. Biol. Med.* **112**, 1037.

Assali, N. S. (1968). "Biology of Gestation," Vol. 1. Academic Press, New York.

Auricchio, S., Ciccimarra, F., Vegnente, A., Andria, G., and Vetrella, M. (1973). *Pediat. Res.* **7**, 95.

Austin, C. R., and Lovelock, J. E. (1958). *Exp. Cell Res.* **15**, 260.

Bäckström, J. (1969). *Acta Pharmacol. Toxicol.* **27**, Suppl. 3, 1.
Bäckström, J., Hansson, E., and Ullberg, S. (1965). *Toxicol. Appl. Pharmacol.* **7**, 90.
Bäckström, J., Hammarström, L., and Nelson, A. (1967). *Acta Radiol. Ther. Phys. Biol.* **6**, 122.
Bakken, A. F. (1969). *Pediat. Res.* **3**, 205.
Balinsky, B. I. (1970). "An Introduction to Embryology." Saunders, Philadelphia, Pennsylvania.
Basu, T. K., Dickerson, J. W. T., and Parke, D. V. (1970). *Biochem. J.* **119**, 54P (abstr.).
Beazley, J. M., Brummer, H. C., and Kurjak, A. (1972). *J. Obstet. Gynaecol. Brit. Commonw.* **79**, 800.
Beck, F., Lloyd, J., and Griffiths, A. (1967). *Science* **157**, 1180.
Behrman, R. E., and Hsia, D. Y.-Y. (1970). *Birth Defects, Orig. Art. Ser.* **6**, 131.
Bellairs, R. (1971). "Development Processes in Higher Vertebrates." Univ. of Miami Press, Coral Gables.
Bengtsson, G. (1963). *Acta Endocrinol. (Copenhagen)* **43**, 581.
Bengtsson, G., and Ullberg, S. (1963). *Acta Endocrinol. (Copenhagen)* **43**, 561.
Bengtsson, G., Ullberg, S., and Perklev, T. (1963). *Acta Endocrinol. (Copenhagen)* **43**, 571.
Bengtsson, G., Ullberg, S., Wiqvist, N., and Diczfalusy, E. (1964). *Acta Endocrinol. (Copenhagen)* **46**, 544.
Benzi, G., Berté, F., Crema, A., and Arrigoni, E. (1968). *J. Pharm. Sci.* **57**, 1031.
Bergeron, M., Fontenelle, A., and Sternberg, J. (1973). *Int. J. Appl. Radiat. Isotop.* **24**, 295.
Bergman, B., and Söremark, R. (1968). *J. Nutr.* **94**, 6.
Berlin, M., and Lewander, T. (1965). *Acta Pharmacol. Toxicol.* **22**, 1.
Berlin, M., and Rylander, A. (1964). *J. Pharmacol. Exp. Ther.* **146**, 236.
Berlin, M., and Ullberg, S. (1963a). *Arch. Environ. Health* **6**, 589.
Berlin, M., and Ullberg, S. (1963b). *Arch. Environ. Health* **6**, 602.
Berlin, M., and Ullberg, S. (1963c). *Arch. Environ. Health* **6**, 610.
Berlin, M., and Ullberg, S. (1963d). *Arch. Environ. Health* **7**, 686.
Berlin, M., and Ullberg, S. (1963e). *Nature (London)* **197**, 84.
Berlin, M., Jerksell, L.-G., and Nordberg, G. (1965). *Acta Pharmacol. Toxicol.* **23**, 312.
Berté, F., and Benzi, G. (1967). *J. Pharm. Pharmacol.* **19**, 608.
Berté, F., Benzi, G., Manzo, L., and Hokari, S. (1968). *Arch. Int. Pharmacodyn. Ther.* **173**, 377.
Bishop, D. W. (1956). *Amer. J. Physiol.* **187**, 347.
Blair, A. H., and Vallee, B. L. (1966). *Biochemistry* **5**, 2026.
Blomquist, L., and Hanngren, Å. (1966). *Biochem. Pharmacol.* **15**, 215.
Bloom, W., and Bartelemez, G. W. (1940). *Amer. J. Anat.* **67**, 21.
Bodin, N. O., Hansson, E., Ramsay, C. H., and Ryrfeldt, A. (1972). *Acta Physiol. Scand.* **84**, 40.
Botte, V., Tramontana, S., and Chieffi, G. (1968). *J. Endocrinol.* **40**, 189.
Bourne, G. L. (1960). *Amer. J. Obstet. Gynecol.* **79**, 1070.
Bourne, G. L. (1962). "The Human Amnion and Chorion." Yearbook Publ., Chicago, Illinois.
Bowman, E. R., Hansson, E., Turnbull, L. B., McKennis, H., Jr., and Schmiterlöw, C. G. (1964). *J. Pharmacol. Exp. Ther.* **143**, 301.

Braithwaite, G. D., Glascock, R. F., and Riazuddin, Sh. (1972). *Brit. J. Nutr.* **27,** 417.

Brambell, F. W. R. (1958). *Biol. Rev. Cambridge Phil. Soc.* **33,** 488.

Brambell, F. W. R., and Halliday, R. (1956). *Proc. Roy. Soc.* **145,** 170.

Brambell, F. W. R., Hemmings, W. A., and Henderson, M. (1951). "Antibodies and Embryos." Oxford Univ. Press (Athlone), London and New York.

Brame, R. G. (1972). *Amer. J. Obstet. Gynecol.* **113,** 1085.

Branch, W. R., and Wild, A. E. (1972). *Z. Zellforsch. Mikrosk. Anat.* **135,** 501.

Bresnick, E., and Stevenson, J. G. (1968). *Biochem. Pharmacol.* **17,** 1815.

Brinsmade, A. B., and Rubsaamen, H. (1957). *Beitr. Pathol. Anat. Allg. Pathol.* **117,** 154.

Brinster, R. L., and Cross, P. C. (1972). *Nature (London)* **238,** 398.

Brown, A. K. (1957). *Amer. J. Dis. Child.* **94,** 510 (abstr.).

Brown, A. K., and Zuelzer, W. W. (1958). *J. Clin. Invest.* **37,** 332.

Brunton, W. J., and Brinster, R. L. (1971). *Amer. J. Physiol.* **221,** 658.

Bryden, M. M., Evans, H. E., and Binns, W. (1972). *J. Morphol.* **138,** 169.

Budreau, C. H., and Singh, R. P. (1973). *Arch. Environ. Health* **26,** 161.

Bürki, K., Seibert, R. A., and Bresnick, E. (1971). *Biochem. Pharmacol.* **20,** 2947.

Bus, J. S., Short, R. D., and Gibson, J. E. (1973). *J. Pharmacol. Exp. Ther.* **184,** 749.

Butt, J. H., II, and Wilson, T. H. (1968). *Amer. J. Physiol.* **215,** 1468.

Calarco, P. G., and Moyer, F. H. (1966). *J. Morphol.* **119,** 341.

Carpenter, S. J., and Ferm, V. H. (1969). *Amer. J. Anat.* **125,** 429.

Cassano, G. B. (1968). *J. Nucl. Biol. Med.* **12,** 13.

Cassano, G. B., and Hansson, E. (1965). *J. Neurochem.* **12,** 851.

Cassano, G. B., and Hansson, E. (1966). *Int. J. Neuropsychiat.* **2,** 269.

Cassano, G. B., and Hansson, E. (1969). *In* "International Conference on Radioactive Isotopes in Pharmacology" (P. G. Waser and B. Glasson, eds.), pp. 421–439. Wiley (Interscience), New York.

Cassano, G. B., Sjöstrand, S. E., and Hansson, E. (1965). *Psychopharmacologia* **8,** 1.

Cassano, G. B., Ghetti, B., Gliozzi, E., and Hansson, E. (1967a). *Brit. J. Anaesth.* **39,** 11.

Cassano, G. B., Placidi, G. F., and Ghetti, B. (1967b). *Riv. Neurobiol.* **13,** 105.

Catz, C., and Yaffe, S. J. (1962). *Amer. J. Dis. Child.* **104,** 116.

Catz, C., and Yaffe, S. J. (1967). *J. Pharmacol. Exp. Ther.* **155,** 152.

Catz, C., and Yaffe, S. J. (1968). *Pediat. Res.* **2,** 361.

Chaube, S., Nishimura, H., and Swinyard, C. A. (1973). *Arch. Environ. Health* **26,** 237.

Chedid, A., and Nair, V. (1974). *Develop. Biol.* **39,** 49.

Christie, G. A. (1968). *J. Anat.* **103,** 91.

Clarkson, T. W., Magos, L., and Greenwood, M. R. (1972). *Biol. Neonate* **21,** 239.

Clemedson, C.-J., Sörbo, G., and Ullberg, S. (1960). *Acta Physiol. Scand.* **48,** 382.

Clemedson, C.-J., Kristoffersson, H., Sörbo, G., and Ullberg, S. (1963a). *Acta Radiol. Ther. Phys. Biol.* **1,** 314.

Clemedson, C.-J., Kristoffersson, H., Sörbo, B., and Ullberg, S. (1963b). *Nord. Hyg. Tidskr.* **44,** 3.

Cohen, E. N., Hood, N., and Golling, R. (1968). *Anesthesiology* **29,** 987.

Conner, E. A., and Miller, J. W. (1973a). *J. Pharmacol. Exp. Ther.* **184,** 285.

Conner, E. A., and Miller, J. W. (1973b). *J. Pharmacol. Exp. Ther.* **184,** 291.

Conney, A. H., Davison, C., Gastel, R., and Burns, J. J. (1960). *J. Pharmacol. Exp. Ther.* **130**, 1.

Conney, A. H., Levin, W., Jacobson, M., and Kuntzman, R. (1973). *Clin. Pharmacol. Ther.* **14**, Part 2, 727.

Curry, H. F., and Ferm, V. H. (1962). *Anat. Rec.* **142**, 21.

Dallner, G., Siekevitz, P., and Palade, G. E. (1965). *Biochem. Biophys. Res. Commun.* **20**, 135.

Dallner, G., Siekevitz, P., and Palade, G. E. (1966a). *J. Cell Biol.* **30**, 73.

Dallner, G., Siekevitz, P., and Palade, G. E. (1966b). *J. Cell Biol.* **30**, 97.

Danforth, D. N., and Hull, R. W. (1958). *Amer. J. Obstet. Gynecol.* **75**, 536.

Dempsey, E. W. (1953). *Amer. J. Anat.* **93**, 331.

Deren, J. J., Padykula, H. A., and Wilson, T. H. (1966a). *Develop. Biol.* **13**, 349.

Deren, J. J., Padykula, H. A., and Wilson, T. H. (1966b). *Develop. Biol.* **13**, 370.

Dixon, R. L., and Willson, V. J. (1968). *Arch. Int. Pharmacodyn. Ther.* **172**, 453.

Done, A. K. (1964). *Clin. Pharmacol. Ther.* **5**, 432.

Done, A. K. (1966). *Annu. Rev. Pharmacol.* **6**, 189.

Douglas, T. A., Renton, J. P., Watts, C., and Ducker, H. A. (1972). *Comp. Biochem. Physiol. A.* **43**, 665.

Duckett, S., and Ellem, K. A. O. (1971). *Exp. Neurol.* **32**, 49.

Dutton, G. J. (1959). *Biochem. J.* **71**, 141.

Dutton, G. J. (1963). *Ann. N.Y. Acad. Sci.* **111**, 259.

Dutton, G. J. (1966a). *Biochem. Pharmacol.* **15**, 947.

Dutton, G. J. (1966b). *In* "Glucuronic Acid: Free and Combined. Chemistry, Biochemistry, Pharmacology, and Medicine" (G. J. Dutton, ed.), pp. 186–299. Academic Press, New York.

Dutton, G. J., Langelaan, D. E., and Ross, P. E. (1964). *Biochem. J.* **93**, 4P (abstr.).

Dyer, N. C., Brill, A. B., Raye, J., Gutberlet, R., and Stahlman, M. (1973). *Radiat. Res.* **53**, 488.

Einer-Jensen, N., and Hansson, E. (1965). *Acta Pharmacol. Toxicol.* **23**, 65.

Eliason, B. C., and Posner, H. S. (1971). *Amer. J. Obstet. Gynecol.* **111**, 925.

Eling, T. E., Harbison, R. D., Becker, B. A., and Fouts, J. R. (1970a). *Eur. J. Pharmacol.* **11**, 101.

Eling, T. E., Harbison, R. D., Becker, B. A., and Fouts, J. R. (1970b). *J. Pharmacol. Exp. Ther.* **171**, 127.

Enders, A. C., and King, B. F. (1970). *Anat. Rec.* **167**, 231.

Ericsson, Y., and Hammarström, L. (1964). *Acta Odontol. Scand.* **22**, 523.

Ericsson, Y., and Hammarström, L. (1965). *Acta Physiol. Scand.* **65**, 126.

Ericsson, Y., and Ullberg, S. (1958). *Acta Odontol. Scand.* **16**, 363.

Ericsson, Y., Santesson, G., and Ullberg, S. (1961). *Arch. Oral Biol.* **4**, 160.

Eriksson, Y., and Larsson, S. (1971). *Acta Pharmacol. Toxicol.* **29**, 256.

Everett, J. W. (1935). *J. Exp. Zool.* **70**, 243.

Ewaldsson, B. (1963). *Arch. Int. Pharmacodyn. Ther.* **142**, 163.

Ewaldsson, B., and Magnusson, G. (1964a). *Acta Radiol. Ther. Phys. Biol.* **2**, 65.

Ewaldsson, B., and Magnusson, G. (1964b). *Acta Radiol. Ther. Phys. Biol.* **2**, 121.

Eyring, E. J., Grosfeld, J. L., and Connelly, P. A. (1973). *Ann. Surg.* **177**, 307.

Fabro, S. (1973). *In* "Fetal Pharmacology" (L. O. Boréus, ed.), pp. 443–461. Raven, New York.

Fabro, S., and Sieber, S. M. (1969a). *In* "The Foeto-Placental Unit" (A. Pecile and C. Finzi, eds.), Int. Congr. Ser. No. 183, pp. 313–320. Excerpta Med. Found., Amsterdam.

Fabro, S., and Sieber, S. M. (1969b). *Nature (London)* **223,** 410.

Fabro, S., Smith, R. L., and Williams, R. T. (1965). *Biochem. J.* **97,** 14P (abstr.).

Fabro, S., Hague, D., and Smith, R. L. (1967). *Biochem. J.* **103,** 26.

Fahim, M. S., Hall, D. G., Jones, T. M., Fahim, Z., and Whitt, F. D. (1970). *Amer. J. Obstet. Gynecol.* **107,** 1250.

Fanska, R., Nemechek, K., Kolb, H., and Grodsky, G. M. (1970). *Clin. Res.* **18,** 128.

Ferm, V. H. (1956). *Anat. Rec.* **125,** 745.

Ferm, V. H., and Carpenter, S. J. (1968). *Lab. Invest.* **18,** 429.

Ferm, V. H., Hanlon, D. W., and Urban, J. (1969). *J. Embryol. Exp. Morphol.* **22,** 107.

Feuer, G., and Liscio, A. (1969). *Nature (London)* **223,** 68.

Feuer, G., and Liscio, A. (1970). *Int. Z. Klin. Pharmakol. Ther. Toxikol.* **3,** 30.

Finster, M., Morishima, H. O., Mark, L. C., Perel, J. M., Dayton, P. G., and James, L. S. (1972a). *Anesthesiology* **36,** 155.

Finster, M., Morishima, H. O., Boyes, R. N., and Covino, B. G. (1972b). *Anesthesiology* **36,** 159.

Fleischner, G., and Arias, I. M. (1970). *Amer. J. Med.* **49,** 576.

Flint, M., Lathe, G. H., Ricketts, T. R., and Silman, G. (1964). *Quart. J. Exp. Physiol. Cog. Med. Sci.* **49,** 66.

Flodh, H. (1968a). *Acta Radiol. Ther. Phys. Biol.* **7,** 121.

Flodh, H. (1968b). *Acta Radiol. Ther. Phys. Biol., Suppl.* **284,** 1.

Forberg, S., Odeblad, E., Söremark, R., and Ullberg, S. (1964). *Acta Radiol. Ther. Phys. Biol.* **2,** 241.

Foreman, P., and Segal, M. B. (1972). *J. Physiol. (London)* **226,** 92P (abstr.).

Fouts, J. R., and Adamson, R. H. (1959). *Science* **129,** 897.

Fouts, J. R., and Devereux, T. R. (1972). *J. Pharmacol. Exp. Ther.* **183,** 458.

Fouts, J. R., and Hart, L. G. (1965). *Ann. N.Y. Acad. Sci.* **123,** 245.

Fouts, J. R., and Rogers, L. A. (1965). *J. Pharmacol. Exp. Ther.* **147,** 112.

Franke, H., and Klinger, W. (1966). *Acta Biol. Med. Ger.* **17,** 507.

Freudenthal, R. I., Martin, J., and Wall, M. E. (1972). *J. Pharmacol. Exp. Ther.* **182,** 328.

Friedler, G., and Cochin, J. (1972). *Science* **175,** 654.

Furner, R. L., McCarthy, J. S., Stitzel, R. E., and Anders, M. W. (1969). *J. Pharmacol. Exp. Ther.* **169,** 153.

Gabler, W. L., and Falace, D. (1970). *Arch. Int. Pharmacodyn. Ther.* **184,** 45.

Gabler, W. L., and Hubbard, G. L. (1972). *Arch. Int. Pharmacodyn. Ther.* **200,** 222.

Garel, J. M., and Dumont, C. (1972). *Horm. Metab. Res.* **4,** 217.

Garrett, N. E., Burriss-Garrett, R. J., and Archdeacon, J. W. (1972). *Toxicol. Appl. Pharmacol.* **22,** 649.

Gartner, L. M., and Arias, I. M. (1963). *Amer. J. Physiol.* **205,** 663.

Garzo, T., Hansson, E., and Ullberg, S. (1962). *Experientia* **18,** 43.

Geddes, I. C., Brand, L., Finster, M., and Mark, L. (1972). *Brit. J. Anaesth.* **44,** 542.

Geelen, J. A. G. (1972). *Teratology* **6,** 19.

Gershon, M. D., and Ross, L. L. (1966). *J. Physiol. (London)* **186,** 477.

Gibson, J. E., and Becker, B. A. (1968). *Teratology* **1,** 393.

Gillette, J. R., Menard, R. H., and Stripp, B. (1973). *Clin. Pharmacol. Ther.* **14,** Part 2, 680.

Gitlin, D., and Perricelli, A. (1970). *Nature (London)* **228,** 995.

3. DISPOSITION OF DRUGS IN THE FETUS

Gitlin, D., Perricelli, A., and Gitlin, G. M. (1972). *Cancer Res.* **32**, 979.

Glass, L. E. (1963). *Amer. Zool.* **3**, 135.

Goldman, A. S. (1969). *Endocrinology* **84**, 1206.

Gottschewski, H. M. (1962). *Naturwiss. Rundsch.* **15**, 257.

Gram, T. E., Guarino, A. M., Schroeder, D. H., and Gillette, J. R. (1969). *Biochem. J.* **113**, 681.

Greengard, O. (1973). *Clin. Pharmacol. Ther.* **14**, Part 2, 721.

Greengard, O., Federman, M., and Knox, W. E. (1972). *J. Cell Biol.* **52**, 261.

Greenhouse, G., Pesetsky, I., and Hamburgh, M. (1969). *J. Exp. Zool.* **171**, 343.

Greenwood, M. R., Clarkson, T. W., and Magos, L. (1972). *Experientia* **28**, 1455.

Gresham, E. L., Simons, P. S., and Battaglia, F. C. (1971). *J. Pediat.* **79**, 809.

Gresham, E. L., James, E. J., Raye, J. R., Battaglia, F. C., Makowski, E. L., and Meschia, G. (1972). *Pediatrics* **50**, 372.

Gripenberg, J., and Penttilä, A. (1970). *Pharmacology* **4**, 287.

Grodsky, G. M., Carone, J. V., and Fanska, R. (1958). *Proc. Soc. Exp. Biol. Med.* **97**, 291.

Gutová, M., Elis, J., and Rašková, H. (1971). *Neoplasma* **18**, 529.

Haar, J. L., and Ackerman, G. A. (1971a). *Anat. Rec.* **170**, 199.

Haar, J. L., and Ackerman, G. A. (1971b). *Anat. Rec.* **170**, 437.

Hakonson, T. E., and Whicker, F. W. (1971). *Health Phys.* **21**, 864.

Hamilton, W. J., and Boyd, J. D. (1960). *J. Anat.* **94**, 297.

Hamilton, W. J., Boyd, J. D., and Mossman, H. W. (1964). "Human Embryology." Williams & Wilkins, Baltimore, Maryland.

Hamilton, W. J., Boyd, J. D., and Mossman, H. W. (1972). "Human Embryology: Prenatal Development of Form and Function." Williams & Wilkins, Baltimore, Maryland.

Hammarström, L. (1966). *Acta Physiol. Scand.* **70**, Suppl. 289, 1.

Hammarström, L., and Nilsson, A. (1970). *Acta Radiol. Ther. Phys. Biol.* **9**, 433.

Hammarström, L., and Ullberg, S. (1966). *Nature (London)* **212**, 708.

Hammarström, L., Neujahr, H., and Ullberg, S. (1966). *Acta Pharmacol. Toxicol.* **24**, 24.

Hamner, C. E., and Fox, S. B. (1969). In "The Mammalian Oviduct" (E. S. E. Hafez and R. J. Blandau, eds.), pp. 333–355. Univ. of Chicago Press, Chicago, Illinois.

Hanngren, Å. (1959). *Acta Radiol., Suppl.* **175**, 1.

Hanngren, Å., Hansson, E., Svartz, N., and Ullberg, S. (1963a). *Acta Med. Scand.* **173**, 61.

Hanngren, Å., Hansson, E., Svartz, N., and Ullberg, S. (1963b). *Acta Med. Scand.* **173**, 391.

Hanngren, Å., Hansson, E., Sjöstrand, S. E., and Ullberg, S. (1964). *Acta Endocrinol. (Copenhagen)* **47**, 95.

Hanngren, Å., Einer-Jensen, N., and Ullberg, S. (1965a). *Acta Endocrinol. (Copenhagen)* **50**, 35.

Hanngren, Å., Einer-Jensen, N., and Ullberg, S. (1965b). *Nature (London)* **208**, 461.

Hansson, E., and Cassano, G. B. (1967). In "Antidepressant Drugs" (S. Garattini and M. N. G. Dukes, eds.), Int. Congr. Ser. No. 122, pp. 10–22. Excerpta Med. Found., Amsterdam.

Hansson, E., and Garzo, T. (1961). *Experientia* **17**, 501.

Hansson, E., and Jacobsson, S.-O. (1966). *Biochim. Biophys. Acta* **115**, 285.

Hansson, E., and Schmiterlöw, C. G. (1961a). *Acta Pharmacol. Toxicol.* **18**, 183.

260   WILLIAM J. WADDELL AND G. CAROLYN MARLOWE

Hansson, E., and Schmiterlöw, C. G. (1961b). *Arch. Int. Pharmacodyn. Ther.* **131**, 309.

Hansson, E., and Schmiterlöw, C. G. (1962). *J. Pharmacol. Exp. Ther.* **137**, 91.

Harbison, R. D., and Becker, B. A. (1971). *Toxicol. Appl. Pharmacol.* **20**, 573.

Harbison, R. D., and Mantilla-Plata, B. (1972). *J. Pharmacol. Exp. Ther.* **180**, 446.

Hart, L. G., Adamson, R. H., Dixon, R. L., and Fouts, J. R. (1962). *J. Pharmacol. Exp. Ther.* **137**, 103.

Hart, L. G., Guarino, A. M., and Adamson, R. H. (1969). *Amer. J. Physiol.* **217**, 46.

Hay, M. F. (1964). *J. Reprod. Fert.* **8**, 59.

Heilbronn, E., Appelgren, L.-E., and Sundwall, A. (1964). *Biochem. Pharmacol.* **13**, 1189.

Henderson, P. T. (1971). *Biochem. Pharmacol.* **20**, 1225.

Herbst, A. L., Ulfelder, H., and Paskanzer, D. C. (1971). *N. Engl. J. Med.* **284**, 878.

Heringová, A., Jirsová, V., and Poláček, K. (1972). *Biol. Neonate* **21**, 303.

Hespe, W., and Prins, H. (1969). *Eur. J. Pharmacol.* **8**, 119.

Hesseldahl, N., and Larsen, J. F. (1969). *Amer. J. Anat.* **126**, 315.

Hidiroglou, M., Hoffman, I., and Jenkins, K. J. (1969). *Can. J. Physiol. Pharmacol.* **47**, 953.

Ho, B. T., Fritchie, G. E., Idänpään-Heikkilä, J. E., and McIsaac, W. M. (1972). *Quart. J. Stud. Alc., Part A* **33**, 485.

Horning, M. G., Waterbury, L. D., Horning, E. C., and Hill, R. M. (1969). In "The Foeto-Placental Unit" (A. Pecile and C. Finzi, eds.), Int. Congr. Ser. No. 183, pp. 305–312. Excerpta Med. Found., Amsterdam.

Horning, M. G., Stratton, C., Nowlin, J., Wilson, A., Horning, E. C., and Hill, R. M. (1973). In "Fetal Pharmacology" (L. Boréus, ed.), pp. 355–373. Raven, New York.

Houston, M. L. (1969a). *Amer. J. Anat.* **126**, 1.

Houston, M. L. (1969b). *Amer. J. Anat.* **126**, 17.

Hoyes, A. D. (1969). *Z. Zellforsch. Mikrosk. Anat.* **99**, 469.

Hoyes, A. D. (1970). *Amer. J. Obstet. Gynecol.* **106**, 557.

Hoyes, A. D. (1971). *J. Anat.* **109**, 17.

Huggert, A., Odeblad, E., Söremark, R., and Ullberg, S. (1961). *Acta Isotop.* **2**, 151.

Hunter, J. A., and Paul, J. (1969). *J. Embryol. Exp. Morphol.* **21**, 361.

Idänpään-Heikkilä, J. E. (1967). *Eur. J. Pharmacol.* **2**, 26.

Idänpään-Heikkilä, J. E, and Schoolar, J. C. (1969). *Science* **164**, 1295.

Idänpään-Heikkilä, J. E., Vapaatalo, H. I., and Neuvonen, P. J. (1968). *Psychopharmacologia* **13**, 1.

Idänpään-Heikkilä, J. E., Jouppila, P. I., and Puolakka, J. O., and Varne, M. S. (1971a). *Amer. J. Obstet. Gynecol.* **109**, 1011.

Idänpään-Heikkilä, J. E., Fritchie, G. E., Ho, B. T., and McIsaac, W. M. (1971b). *Amer. J. Obstet. Gynecol.* **110**, 426.

Idänpään-Heikkilä, J. E., Taska, R. J., Allen, H. A., and Schoolar, J. C. (1971c). *J. Pharmacol. Exp. Ther.* **176**, 752.

Idänpään-Heikkilä, J., Jouppila, P., Åkerblom, H. K., Isoaho, R., Kauppila, E., and Koivisto, M. (1972). *Amer. J. Obstet. Gynecol.* **112**, 387.

Iffy, L., Shepard, T. H., Jakobovits, A., Lemine, R. J., and Kerner, P. (1967). *Acta Anat.* **66**, 178.

Inscoe, J. K., and Axelrod, J. (1960). *J. Pharmacol. Exp. Ther.* **129**, 128.

Jackson, B. T., Smallwood, R. A., Piasecki, G. J., Brown, A. S., Rauschecker, H. F. J., and Lester, R. (1971). *J. Clin. Invest.* **50**, 1286.

Jacobsson, S. O., and Hansson, E. (1965). *Acta Vet. Scand.* **6**, 287.

Jaszczak, S., Choroszewska, A., and Bentyn, K. (1970). *Pol. Med. J.* **9**, 1308.

Jóhannesson, T., Steele, W. J., and Becker, B. A. (1972). *Acta Pharmacol. Toxicol.* **31**, 353.

Jollie, W. P., and Jollie, L. G. (1967). *J. Ultrastruct. Res.* **18**, 102.

Jondorf, W. K., Maickel, R. P., and Brodie, B. B. (1958). *Biochem. Pharmacol.* **1**, 352.

Jori, A., and Briatico, G. (1973). *Biochem. Pharmacol.* **22**, 543.

Juchau, M. R. (1971). *Arch. Int. Pharmacodyn. Ther.* **194**, 346.

Juchau, M. R., and Pedersen, M. G. (1973). *Life Sci., Part II* **12**, 193.

Juchau, M. R., Pedersen, M. G., and Symms, K. G. (1972). *Biochem. Pharmacol.* **21**, 2269.

Kalberer, F. (1966a). *Advan. Tracer Methodol.* **3**, 139.

Kalberer, F. (1966b). *Atomlight* **51**, 1.

Kardish, R., and Feuer, G. (1972). *Biol. Neonate* **20**, 58.

Kato, R., Chiesara, E., and Frontino, G. (1961). *Experientia* **17**, 520.

Kato, R., Vassanelli, P., Frontino, G., and Chiesara, E. (1964). *Biochem. Pharmacol.* **13**, 1037.

Katz, J. (1969). *Brit. J. Anaesth.* **41**, 929.

Katz, J., Gershwin, M. E., and Hood, N. L. (1968). *Arch. Int. Pharmacodyn. Ther.* **175**, 339.

Keberle, H., Faigle, J. W., Fritz, H., Knusel, F., Loustalot, P., and Schmid, K. (1965). *In* "Embryopathic Activity of Drugs" (J. M. Robson, F. M. Sullivan, and R. L. Smith, eds.), p. 210. Little, Brown, Boston, Massachusetts.

Keberle, H., Schmid, K., Faigle, J. W., Fritz, H., and Loustalot, P. (1966). *Bull. Schweiz. Akad. Med. Wiss.* **22**, 134.

Kennedy, J. S., and Waddell, W. J. (1972). *Toxicol. Appl. Pharmacol.* **22**, 252.

Kernis, M. M. (1971). *Experientia* **27**, 1329.

Kernis, M. M., and Johnson, E. M. (1969). *J. Embryol. Exp. Morphol.* **22**, 115.

King, B. F., and Enders, A. C. (1970). *Amer. J. Anat.* **129**, 261.

Kirby, L., and Hahn, P. (1973). *Pediat. Res.* **7**, 75.

Kivalo, I., and Saarikoski, S. (1972). *Brit. J. Anaesth.* **44**, 557.

Klaassen, C. D. (1972). *J. Pharmacol. Exp. Ther.* **183**, 520.

Klaassen, C. D. (1973). *J. Pharmacol. Exp. Ther.* **184**, 721.

Klein, D. C. (1972). *Nature (London), New Biol.* **237**, 117.

Koransky, W., and Ullberg, S. (1964). *Proc. Soc. Exp. Biol. Med.* **116**, 512.

Kristerson, L., Hoffmann, P., and Hansson, E. (1965). *Acta Pharmacol. Toxicol.* **22**, 205.

Krzyzowska-Gruca, S., and Schiebler, T. H. (1967). *Z. Zellforsch. Mikrosk. Anat.* **79**, 157.

Kulangara, A. C., Krishna Menon, M. K., and Willmott, M. (1965). *Nature (London)* **206**, 1259.

Kulay, L., and Fava De Moraes, F. (1965). *Acta Histochem.* **22**, 309.

Lal, H., Barlow, C. F., and Roth, L. J. (1964). *Arch. Int. Pharmacodyn. Ther.* **149**, 25.

Lambson, R. O. (1966). *Amer. J. Anat.* **118**, 21.

Lambson, R. O. (1970). *Amer. J. Anat.* **129**, 1.

Landauer, W., and Wakasugi, N. (1967). *J. Exp. Zool.* **164**, 499.

Lathe, G. H., and Walker, M. (1957). *Biochem. J.* **67,** 9P (abstr.).
Lathe, G. H., and Walker, M. (1958a). *Biochem. J.* **70,** 705.
Lathe, G. H., and Walker, M. (1958b). *Quart. J. Exp. Physiol. Cog. Med. Sci.* **43,** 257.
Leder, O., and Paschen, S. (1965). *Pfluegers Arch. Gesamte Physiol. Menschen Tiere* **285,** 147.
Leitman, P. S. (1972). *Fed. Proc., Fed. Amer. Soc. Exp. Biol.* **31,** 62.
Lester, R., Jackson, B. T., and Smallwood, R. A. (1970). *Birth Defects, Orig. Artic. Ser.* **6,** 16.
Levi, A. J., Gatmaitan, Z., and Arias, I. M. (1969). *J. Clin. Invest.* **48,** 2156.
Levy, G., and Ertel, I. J. (1971). *Pediatrics* **47,** 811.
Lindquist, N. G., and Ullberg, S. (1971). *Experientia* **27,** 1439.
Lindquist, N. G., and Ullberg, S. (1972). *Acta Pharmacol. Toxicol.* **31,** Suppl. 2, 1.
Lister, V. M. (1968). *J. Obstet. Gynaecol. Brit. Commonw.* **75,** 327.
Logothetopoulus, J. H., and Myant, N. B. (1956). *J. Physiol. (London)* **133,** 213.
Lüders, D. (1971). *Monatsschr. Kinderheilk* **119,** 320.
Luse, S. A. (1957). *Macy Found. Conf. Gestation* **4,** 115.
Lutwak-Mann, C. (1954). *J. Embryol. Exp. Morphol.* **2,** 1.
Lutwak-Mann, C. (1962). *Nature (London)* **193,** 653.
Lutwak-Mann, C. (1973). *In* "Fetal Pharmacology" (L. O. Boréus, ed.), pp. 419–442. Raven, New York.
Lutwak-Mann, C., and Hay, M. F. (1962). *Brit. Med. J.* **2,** 944.
McDowell, R. W., Landolt, R. R., Kessler, W. V., and Shaw, S. M. (1971). *J. Pharm. Sci.* **60,** 695.
McLachlan, J. A., Sieber, S. M., and Fabro, S. (1969). *Fed. Proc., Fed. Amer. Soc. Exp. Biol.* **28,** 744 (abstr.).
MacLeod, S. M., Renton, K. W., and Eade, N. R. (1972). *J. Pharmacol. Exp. Ther.* **183,** 489.
Maeyama, M., Matuoka, H., Tuchida, Y., and Hashimoto, Y. (1969). *Steroids* **14,** 144.
Manzo, L., Berté, F., and de Bernardi, M. (1969). *Boll. Chim. Farm.* **108,** 19.
Marks, P. A., and Rifkind, R. A. (1972a). *Science* **175,** 955.
Marks, P. A., and Rifkind, R. A. (1972b). *Science* **177,** 187.
Mascherpa, P. (1968). *Boll. Chim. Farm.* **107,** 589.
Mastroianni, L., and Wallach, R. C. (1961). *Amer. J. Physiol.* **200,** 815.
Mastroianni, L., Beer, F., Shah, U., and Cleuse, T. H. (1961). *Endocrinology* **68,** 92.
Masuoka, D., and Hansson, E. (1967). *Acta Pharmacol. Toxicol.* **25,** 447.
Maurer, H. M., Wolff, J. A., Finster, M., Poppers, P. J., Pantuck, E., Kuntzman, R., and Conney, A. H. (1968). *Lancet* **2,** 122.
Midgley, A. R., and Pierce, G. B. (1963). *Amer. J. Anat.* **63,** 929.
Miller, R. K., Ferm, V. H., and Mudge, G. H. (1972). *Amer. J. Obstet. Gynecol.* **114,** 259.
Mirkin, B. L. (1971a). *Amer. J. Obstet. Gynecol.* **109,** 930.
Mirkin, B. L. (1971b). *J. Pediat.* **78,** 329.
Mirkin, B. L. (1973). *In* "Fetal Pharmacology" (L. O. Boréus, ed.), pp. 1–27. Raven, New York.
Molinaro, M., Siracusa, G., and Monesi, V. (1972). *Exp. Cell Res.* **71,** 261.
Moore, M. A. S., and Metcalf, D. (1970). *Brit. J. Haematol.* **18,** 279.

Mosier, H. D., Jr., and Jansons, R. A. (1972). *Teratology* **5**, 303.

Mossman, H. W. (1937). *Contrib. Embryol. Carnegie Inst.* **26**, 133.

Murthy, V. V., Becker, B. A., and Steele, W. J. (1973). *Cancer Res.* **33**, 664.

Naharin, A., Lubin, E., and Feige, Y. (1969). *Health Phys.* **17**, 717.

Nasjleti, C. E., Avery, J. K., Spencer, H. H., and Walden, J. M. (1967). *J. Oral Ther. Pharmacol.* **4**, 71.

Nebert, D. W. (1973). *Clin. Pharmacol. Ther.* **14**, Part 2, 693.

Nebert, D. W., and Gelboin, H. V. (1969). *Arch. Biochem. Biophys.* **134**, 76.

Nelson, A., and Ullberg, S. (1960). *Acta Radiol.* **53**, 305.

Nelson, A., Ullberg, S., Kristoffersson, H., and Rönnbäck, C. (1961). *Acta Radiol.* **55**, 374.

Nelson, A., Ullberg, S., Kristoffersson, H., and Rönnbäck, C. (1962). *Acta Radiol.* **58**, 353.

New, D. A. T., and Brent, R. L. (1972). *J. Embryol. Exp. Morphol.* **27**, 543.

Nishimura, M., Urakawa, N., and Ikeda, M. (1971). *Jap. J. Pharmacol.* **21**, 651.

Nitowsky, H. M., Matz, L., and Berzofsky, J. A. (1966). *J. Pediat.* **69**, 1139.

Olsson, K. Å., Söremark, R., and Wing, K. R. (1969). *Acta Physiol. Scand.* **77**, 322.

Östlund, K. (1969). *Acta Pharmacol. Toxicol.* **27**, Suppl. 1, 1.

Padykula, H. A., Deren, J. J., and Wilson, T. H. (1966). *Develop. Biol.* **13**, 311.

Pantuck, E., Conney, A. H., and Kuntzman, R. (1968). *Biochem. Pharmacol.* **17**, 1441.

Past, W. L. (1963). *Amer. J. Pathol.* **42**, 285.

Patton, B. M. (1968). "Human Embryology," 3rd ed. McGraw-Hill, New York.

Payne, G. S., and Deuchar, E. M. (1972). *J. Embryol. Exp. Morphol.* **27**, 533.

Pecile, A., Chiesara, E., and Conti, F. (1969). *In* "The Foeto-Placental Unit" (A. Pecile and C. Finzi, eds.), Int. Congr. Ser. No. 183., pp. 255–259. Excerpta Med. Found., Amsterdam.

Pelkonen, O. (1973). *Arch. Int. Pharmacodyn. Ther.* **202**, 281.

Pelkonen, O., Vorne, M., and Kärki, N. T. (1969). *Acta Physiol. Scand.* **69**, Suppl. 330, 69 (abstr.).

Pelkonen, O., Vorne, M., Jouppila, P., and Kärki, N. T. (1971a). *Acta Pharmacol. Toxicol.* **29**, 284.

Pelkonen, O., Arvela, P., and Kärki, N. T. (1971b). *Acta Pharmacol. Toxicol.* **30**, 385.

Pelkonen, O., Jouppila, P., and Kärki, N. T. (1972). *Toxicol. Appl. Pharmacol.* **23**, 399.

Peters, M. A., Turnbow, M., and Buchenauer, D. (1972). *J. Pharmacol. Exp. Ther.* **181**, 273.

Pierce, G. B., Midgley, A. R., Sci Ram, J., and Feldman, J. D. (1962). *Amer. J. Pathol.* **41**, 549.

Pikkarainen, P. H. (1971). *Life Sci., Part II* **10**, 1359.

Pikkarainen, P. H., and Räihä, N. C. R. (1967). *Pediat. Res.* **1**, 165.

Pitkin, R. M., Reynolds, W. A., and Filler, L. J., Jr. (1970). *Amer. J. Obstet. Gynecol.* **108**, 1043.

Pitkin, R. M., Reynolds, W. A., Filler, L. J., Jr., and King, T. G. (1971). *Amer. J. Obstet. Gynecol.* **111**, 280.

Pitkin, R. M., Connor, W. E., and Lin, D. S. (1972). *J. Clin. Invest.* **51**, 2584.

Plaa, G. L. (1968). *Lancet* **2**, 1348.

Placidi, G. F., and Cassano, G. B. (1968). *Int. J. Neuropharmacol.* **7**, 383.

Placidi, G. F., Masuoka, D. T., Alcaraz, A., Taylor, J., and Earle, R. W. (1968). *Proc. West. Pharmacol. Soc.* **11**, 53.

Pomp, H., Schnoor, M., and Netter, K. J. (1969). *Deut. Med. Wochenschr.* **94,** 1232.
Potter, E. L. (1961). "Pathology of the Fetus and Infant," 2nd ed. Yearbook Publ., Chicago, Illinois.
Proffit, W. R., and Edwards, L. E. (1962). *J. Exp. Zool.* **151,** 53.
Puolakka, J., Vorne, M., and Idänpään-Heikkilä, J. (1971). *Scand. J. Clin. Lab. Invest.* **27,** Suppl. 116, 57 (abstr.).
Quinones, J. D., Boyd, C. M., Beierwaltes, W. H., and Poissant, G. R. (1972). *J. Nucl. Med.* **13,** 148.
Rane, A., and Ackermann, E. (1972). *Clin. Pharmacol. Ther.* **13,** 663.
Rane, A., and Sjöqvist, F. (1972). *Pediat. Clin. N. Amer.* **19,** 37–49.
Rane, A., Sjöqvist, F., and Orrenius, S. (1971). *Chem.-Biol. Interact.* **3,** 305.
Rane, A., Sjöqvist, F., and Orrenius, S. (1973a). *Clin. Pharmacol. Ther.* **14,** Part 2, 666.
Rane, A., von Bahr, C., Orrenius, S., and Sjöqvist, F. (1973b). *In* "Fetal Pharmacology" (L. Boréus, ed.), pp. 287–302. Raven, New York.
Reminga, T. A., and Avery, J. K. (1972). *J. Dent. Res.* **51,** 1426.
Reynolds, J. W., and Mirkin, B. L. (1973). *Clin. Pharmacol. Ther.* **14,** 891.
Ritzén, M., Hammarström, L., and Ullberg, S. (1965). *Biochem. Pharmacol.* **14,** 313.
Roberts, R. J., and Plaa, G. L. (1967). *Biochem. Pharmacol.* **16,** 827.
Rogers, L. A., Dixon, R. L., and Fouts, J. R. (1963). *Biochem. Pharmacol.* **12,** 341.
Rosell, S., Sedvall, G., and Ullberg, S. (1963). *Biochem. Pharmacol.* **12,** 265.
Rugh, R. (1968). "The Mouse; Its Reproduction and Development." Burgess, Minneapolis, Minnesota.
Saarikoski, S., and Castrén, O. (1971). *Acta Obstet. Gynecol. Scand.* **50,** Suppl. 9, 60.
Saarikoski, S., and Seppälä, M. (1973). *Amer. J. Obstet. Gynecol.* **115,** 1100.
Sakuma, M., Yoshikawa, M., and Sato, Y. (1971). *Chem. Pharm. Bull.* **19,** 995.
Scammon, R. E., and Calkins, L. A. (1929). "Growth in the Fetal Period." Univ. of Minnesota Press, Minneapolis.
Schachter, D., Kass, D. J., and Lannon, T. J. (1958). *Fed. Proc., Fed. Amer. Soc. Exp. Biol.* **17,** 304 (abstr.).
Schachter, D., Kass, D. J., and Lannon, T. J. (1959). *J. Biol. Chem.* **234,** 201.
Scharpf, L. G., Jr., Hill, I. D., Wright, P. L., Plank, J. B., Keplinger, M. L., and Calandra, J. C. (1972). *Nature (London)* **239,** 231.
Schechter, P. J., and Roth, L. J. (1967). *J. Pharmacol. Exp. Ther.* **158,** 164.
Schechter, P. J., and Roth, L. J. (1971). *Toxicol. Appl. Pharmacol.* **20,** 130.
Schenker, S., and Schmid, R. (1964). *Proc. Soc. Exp. Biol. Med.* **115,** 446.
Schenker, S., Dawber, N. H., and Schmid, R. (1964). *J. Clin. Invest.* **43,** 32.
Schlede, E., and Merker, H.-J. (1972). *Naunyn-Schmiedebergs Arch. Pharmakol.* **272,** 89.
Schmid, R., and Lester, R. (1966). *In* "Glucuronic Acid: Free and Combined. Chemistry, Biochemistry, Pharmacology, and Medicine" (G. J. Dutton, ed.), pp. 493–506. Academic Press, New York.
Schmid, R., Buckingham, S., and Hammaker, L. (1959). *Amer. J. Dis. Child.* **98,** 631.
Schmidt, R., and Dedek, W. (1972). *Experientia* **28,** 56.
Schmiterlöw, C. G. (1965). *Amer. J. Vet. Res.* **26,** 539.
Schmiterlöw, C. G., Hansson, E, Appelgren, L.-E., and Hoffman, P. C. (1965). *In* "Isotopes in Experimental Pharmacology" (L. J. Roth, ed.), pp. 75–89. Univ. of Chicago Press, Chicago, Illinois.

Schröter, W., and Eggeling, U. (1965). *Klin. Wochenschr.* **43**, 116.
Scott, T., Seakula, E., and Duckett, S. (1971). *Stain Technol.* **46**, 95.
Seeds, A. E. (1970). *Amer. J. Physiol.* **219**, 551.
Sereni, F. (1973). *Clin. Pharmacol. Ther.* **14**, Part 2, 662.
Shah, N. S., Neely, A. E., Shah, K. R., and Lawrence, R. S. (1973). *J. Pharmacol. Exp. Ther.* **184**, 489.
Sharp, H. L., and Mirkin, B. L. (1970). *Clin. Res.* **18**, 344 (abstr.).
Shindo, H., Takahashi, I., and Nakajima, E. (1971). *Chem. Pharm. Bull.* **19**, 513.
Shoeman, D. W., Kauffman, R. E., Azarnoff, D. L., and Boulos, B. M. (1972). *Biochem. Pharmacol.* **21**, 1237.
Short, C. R., and Davis, L. E. (1970). *J. Pharmacol. Exp. Ther.* **174**, 185.
Short, C. R., Maines, M. D., and Westfall, B. A. (1972). *Biol. Neonate* **21**, 54.
Sieber, S. M., and Fabro, S. (1971). *J. Pharmacol. Exp. Ther.* **176**, 65.
Sinha, A. A. (1971). *Z. Zellforsch Mikrosk. Anat.* **122**, 1.
Sjöqvist, F., Bergfors, P. G., Borgå, O., Lind, M., and Ygge, H. (1972). *J. Pediat.* **80**, 496.
Sjöstrand, S. E., and Schmiterlöw, C. G. (1968). *Arzneim.-Forsch.* **18**, 62.
Sjöstrand, S. E., Cassano, G. B., and Hansson, E. (1965). *Arch. Int. Pharmacodyn. Ther.* **156**, 34.
Skalko, R. G., and Morse, J. M. D. (1969). *Teratology* **2**, 57.
Slade, B. S. (1970). *J. Anat.* **107**, 531.
Slade, B., and Budd, S. (1972). *Biol. Neonate* **21**, 309.
Slade, B. S., and Wild, A. E. (1971). *Immunology* **20**, 217.
Smallwood, R. A., Lester, R., Piasecki, G. J., Klein, P. D., Greco, R., and Jackson, B. T. (1972). *J. Clin. Invest.* **51**, 1388.
Smith, M. W. (1970). *Experientia* **26**, 736.
Smith, N. C., and Brush, M. G. (1971). *J. Endocrinol.* **51**, 409.
Snell, G. D. (1941). *In* "Biology of the Laboratory Mouse" (G. D. Snell, ed.), 1st ed., pp. 1–54. McGraw-Hill (Blakiston Div.), New York.
Snell, G. D., and Stevens, L. C. (1966). *In* "Biology of the Laboratory Mouse" (E. L. Green, ed.), 2nd ed., pp. 205–245. McGraw Hill (Blakiston Div.), New York.
Söremark, R. (1960). *Acta Radiol., Suppl.* **190**, 1.
Söremark, R., and Hunt, V. R. (1966). *Int. J. Radiat. Biol.* **11**, 43.
Söremark, R., and Ullberg, S. (1960). *Int. J. Appl. Radiat. Isotop.* **8**, 192.
Söremark, R., and Ullberg, S. (1962). *In* "Use of Radioisotopes in Animal Biology and the Medical Sciences" (M. Fried, ed.), Vol. 2, pp. 103–114. Academic Press, New York.
Soyka, L. F. (1969). *Biochem. Pharmacol.* **18**, 1029.
Soyka, L. F. (1970). *Biochem. Pharmacol.* **19**, 945.
Stålhanske, T., Slanina, P., Tjälve, H., Hansson, E., and Schmiterlöw, C. G. (1969). *Acta Pharmacol. Toxicol.* **27**, 363.
Stephens, R. J., and Cabral, L. J. (1971). *Anat. Rec.* **171**, 293.
Stephens, R. J., and Easterbrook, N. (1968). *J. Ultrastruct. Res.* **24**, 239.
Stephens, R. J., and Easterbrook, N. (1969). *Amer. J. Anat.* **124**, 47.
Stephens, R. J., and Easterbrook, N. (1971). *Anat. Rec.* **169**, 207.
Stevens, L. (1962). *Comp. Biochem. Physiol.* **6**, 129.
Stiehl, A., Admirand, W. H., and Thaler, M. M. (1971). *Gastroenterology* **60**, 183 (abstr.).
Streeter, G. L. (1920). *Contrib. Embryol. Carnegie Inst.* **11**, 143.

Stumpf, W. E. (1968). *Science* **163,** 958.

Svartz, N. (1964). *Gastroenterologia* **101,** 145.

Sy, W. M., Rosen, H., Griffin, N. E., Fink, H., Vasicka, A., Lorber, S. A., and Solomon, N. A. (1972). *Radiology* **103,** 139.

Takahashi, G., and Yasuhira, K. (1973). *Cancer Res.* **33,** 23.

Takahashi, T., and Sato, Y. (1968). *Radioisotopes* **17,** 1.

Takahashi, T., Kimura, T., and Sato, Y. (1969). *Bitamin* **39,** 236.

Takahashi, T., Kimura, T., Sato, Y., Shiraki, H., and Ukita, T. (1971). *Eisei Kagaku* **17,** 93.

Taska, R. J., and Schoolar, J. C. (1972). *J. Pharmacol. Exp. Ther.* **183,** 427.

Taylor, I. M. (1972). *Experientia* **28,** 560.

Thaler, M. M. (1969). *Pediat. Res.* **3,** 355 (abstr.).

Thaler, M. M. (1970). *Science* **170,** 555.

Thaler, M. M., Gemes, D. L., and Bakken, A. F. (1972). *Pediat. Res.* **6,** 197.

Tjälve, H. (1972). *Toxicol. Appl. Pharmacol.* **23,** 216.

Tjälve, H., Hansson, E., and Schmiterlöw, C. G. (1968). *Acta Pharmacol. Toxicol.* **26,** 539.

Tomatis, L., Turusov, V., Guibbert, D., Duperray, B., Malaveille, C., and Pacheco, H. (1971). *J. Nat. Cancer Inst.* **47,** 645.

Tomlinson, G. A., and Yaffe, S. J. (1966). *Biochem. J.* **99,** 507.

Tubaro, E., and Bulgini, M. J. (1971). *Naunyn-Schmiedebergs Arch. Pharmakol.* **270,** 18.

Uher, J. (1969). *In* "The Foeto-Placental Unit" (A. Pecile and C. Finzi, eds.), Int. Congr. Ser. No. 183, pp. 240–254. Excerpta Med. Found., Amsterdam.

Ukita, T., Takeda, Y., Takahashi, T., Yoshikawa, M., Sato, Y., and Shiraki, H. (1969). *Symp. Drug Metab. Action, 1st, 1967,* pp. 32–42.

Ullberg, S. (1954a). *Acta Radiol., Suppl.* **118,** 1.

Ullberg, S. (1954b). *Proc. Soc. Exp. Biol. Med.* **85,** 550.

Ullberg, S. (1959). *Progr. Nucl. Energy* **2,** 29.

Ullberg, S. (1962). *Biochem. Pharmacol.* **9,** 29.

Ullberg, S. (1965). *In* "Isotopes in Experimental Pharmacology" (L. J. Roth, ed.), pp. 63–74. Univ. of Chicago Press, Chicago, Illinois.

Ullberg, S. (1973). *In* "Fetal Pharmacology" (L. O. Boréus, ed.), pp. 55–73. Raven, New York.

Ullberg, S., and Bengtsson, G. (1963). *Acta Endocrinol. (Copenhagen)* **43,** 75.

Ullberg, S., and Blomquist, L. (1968). *Acta Pharm. Suecica* **5,** 45.

Ullberg, S., and Ewaldsson, B. (1964). *Acta Radiol., Ther., Phys., Biol.* **2,** 24.

Ullberg, S., and Hammarström, L. (1969). *In* "Radioactive Isotopes in Pharmacology" (P. G. Waser and B. Glasson, eds.), pp. 225–241. Wiley (Interscience), New York.

Ullberg, S., Sörbo, B., and Clemedson, C.-J. (1961). *Acta Radiol.* **55,** 145.

Ullberg, S., Nelson, A., Kristoffersson, H., and Engstrom, A. (1962). *Acta Radiol.* **58,** 459.

Ullberg, S., Applegren, L.-E., Clemedson, C.-J., Ericsson, Y., Ewaldsson, B., Sörbo, G., and Söremark, R. (1964). *Biochem. Pharmacol.* **13,** 407.

Ullberg, S., Kristoffersson, H., Flodh, H., and Hanngren, Å. (1967). *Arch. Int. Pharmacodyn. Ther.* **167,** 431

Ullberg, S., Lindquist, N. G., and Sjöstrand, S. E. (1970). *Nature (London)* **227,** 1257.

Van der Kleijn, E. (1969a). *Arch. Int. Pharmacodyn. Ther.* **178,** 193.

Van der Kleijn, E. (1969b). *Arch. Int. Pharmacodyn. Ther.* **178**, 457.

Van der Kleijn, E. (1969c). *Arch. Int. Pharmacodyn. Ther.* **182**, 433.

Van der Kleijn, E., and Wijffels, C. C. G. (1971). *Arch. Int. Pharmacodyn. Ther.* **192**, 255.

van Leusden, H. A. I. M., Bakkeren, J. A. J. M., Zilliken, F., and Stolte, L. A. M. (1962). *Biochem. Biophys. Res. Commun.* **7**, 67.

Vapaatalo, H. I., Idänpään-Heikkilä, J. E., and Neuvonen, P. J. (1968). *Psychopharmacologia* **13**, 14.

Vest, M. F., and Rossier, R. (1963). *Ann. N.Y. Acad. Sci.* **111**, 183.

Vest, M. F., and Streiff, R. R. (1959). *Amer. J. Dis. Child.* **98**, 688.

Vishwakarma, P. (1962). *Fert. Steril.* **13**, 481.

Waddell, W. J. (1968). *J. Appl. Physiol.* **24**, 828.

Waddell, W. J. (1971a). *Teratology* **4**, 355.

Waddell, W. J. (1971b). *In* "Fundamentals of Drug Metabolism and Drug Disposition" (B. N. LaDu, H. G. Mandel, and E. L. Way, eds.), pp. 505–514. Williams & Wilkins, Baltimore, Maryland.

Waddell, W. J. (1972a). *Fed. Proc., Fed. Amer. Soc. Exp. Biol.* **31**, 52.

Waddell, W. J. (1972b). *Teratology* **5**, 219.

Waddell, W. J. (1973a). *Annu. Rev. Pharmacol.* **13**, 153.

Waddell, W. J. (1973b). *Drug. Metab. Disposition* **1**, 598.

Waddell, W. J., and Bates, R. G. (1969). *Physiol. Rev.* **49**, 285.

Waddell, W. J., and Marlowe, G. C. (1973). *Teratology* **7**, A29 (abstr.).

Waddell, W. J., and Mirkin, B. (1972). *Biochem. Pharmacol.* **21**, 547.

Waddell, W. J., Ullberg, S., and Marlowe, C. (1969). *Arch. Int. Physiol. Biochim.* **77**, 1.

Weiss, C. F., Glazko, A. J., and Weston, J. K. (1960). *N. Engl. J. Med.* **262**, 787.

Welch, R. M., Gommi, B., Alvares, A. P., and Conney, A. H. (1972). *Cancer Res.* **32**, 973.

Werner, H. (1971a). *Strahlentherapie* **141**, 86.

Werner, H. (1971b). *Strahlentherapie* **141**, 221.

Widdowson, E. M., Chan, H., Harrison, G. E., and Milner, R. D. G. (1972). *Biol. Neonate* **20**, 360.

Wild, A. E. (1970). *J. Embryol. Exp. Morphol.* **24**, 313.

Wild, A. E. (1971). *Immunology* **20**, 789.

Wild, A. E., Stauber, V. V., and Slade, B. S. (1972). *Z. Zellforsch. Mikrosk. Anat.* **123**, 168.

Wilson, J. (1967). "Conference on Pediatric Pharmacology," p. 34. U.S. Govt. Printing Office, Washington, D.C.

Wislocki, G. B., and Dempsey, E. W. (1955). *Anat. Rec.* **123**, 33.

Wislocki, G. B., and Padykula, H. A. (1953). *Amer. J. Anat.* **92**, 117.

Witschi, E. (1956). "Development of Vertebrates," pp. 405 and 498. Saunders, Philadelphia, Pennsylvania.

Woolley, D. E., and Talens, G. M. (1971). *Toxicol. Appl. Pharmacol.* **18**, 907.

Wykoff, M. H. (1971a). *Radiat. Res.* **47**, 628.

Wykoff, M. H. (1971b). *Radiat. Res.* **48**, 394.

Wynn, R. M., and French, G. L. (1968). *Obstet. Gynecol.* **31**, 759.

Wynn, R. M., Panigel, M., and MacLennon, A. H. (1971). *Amer. J. Obstet. Gynecol.* **109**, 638.

Yaffe, S. J., and Back, N. (1966). *Pediat. Clin. N. Amer.* **13**, 527.

Yaffe, S. J., Levy, G., Matsuzawa, T., and Baliah, T. (1966). *N. Engl. J. Med.* **275**, 1461.

Yaffe, S. J., Krasner, J., and Catz, C. S. (1968). *Ann. N.Y. Acad. Sci.* **151,** 887.
Yaffe, S. J., Rane, A., Sjöqvist, F., Boréus, L.-O., and Orrenius, S. (1970). *Life Sci.,* *Part II* **9,** 1189.
Yang, M. G., Krawford, K. S., Garcia, J. D., Wang, J. H. C., and Lei, K. Y. (1972). *Proc. Soc. Exp. Biol. Med.* **141,** 1004.
Yeh, S. Y., and Woods, L. A. (1970). *J. Pharmacol. Exp. Ther.* **174, 9.**
Yoshikawa, M., Takahashi, T., and Sato, Y. (1971). *Yakugaku Zasshi* **91,** 109.
Young, L. M., Mukherjee, A. B., Cohen, M. M., and Yaffe, S. J. (1972). *Res. Commun. Chem. Pathol. Pharmacol.* **3,** 579.
Zamboni, L. (1965). *J. Ultrastruct. Res.* **12,** 509.
Zarrow, M. X., Philpott, J. E., and Denenberg, V. H. (1970). *Nature (London)* **226,** 1058.
Zimmerman, E. F., and Bowen, D. (1972). *Teratology* **5,** 335.

4

Pharmacologically Induced Modifications of Behavioral and Neurochemical Development

John E. Thornburg
Kenneth E. Moore

I. Introduction

Do drugs which are administered (1) to the pregnant mother before or during delivery, (2) to the newborn infant, or (3) to the young child influence the subsequent behavior of the child? The initial aim in writing this chapter was to answer this question, but as will become evident an unequivocal answer is not possible at the present time. Teratological and perinatal toxicological effects of drugs in the central nervous system (CNS) are relatively easy to discern compared with potential subtle behavioral effects.* Nevertheless, drug-induced alterations of behavioral development may have important medical consequences.

Clinical studies in developmental neuro- or behavioral pharmacology are plagued by a variety of confounding variables—a small population base, ethical considerations, and inadequate controls. Except for experiments involving drugs which are used during labor and delivery most of the studies are retrospective in nature. Controlled experiments in animals, however, do suggest that perinatal drug administration can influence brain development and behavior in the developing animal. The overall objective of this chapter, therefore, has been to review information on the effects of drugs which, when administered during the pre- or postnatal periods, alter neuronal development and associated behavioral patterns in experimental animals and in man.

II. Developmental Brain Morphology

Morphological changes in the developing brain are, primarily, a result of genetically determined maturational processes. The brains of most species (e.g., mouse, rat, cat, rabbit, man) are morphologically immature at birth and increase in both weight and complexity during the postnatal period. These changes may be related, in part, to the development of sensory and motor capacities that necessitate more complex processing by neural circuits and an enlarged storage capacity for memory. The plasticity of the nervous system is most evident during these pre- and postnatal periods when the brain is susceptible to reorganization by external or internal factors. External events, in the form of sensory stimuli produced by the environment, can apparently influence the organization of neural circuits as reflected by environmentally induced morphological,

---

* The teratological and perinatal toxicological effects of drugs on the CNS were reviewed by Becker (1970) and are not considered here. No effort has been made to review the effects of hormones on brain development and behavior; readers interested in this topic should consult reviews by Levine and Mullins (1968), Schapiro (1971), Balazs *et al.* (1971), and Earys (1971).

chemical, and behavioral changes (Geller, 1971). Similar changes can be produced by exogenous chemicals; these are most dramatically evidenced by the teratological actions of chemical agents (Becker, 1970). As a background for discussion of the factors that alter behavior, a cursory review of morphological events that occur during the growth of the brain in the pre- and postnatal periods is presented.

Development of the central nervous system consists of a parallel series of morphological and biochemical events occurring in a genetically controlled sequential fashion. These events are remarkably similar from species to species, the major difference being the extent of maturation of the brain at the time of birth (Davison and Dobbing, 1968). Primitive, undifferentiated embryonic cells in the neural plate display no specialization or complexity but proliferate to form the neural tube. The posterior portion of this tube forms the spinal cord, the anterior portion forms the brain with the central lumen evolving into the central canal of the spinal cord and the cerebroventricular system of the brain. At the earliest stages of development, primitive matrix cells lining the neural tube produce only cells of their own type, but as development proceeds they give rise to early neuroblasts and subsequently to spongioblasts. Spongioblasts will eventually develop into glial cells whereas neuroblasts differentiate to form neurons. In the latter process initial changes occur in the nucleus and cytoplasm of the apolar neuroblasts. These cells become unipolar or bipolar and eventually dendrites and axons grow out of their perikarya. They develop synaptic contacts with other neurons and thereby establish the circuitry within the CNS. Differentiation of spongioblasts into astrocytes and oligodendrocytes occurs after neuronal formation is well advanced. A more detailed discussion of the ultrastructure of the developing nervous system is available in the review by Tennyson (1970).

The development of the brain may be broken down into fairly distinct but overlapping periods which are generally similar from species to species but differ with respect to time scale. The first period is one of cell multiplication, so that by the time of birth more than 90% of the adult complement of brain cells have been formed. These cells migrate to specific loci; their route of migration and eventual destination are fixed. The second period begins with accelerated growth of the nucleus and soma of the neuroblasts followed by the characteristic growth of axons and dendrites. This latter growth is directional and shows specificity with respect to the connections which are established between the terminals and the innervated structures. It is not clear what controls the migration of the neuroblasts and the subsequent growth of the axons, although some type of chemotaxis is generally proposed. The next step consists of the establishment of neural connections (synaptogenesis) and the formation of the circuitry of the CNS. This takes place in the neuropil, which makes up the major volume of the brain, and is composed of terminals, dendrites, and glial fibers.

The final period of CNS development is characterized by the growth of glial cells. Astrocytes, which are intermediary between nerve cells and capillaries, presumably play a role in the transportation of nutrients and waste products into and out of the brain. The postnatal increase in astrocytes may be related to the increasing metabolic demands of the maturing brain; maturation of these cells is related temporally with the reduction of the extracellular spaces, vascularization of the brain, and development of the blood–brain barrier (the barrier that serves to limit the transfer of many chemicals into and out of the brain). Oligodendroglial cells are responsible for the myelination of axons, and their increase is related to the progressive myelination of the brain after birth. Myelination, the process by which axons become enveloped by a proteolipid sheath, confers on the nerve fiber a lowered threshold, an increased conduction velocity, and an ability to carry repetitive impulses. It is associated temporally with an increase in the lipid content and a decrease in the water content of the brain. The chemistry of the brain after myelination closely resembles that of the adult brain, although there is continued growth of some brain regions, particularly of the spinal cord, to keep pace with the growth of body size. The time at which maturation stops and increase in size exclusively begins is approximately the fifth week in the rat and the first week in the guinea pig. Growth of the brain occurs primarily before growth of the body as a whole, so that the brain weight/body weight ratio decreases as the animal matures.

The growth of the rat cerebral cortex following birth has been studied in detail (see Caley and Maxwell, 1971); a brief review of these findings can serve as an example of a relationship of morphological structures to physiological activity in a developing brain structure. (For a similar account of the growth of the human brain, see Timiras et al., 1968.) During the first 10 days after birth the sizes of the perikaryon and the nucleus increase considerably. At the same time the packing density of the neurons decreases because of the extensive proliferation of the dendritic tree of pyramidal neurons and the invasion of axons. During this period the cerebral cortex contains few blood vessels although there are clusters of epithelial cells which by 10 days form primitive blood vessels filled with blood; by 12 days the blood vessels are covered with astrocytic feet which probably account, at least in part, for the characteristics of the blood–brain barrier. It is assumed that, before opening of the blood vessels, large extracellular spaces (approximately 10% of tissue volume from days 1–10) provide nutrition for the developing cortex. By 21 days the extracellular spaces are reduced to very narrow clefts between nerve processes by the growth of glia, and nutrition must be provided for by the blood vessels.

It is difficult to correlate the appearance of particular morphological structures with function, because the development of the cortex consists of progressive and parallel development of many structures. Action potential discharges can be detected by the fourth day. EEG activity, probably related to the development of the dendritic tree of cortical neurons, becomes demonstrable by day 6. During the first week of life, rats display integrated bulbospinal reflexes involved with respiration, cardiovascular control, breathing, crawling, sucking, and righting; these reflexes are due to the circuitry in the brain stem reticular formation which is relatively mature at birth (Scheibel and Scheibel, 1971). During the second week, behavior becomes more complex and spinal reflexes are diminished as a result of influences of inhibitory fibers descending from the cortex. By the third week, the cortex has developed into the adult form with tightly packed axons, dendrites, and glial processes.

The increase in dendritic growth of cells during brain development probably represents an increase in connections of neurons and, hence, an increase in functional capacity. Do these postnatal changes in brain morphology represent a late phase of maturation which is under strict genetic control or a plastic phase of structural organization contingent upon sensory input? Some studies suggest that the growth of the cortex can be influenced by the external (rats in enriched environment) and the internal (thyroid hormone) environment (Geller, 1971; Schapiro, 1971). Thus, chemical manipulation of the environment of growing dendritic connections can apparently influence synaptic connections, and this may be a mechanism by which drugs can alter behavior.

III. Developmental Brain Biochemistry

Much has been written about the general chemistry of the brain during development, particularly with regard to lipid and energy metabolism. Only a cursory review of general chemical events that accompany functional maturation of the CNS will be presented here, although the chemistry of putative transmitter substances will be considered in some detail (see Section VI). A few general points should be made, however, concerning the difficulties in interpreting chemical changes in the brain during development.

Interpretations of biochemical analyses of the adult brain are complicated by the morphological heterogeneity of the CNS, by the inaccessibility of the brain afforded by the skull and by the extreme lability of certain chemical elements (Moore, 1971). These problems are compounded in the development brain because of the changing characteristics in the local composition of cell bodies, axons, and glia, as a result of growth and myelination processes. Accordingly, it is difficult to decide upon the units that should be used to express chemical data—whole brain, wet weight, protein content, lipid content, or DNA content. There are disadvantages associated with the use of any single unit so that data are frequently reported on the basis of several different units. Other problems related to the biochemistry of the CNS in adult and infant organisms result from changes in diurnal or circadian rhythms and from different forms of enzymes and cofactors (Yuwiler, 1971).

A. Carbohydrates

During development there is a shift from anaerobic to aerobic metabolism of glucose, and this is mirrored by a change in the sensitivity of the brain to anoxia. Whereas the adult is extremely sensitive to oxygen deprivation, the newborn is resistant.

B. Lipids

In the fetus there is little difference between the lipid content of gray and white matter. The adult pattern of lipid content is attained after myelination during which glycosphingolipids markedly increase, particularly in white matter. Myelination does not occur in all regions of the brain concurrently; the spinal cord is myelinated before the medulla which in turn is myelinated before the cerebrum and cerebellum. The rat brain content of gangliosides, which are located predominantly within neurons, increases markedly from 4 days before birth until 18 days after birth; this corresponds to the period of enlargement of neurons and proliferation of dendrites and synaptic connections. Cerebrosides, which are concentrated in myelin, exhibit their major increase after the increase in gangliosides.

C. Nucleic Acids

The whole brain concentration of RNA and DNA is high during the early phase of development but gradually decreases as maturation proceeds. This decrease is attributable to a reduction in cell density as the neuropil increases in mass. The DNA content, since it is located almost exclusively within the nucleus, has been used to calculate the number and size of cells.

D. Proteins

There is a small increase in the protein concentration of the brain during development. This reflects, to some extent, brain growth but also a reduction in the water concentration and, therefore, an increase in the percentage of solid material in the brain.

E. Amino Acids

The brain contains a particularly high concentration of free amino acids. The functional significance of these amino acids is not known, although they do not appear to be exclusively concerned with protein synthesis. They may play a special role in the functioning of the fully integrated adult CNS. The free amino acid pool can be divided into groups depending on whether the amino acids increase, decrease, or show no change in concentration during development. The amino acids which decrease during development (tyrosine, tryptophan, phosphoethanolamine) are believed to participate in tissue protein synthesis, the reduction in concentration being an indication of utilization during protein synthesis. Amino acids which increase during development include glutamic acid, glutamine, aspartic acid, and γ-aminobutyric acid (GABA). In addition to participating to a small extent in protein synthesis these amino acids exert some control over the operation of the tricarboxylic acid cycle and perhaps have transmitter functions. Glycine, alanine, threonine, and glutamine concentrations do not change markedly during development. Changes in GABA content occurring during development will be considered in detail in Section VI,C, which deals with putative transmitter substances.

F. Electrolytes

Concentrations of sodium and chloride ions in extracellular spaces decrease progressively after birth whereas that of potassium, an intracellular ion, increases.

IV. Brain Plasticity and Critical Periods

Prior to the twentieth century, structural plasticity of the brain was a generally accepted phenomenon. It was felt that growth of brain regions could be altered by "exercise" or "mental activity." Since the beginning of the twentieth century maturation of the brain has been generally believed to be under the primary control of genetic factors. Nevertheless, physical and chemical influences appear to alter morphological features of the brain throughout adult life (Rosenzweig et al., 1968). Altman (1970) has suggested that although cell proliferation, migration, and differentiation are primarily active in the pre- and early postnatal periods, this activity continues in glia and microneurons in some brain regions into adulthood. Altman divided the construction of the CNS into stages of plasticity and stability. Prenatal differentiation of large neurons is morphogenetically determined with fixed afferent, relay, and efferent connections; this represents a rather rigid or stable phase of development. The subsequent postnatal formation of dendrites, terminals, and synaptic contacts represents a dynamic and flexible feature of structural organization which can be influenced by a variety of internal and external factors. Upon the envelopment of these neuronal processes with glia and myelin, relatively stable interrelationships are established which are more resistant to modifying influences. Nevertheless, some plasticity, which accounts for modifications associated with learning, must continue throughout life.

The concept of brain plasticity is often discussed in terms of "critical periods," intervals of time during which there are rapid changes in morphological, biochemical, and physiological maturation of the brain occurring in a temporally related fashion. Intervals of rapid change have also been described as "vulnerable periods," because some components of the brain are particularly sensitive to internal and environmental influences at these times (e.g., nutritional deficiencies—Davison and Dobbing, 1968; hormonal influences—Schapiro, 1971). Although this concept is useful in some contexts (imprinting of following behavior in precocial birds can be established only during a brief period shortly after hatching), patterns of most chemical events occur in a smooth sequential manner. Critical periods of chemical maturation are most clearly defined in small animals that have short life spans and correspondingly rapid periods of development; in other animals that have long development periods, such as man, critical periods are not as prominent. Critical periods of behavioral development may (Schapiro, 1971) or may not (Werboff, 1970) be valid.

Critical periods of chemical development in the CNS may be masked as a result of the heterogeneity of the brain. Heterogeneity results from regional gross anatomic differences, and, at a very local level, from the intermingling of many cell types and structures in even the smallest circumscribed locus. This poses special problems when the ontogeny of the

CNS is examined. At the local level, various cellular components mature at different times (e.g., axons before dendrites, neurons before glia). There are also marked regional differences; neuronal maturation in the reticular formation of the medulla occurs before maturation in subcortical and cortical regions. In addition to artifacts that are inherent in the chemical analysis of the brain resulting from heterogeneity, complications due to circadian rhythm must also be considered. It is now recognized that enzyme activities and the contents of certain chemicals in the brain change in rhythmic cycles. Thus, superimposed upon changes in ontogeny are the changes resulting from circadian rhythms which, unless they are recognized and accounted for, may mask "critical periods" and confound the interpretation of chemical measurements during various periods of development.

Although heterogeneity of the brain poses special problems for chemical analyses, it becomes more of a problem when attempts are made to relate chemical changes with physiological or behavioral events. For example, with electrical recordings from circumscribed regions it is not always possible to identify the cells responsible for the recorded electrical events. This difficulty is magnified manyfold when attempts are made to relate chemical changes in the whole brain or even in various regions with behavioral activity of the whole animal.

V. Memory

If the administration of drugs during pre- or postnatal periods alters subsequent behavior patterns, then some long-lasting change must have taken place in the brain to effect these alterations. "Engram" or "memory trace" are terms used to describe changes in the characteristics of nerve cells which account for the persistence of memory. Hypothetical engrams can be divided into two major categories: functional and structural. (For other classifications see Nelson, 1967.)

The functional hypothesis assumes that information is stored by changes in neural activity without accompanying changes in morphological structure of the neuron or of neuronal interconnections. For example, sensory input could establish reverberating circuits of neuronal activity which would persevere and thereby cause information to be retained. Such a process may be important for the consolidation of newly acquired information since interruption of electrical activity in these postulated circuits by anesthesia or electroconvulsive shock can influence short-term memory. Similar interruptions do not interfere with long-term memory.

The structural hypothesis of engram assumes that memory is dependent upon some permanent alteration in the structural characteristics of nerve cells; this change may involve an internal alteration in an individual neuron (molecular or chemical hypothesis) or an alteration in the interrelationships of neurons (morphological hypothesis). The molecular hypothesis proposes that there is a conformational change in stable macromolecules within nerve cells in response to learning procedures. For example, information may be initially coded in chromosomal DNA and subsequently transferred to cytoplasmic RNA and protein. Thus, the molecular hypothesis assumes that lasting molecular transformations are the basis for the preservation of memory; presumably these changes influence the activity of the neuron and thereby induce alterations in behavior patterns. The morphological hypothesis, on the other hand, suggests that during the consolidation of memory there are structural changes in the neural elements of cells or in the interrelationships of the neurons with other neurons and glial cells. Glial cells separate and support nerve cells and probably play a role in regulating the exchange of metabolites, electrolytes, and water between various compartments of the brain. Any change in glial function could alter the activity of neurons and thereby mediate memory functions. Other hypotheses propose that sensory information establishes new neural circuits as a result of altered synaptic contacts among neurons. Depending on the use or disuse of certain neurons or neural pathways there may be shrinking or swelling of nerve processes; synaptic contacts may change by the growth or withdrawal of dendritic spines or terminal boutons. Changes in pre- and postsynaptic membranes and in the short axon nerve cells located between various neuronal elements may be important (see Altman, 1967, 1970). Synaptic changes may not involve morphological alterations exclusively but may be explained on the basis of changing dynamics of chemical transmitter substances in the presynaptic terminals or altered transmitter receptor sensitivity on the postsynaptic membrane. At the present time, however, there is no unequivocal evidence in support of any particular hypothesis to explain memory; indeed the various hypotheses need not be mutually exclusive.

Antimetabolites have been used to block protein synthesis in an effort to disrupt the consolidation and retention of learned behavior (Agranoff, 1967). Experiments with these drugs are complex and difficult to interpret, because these drugs can cause generalized dysfunction of the brain (antimetabolites and alkylating agents have marked teratogenic effects but there is little evidence to suggest they produce specific behavioral effects).

Section VI focuses upon the ontogenetic development of processes involved with the transfer of information from one neuron to the next and thus with the dynamic properties of various putative transmitter substances in the CNS. There is much current interest in the involvement of these transmitter substances in the mediation of behavioral patterns and in drug effects, although there is little evidence to suggest that transmitter dynamics are altered as a consequence of learning.

VI. Putative Neurotransmitters in the Developing Brain

Neurotransmitter metabolism in the developing CNS is being actively investigated in many laboratories. The purposes of this discussion are (1) to evaluate the developmental data with respect to current concepts of normal, adult neurotransmitter metabolism and function; (2) to indicate the many problems facing researchers in this field; (3) to suggest directions for future research, particularly the need for correlative studies of behavioral and neurochemical development.

In general, this discussion considers only data pertaining to the developing mammalian CNS; data from human brain, however, are so limited as to preclude meaningful interpretation and are excluded. The many studies of neurotransmitter metabolism in the developing chick embryo and brain are included in Tables I and III–V but are discussed only in special instances.

A. Catecholamines (Dopamine and Norepinephrine)

The present knowledge of the development of central catecholaminergic neuronal systems, although primarily descriptive in nature, is more advanced than that of any other developing neurotransmitter system. Moreover, several investigators are now examining the biochemical dynamics and functional relationships of brain norepinephrine and dopamine in the developing nervous system. This discussion attempts to summarize the present state of knowledge, to point out critical information gaps regarding the catecholaminergic systems, and to indicate the possible utility of developing noradrenergic and dopaminergic neuronal systems as "models" in studies of mechanisms of drug action and basic neuronal regulation.

1. DISTRIBUTION AND LOCALIZATION

The availability of specific, sensitive techniques for estimating and visualizing catecholamine contents in the CNS is the primary reason for the relatively greater advances in the study of catecholamine function than of other proposed neurotransmitters. The applications of bioassay, spectrophotofluorometric and gas chromatographic techniques, as well as histochemical fluorescence, electron microscopy–autoradiography, and density gradient centrifugation methodology to studies of catecholamines, have been adequately reviewed (Cooper et al., 1970).

Both dopamine and norepinephrine are localized within specific neurons in the CNS where they are stored in synaptic vesicles. Dopamine serves both as a precursor to norepinephrine and as a specific neurotransmitter substance in certain neuronal tracts. Both dopamine and norepinephrine have selective regional distributions within the brain. Norepinephrine is found in highest concentrations in the hypothalamus and limbic system, whereas about 85% of the brain content of dopamine is concentrated in the caudate nucleus and globus pallidus.

Dahlström and co-workers (Dahlström and Fuxe, 1965; Hillarp et al., 1966), by combining histochemical fluorescence techniques with the use of discrete brain lesions, have succeeded in mapping most monoamine-containing neurons in the CNS (also see Ungerstedt, 1971a). Most noradrenergic cell bodies lie in the medulla and pons with axons projecting both distally and rostrally. Although the absolute concentration of norepinephrine is apparently higher in nerve terminals than in cell bodies, the small and diffuse nature of many forebrain nerve terminals with norepinephrine contents below the resolving power of the technique has precluded their complete mapping. The nigrostriatal pathway is the major dopaminergic pathway in the brain. The cell bodies and nerve terminals of this pathway lie in the substantia nigra and basal ganglia (caudate nucleus, putamen, and globus pallidus), respectively (Ungerstedt, 1971a). Marked degeneration of this pathway is a major characteristic of Parkinson's disease. The tuberoinfundibular pathway is a dopaminergic system which may be important in the regulation of certain hormones of the pituitary gland.

The developmental patterns of whole brain catecholamine contents and enzymes involved in their synthesis and metabolism have been reported for the rat, mouse, cat, rabbit, guinea pig, and chick (Table I). There is a major species-dependent maturational pattern; the precocial guinea pig and chick have nearly adult brain contents of norepinephrine and dopamine at birth, whereas the newborn rat, mouse, cat, and rabbit are relatively immature and have correspondingly low brain amine contents. In the rat, (Fig. 1) the brain concentrations of norepinephrine, expressed as $\mu g/gm$, were about 20% of adult values in the newborn and gradually increased to adult values by 5–7 weeks (Karki et al., 1962; Agrawal et al., 1966a; Breese and Taylor, 1972). When norepinephrine values were expressed as absolute amounts per brain rather than as concentrations,

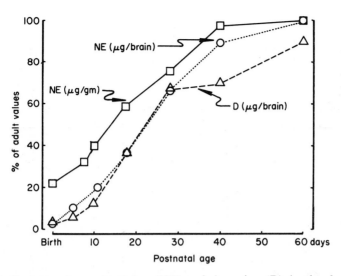

FIG. 1. Contents of norepinephrine (NE) and dopamine (D) in the developing rat brain. (After Breese and Traylor, 1972.)

adult values were attained somewhat later. Using a radiometric catechol-O-methyltransferase assay capable of detecting 100 pg of catecholamines, Coyle and Henry (1973) were able to detect these amines in the rat brain as early as day 15 of gestation. Both norepinephrine and dopamine increased 15-fold during the last week of gestation.

Maturation of the dopamine and norepinephrine contents of rat brain progresses in a distinct caudal to rostral direction. As indicated in Fig. 2, the adult concentration of norepinephrine in the medulla pons was attained earlier than in the more rostral mes–diencephalon and telencephalon (Loizou and Salt, 1970). Similar patterns of regional development have been reported for the cat (Pscheidt and Himwich, 1966) and rabbit (Himwich et al., 1967). Other putative neurotransmitters and their respective biosynthetic enzymes all exhibit caudal to rostral patterns of maturation in the brain. Clearly then, analysis of whole brain contents of norepinephrine and other substances may mask important differences among brain regions.

With respect to noradrenergic neurons, a caudal to rostral pattern suggests that maturation of cell bodies localized primarily in the pons medulla precedes that of nerve terminals, which are found mainly in the forebrain. Assuming that functional activity of the neurons is dependent on operational nerve terminals, it is of critical importance to distinguish between the presence of norepinephrine in terminals as opposed to cell

TABLE I Summary of Developmental Studies of Central Catecholaminergic Neuronal Systems

	Parameter measured[a]									
Species	NE	DA	T-OH	AAD	D-βH	MAO	COMT	NE*	Tissue analyzed	Reference
Rat	+			+		+			Whole brain	Karki et al., 1962
				+		+			Whole brain; 5HT as substrate	Bennett and Giarman, 1965
	+	+							Whole brain	Agrawal et al., 1966a
								+	Hypothalmohypophyseal system	Björklund et al., 1968
								+	Hypothalmohypophyseal system	Hyyppä, 1969
	+								Whole brain	Agrawal and Himwich, 1970
	+	+							Brain regions	Hyyppä, 1971
								+	Hypothalmohypophyseal system	Smith and Simpson, 1970
	+	+							Medulla pons, telencephalon	Loizou and Salt, 1970
	+								Whole brain; circadian rhythm	Asano, 1971
								+	Hypothalmohypophyseal system	Loizou, 1971b
		+	+						Caudate nucleus	McGeer et al., 1971
	+	+	+	+	+	+			Whole brain; regions	Porcher and Heller, 1972
			+			+	+		Whole brain; electrophoretic patterns	Shih and Eiduson, 1971
	+	+							Whole brain	Breese and Traylor, 1972
	+	+			+				Brain regions	Coyle and Axelrod, 1972a
	+	+							Brain regions	Coyle and Henry, 1973

	Measurement	Reference
	Brain regions; subcellular distribution	Coyle and Axelrod, 1972b
	Whole brain	Ghosh and Guha, 1972
	Brain regions	Weiner and Ganong, 1972
	Brain stem	Robinson, 1968
	Brain regions	Kellogg et al., 1973
	Brain regions	Lamprecht and Coyle, 1972
Mouse	Whole brain	Agrawal et al., 1968a
	Hypothalamus	Enemar and Falck, 1968
	Whole brain	Pryor, 1968
Rabbit	Brain regions	McCaman and Aprison, 1964
	Brain regions	Himwich et al., 1967
Guinea pig	Newborn vs adult whole brain	Karki et al., 1962
Cat	Brain regions	Pscheidt and Himwich, 1966
	Brain regions	McGeer et al., 1967
	Brain regions	Himwich et al., 1967
	Caudate nucleus	Connor and Neff, 1970
Chick	Whole brain	Bourne, 1965
	Whole brain	Pscheidt and Taimimie, 1966
	Whole brain	Ignarro and Shideman, 1968
	Whole brain	Watts et al., 1969
	Brain regions	Eiduson, 1971
	Brain regions	Kobayashi and Eiduson, 1970
	Spinal cord	Filogamo et al., 1971

a +, indicates that data were presented for the respective amine or enzyme activity. NE, norepinephrine; DA, dopamine; T-OH, tyrosine hydroxylase; AAD, aromatic-L-amino acid decarboxylase; D-βH, dopamine-β-hydroxylase; MAO, monoamine oxidase; COMT, catechol-O-methyltransferase; NE*, histochemical fluorescent localization of norepinephrine.

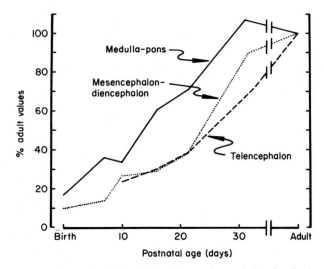

FIG. 2. Contents of norepinephrine in various regions of the developing rat brain. (After Loizou and Salt, 1970.)

bodies. Even so, the mere presence of the amine in nerve terminals cannot, on that basis alone, be equated with functional activity. Thus, the question of how to best express norepinephrine concentrations in developing animals may be of academic interest only.

Histochemical fluorescence studies of the ontogenesis of norepinephrine in the hypothalamohypophyseal systems of rat (Björklund et al., 1968; Hyyppä, 1969; Smith and Simpson, 1970; Loizou, 1971b) and mouse (Enemar and Falck, 1968) showed that norepinephrine was first detectable at birth, that cell bodies exhibited the earliest strong fluorescence, and that adult patterns were attained by 2–4 weeks. Loizou (1971b) found that adult fluorescence patterns occurred earlier in the pons medulla than in the forebrain regions of rat. All areas of the brain had attained the adult pattern by the fourth to fifth postnatal week. Thus, comparable ontogenetic patterns of brain norepinephrine contents are obtained by chemical and histochemical techniques. Histochemical fluorescent patterns of dopaminergic, noradrenergic, and serotonergic neuronal systems in discrete regions of the developing rat brain have been described (Loizou, 1971).

Eighty to ninety percent of the dopamine content in the CNS is located in dopaminergic nerve terminals in the basal ganglia, primarily in the caudate nucleus. Analysis of dopamine contents of whole rat brain suggests a time sequence of development that is slightly delayed but nevertheless similar to that for norepinephrine (Fig. 1). Loizou and Salt (1970) reported that rat mesencephalon had attained adult concentrations of dopamine at postnatal day 30, although the telencephalon contained only 50% of the adult concentration.

Using the Falck–Hillarp histochemical fluorescence technique, the nigrostriatal dopaminergic projection cannot be clearly discerned in adult brain. This projection can be distinguished, however, in the 14- to 17-day rat embryo (Golden, 1972; Olson et al., 1972; Loizou, 1972). By using the histochemical fluorescence technique in developing brain, it may be possible to better define other discrete monoaminergic pathways. In electron microscopic studies, Hattori and McGeer (1973) and Tennyson et al. (1972, 1973) were able to characterize morphological changes in numbers and types of synapses occurring during different stages of development of the nigrostriatal system.

Diurnal variations in norepinephrine and dopamine contents have been demonstrated in various brain regions of the rat (Manshardt and Wurtman, 1968; Friedman and Walker, 1968; Scheving et al., 1968) and cat (Reis and Wurtman, 1968; Reis et al., 1968). The rhythms in norepinephrine contents among several regions of cat brain are asynchronous and may show either a circadian or ultradian pattern (Reis et al., 1968). The mechanisms regulating such diurnal variation in amine contents are not understood. Nor it is clear whether or not the rhythms in norepinephrine and dopamine contents are related functionally to rhythmic physiological processes such as sleep, locomotor activity, and plasma concentrations of corticosterone and other hormones. Correlative studies on the developmental patterns of the diurnal variation in brain amine contents and rhythmic physiological processes are one means of examining such questions. Asano (1971) used this approach to examine the relationship between metabolism of brain norepinephrine and 5-hydroxytryptamine and the mechanisms for spontaneous locomotor activity and sleep–wakefulness patterns in the rat. Unfortunately, Asano analyzed only whole brain contents of norepinephrine and 5-hydroxytryptamine and only superficially examined the sleep and locomotor activity patterns. To date no other study has examined the development of diurnal rhythms of either norepinephrine or dopamine contents of brain.

2. SYNTHESIS

The biosynthetic pathway of norepinephrine and dopamine is illustrated in Fig. 3. Tyrosine hydroxylase and dopamine-β-hydroxylase are located exclusively in catecholamine-containing neurons, whereas aromatic L-amino acid decarboxylase is not so restricted in distribution. Tyrosine hydroxylase is the rate-limiting enzyme in the pathway and is

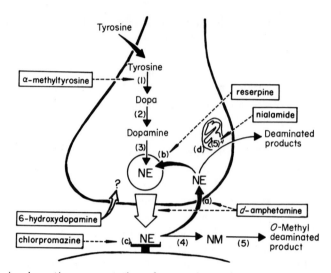

Fig. 3. A schematic representation of a noradrenergic synapse depicting probable sites of action of some of the drugs discussed in the text. Numbers represent reactions catalyzed by the following enzymes: (1) tyrosine hydroxylase, (2) aromatic L-amino acid decarboxylase, (3) dopamine-β-hydroxylase, (4) catechol-O-methyltransferase, (5) monoamine oxidase. The letters identify sites of (a) NE transport mechanism in the membrane of the presynaptic nerve terminal, (b) NE transport mechanism in the synaptic vesicle, (c) NE receptor on the postsynaptic neuronal membrane, (d) mitochondrion. NE, norepinephrine; NM, normetanephrine. For additional details, see text or Moore, 1971.

controlled, in part, by end-product inhibition (Udenfriend, 1966; Weiner and Rabadjija, 1968). The properties of tyrosine hydroxylase were reviewed by Moore and Dominic (1971). Coyle and Axelrod (1972a) have adapted a specific and sensitive assay for dopamine-β-hydroxylase activity (Molinoff et al., 1971) to brain tissue. In rat brain, 95% of dopamine-β-hydroxylase activity was found tightly bound to noradrenergic synaptic vesicular membranes (Coyle and Axelrod, 1972a).

Both tyrosine hydroxylase and dopamine-β-hydroxylase activities were detected by day 15 of gestation in the rat using the sensitive assays recently developed by Coyle and Axelrod (1972a,b). During this early developmental period (up to postnatal day 5), increases in tyrosine hydroxylase and dopamine-β-hydroxylase preceded those in norepinephrine contents. Subsequent development of both enzyme activities, however, paralleled the increases of norepinephrine contents (Coyle and Axelrod, 1972a,b). McGeer et al. (1967) found that the brain concentration of tyrosine remained constant throughout postnatal life, suggesting that substrate availability is not the rate-limiting factor in norepinephrine synthesis in the neonate.

Analysis of the regional distributions of tyrosine hydroxylase and dopamine-β-hydroxylase in rat brain showed that the maturation of these enzymes, like that of the norepinephrine contents, proceeded in a caudal to rostral direction (Coyle and Axelrod, 1972a,b). For example, tyrosine hydroxylase activity of the brain stem had attained adult values at post-natal day 14, whereas activities of the cortex and corpus striatum were 43 and 74%, respectively, of adult values even at 28 days. The slow development of tyrosine hydroxylase in the corpus striatum observed by Coyle and Axelrod (1972b) contrasts with the report of McGeer et al. (1971) that the rat caudate nucleus achieved adult tyrosine hydroxylase activity by 20 days postnatally.

Changing ratios of the relative contributions of caudate nucleus and cerebral cortex to total kitten brain tyrosine hydroxylase activity during development emphasize the necessity to analyze specific brain regions in order to avoid gross errors in interpretation (McGeer et al., 1967). At birth, the cortex and caudate enzyme activities accounted for 20 and 40%, respectively, of total kitten brain tyrosine hydroxylase activity. By 10 days of age, each area contained 30% of total brain activity, and by 60 days, the caudate and cortex accounted for 55 and 30%, respectively. Importantly, tyrosine hydroxylase activities of the caudate and cortex represent those of dopaminergic and noradrenergic neurons, respectively.

Coyle and Axelrod (1972a,b) found that during development the proportions of total brain dopamine-β-hydroxylase and tyrosine hydroxylase activities found in the synaptosome (nerve-ending) fraction of brain increased markedly. Possibly, neuronal membranes were more fragile or labile in the newborn and, therefore, did not form intact, stable synaptosomes upon homogenization. Alternatively, the major fraction of dopamine-β-hydroxylase activity in the newborn was confined to cell bodies in the brain stem which do not form synaptosomes. Thus, the increasing proportion of bound, synaptosomal dopamine-β-hydroxylase activity occurring during development primarily reflects increasing neuronal differentiation with concomitant proliferation of nerve terminals. Although other evidence (see Section VI,A,6) suggests that noradrenergic and dopaminergic neuronal systems in the rat are partially functional at birth or shortly thereafter, one should not equate tyrosine hydroxylase or dopamine hydroxylase activities with functionality.

The development of aromatic L-amino acid decarboxylase has been examined in the rat, mouse, rabbit, and chick using L-dihydroxyphenylalanine (dopa) as substrate (Table I). Some error could result if different decarboxylase-containing neurons (5-hydroxytryptamine versus norepinephrine) develop at markedly different rates, since measurement of in vitro decarboxylation of dopa reflects general decarboxylase activity.

Nevertheless, since aromatic L-amino acid decarboxylase is probably never rate limiting, the consequences of such error are probably of little importance.

Bennett and Giarman (1965) first demonstrated that the developmental pattern of aromatic L-amino acid decarboxylase resembled that of many brain enzymes (see Flexner, 1955). A sharp rise in enzyme activity to 80% of adult activity at birth was followed by a slight fall and then a gradual rise to adult activity at about 6 weeks of age. Nevertheless, at birth, decarboxylase activities varied from 100% in the pons medulla and mes–diencephalon to 30 to 50% of adult values in the telencephalon.

3. Catabolism

Enzymatic inactivation is one means of terminating the postsynaptic actions of dopamine and norepinephrine, although reuptake into the presynaptic terminal is probably the primary mechanism under normal conditions. Passive diffusion of catecholamines away from the receptor region may also serve to limit the postsynaptic actions of these amines.

The major degradative enzymes for the catecholamines are monoamine oxidase and catechol-O-methyltransferase, which catalyze oxidative deamination and O-methylation reactions, respectively (Fig. 3). The unstable aldehyde product of the monoamine oxidase-catalyzed reaction is then further oxidized or reduced to the corresponding acid or alcohol products, the predominance of which can vary with the metabolic conditions but which is primarily species dependent. In rat brain, the major end products of norepinephrine metabolism are the alcohols, 3-methoxy-4-hydroxphenylethylglycol and 3,4-dihydroxyphenylglycol; dopamine is converted to the acid metabolites, homovanillic acid and 3,4-dihydroxyphenylacetic acid.

The functional importance of these enzymes remains poorly understood. Inactivation of either monoamine oxidase or catechol-O-methyltransferase does not drastically alter the synaptic actions of norepinephrine at sympathetic neuroeffector junctions, suggesting that enzymatic inactivation is not important for terminating the synaptic actions of this amine. Particularly in the CNS, the anatomic localizations of monoamine oxidase and catechol-O-methyltransferase are poorly understood. Moreover, recent evidence suggesting several isozymic forms of monoamine oxidase further complicates the situation (Eiduson, 1966).

The ontogenesis of monoamine oxidase activity of brain has been studied by several investigators (see Table I). Bennett and Giarman (1965) found that monoamine oxidase activity in rat brain increased threefold after birth to attain adult activity by postnatal day 21. In the pons medulla of the rat, enzyme activity was equal to or greater than adult values throughout the postnatal period, suggesting a caudal to rostral pattern of development (Porcher and Heller, 1972). Loizou (1971a) demonstrated that treatment with nialamide, a monoamine oxidase inhibitor, increased norepinephrine-related fluorescence in the newborn rat brain, suggesting that monoamine oxidase is important functionally in the newborn. In the precocial guinea pig and chick, brain monoamine oxidase activity was equivalent to adult activity (Eiduson, 1966).

Shih and Eiduson (1969, 1971), using a disc gel electrophoresis technique, detected more isozymes of monoamine oxidase in adult than in embryonic or newborn chick brain regardless of the amine employed as substrate. Marked differences in substrate specificity were noted, however. As Shih and Eiduson pointed out, it remains to be proved that multiple forms of monoamine oxidase are not artifacts of the methodology. Further analysis of the developmental patterns of the isozymes may substantiate or disprove their authenticity and aid in defining their functional roles.

Porcher and Heller (1972) studied the developmental pattern of catechol-O-methyltransferase in rat brain. The enzyme activity was similar in all brain regions examined and, if expressed as activity per milligram protein, was equal to or greater than adult activity throughout the postnatal period. Thus, maturation of catechol-O-methyltransferase activity preceded that of monoamine oxidase activity. The formation of norepinephrine metabolites in the developing brain has been reported only in the chick (Kellogg et al., 1971).

4. STORAGE, UPTAKE, AND RELEASE

Current concepts of catecholamine storage, uptake, and release in the CNS are based on studies at peripheral sympathetic sites and the adrenal medulla. The available information, however, suggests that these concepts apply to dopaminergic and noradrenergic neurons in the CNS (see review by Glowinski, 1970).

At least two separate uptake processes occur at catecholamine-containing synapses. Uptake at the neuronal membrane is an energy-requiring, stereospecific, reserpine-insensitive process and is considered the chief mechanism for terminating the postsynaptic actions of norepinephrine and dopamine; this process is blocked by cocaine, imipramine, amphetamine, and many other drugs (Fig. 3). The synaptic vesicular membrane possess a distinct uptake mechanism, which also requires adenosine triphosphate (ATP) but is reserpine sensitive.

In the developing CNS, uptake of labeled norepinephrine has been examined using *in vitro* preparations of developing rat brain (Coyle and Axelrod, 1971) and of chicken embryo cerebral cortex (Kellogg et al., 1971). In the rat brain preparation, a saturable uptake was first demonstrable at 18 days of gestation. The K_m for uptake remained constant after this time, whereas the V_{max} for uptake increased fivefold between 18 days of gestation and 28 days postnatally. Thus, the developmental pattern of saturable uptake paralleled but slightly preceded that of the endogenous norepinephrine contents. Both the increasing V_{max}, which may represent the number of available transport sites, and the norepinephrine content may reflect an increased proliferation of noradrenergic terminals. Using a histochemical fluorescence technique, Loizou (1971a) found that rat hypothalamic neurons were capable of storing exogenous dopa or norepinephrine at 2–3 days postnatal age.

Data of Coyle and Axelrod indicate that development of the norepinephrine uptake mechanism at the neuronal membrane occurs earlier than development of the intraneuronal storage capacity. For example, reserpine exerted a progressively greater inhibition of norepinephrine accumulation up to 28 days postnatally in the rat. In contrast, the degree of desipramine- or cocaine-induced inhibition of norepinephrine uptake was constant after 18 days gestational age. Also, the development of the storage mechanism for norepinephrine and the endogenous norepinephrine contents of brain occurred in close parallel. The intraneuronal binding of norepinephrine may require the presence of a specific binding protein as suggested by the studies of Mirkin (1972, 1974) in fetal and neonatal rats. These proteins are not detectable prior to the time uptake can be demonstrated, however their definitive role in the storage process remains to be defined.

5. DYNAMICS

Measurement of the endogenous steady-state concentrations of catecholamines yields little insight into the dynamic state of the neuronal metabolism of the amines. Recognition of this fact spurred the development of several techniques for estimating *in vivo* the synthesis or turnover rates of norepinephrine and dopamine in the CNS. The turnover rate of an amine appears to be related to the functional activity of a neuronal population that utilizes the amine as a neurotransmitter. Brain catecholamine turnover rates may be calculated by determining (1) the initial rate of decline in the concentration of catecholamines following inhibition of synthesis by α-methyltyrosine, (2) the rate of decay of specific activity of catecholamines following intraventricular administration of labeled dopamine and norepinephrine, (3) the rate of conversion of labeled tyrosine to catecholamines. A critical discussion of the advantages and disadvantages of each method can be found in a review (Costa, 1969).

Little is known about the dynamics of catecholaminergic neuronal populations in the CNS at various stages of development. An attempt to label endogenous brain catecholamine stores of 20-day-old rat fetuses by administering ^{3}H-tyrosine to the mother resulted in negligible formation of norepinephrine. Similar administration of ^{3}H-dopa, however, resulted in greater formation of labeled norepinephrine and dopamine in fetal brains than in the brain of the mother (Lundborg and Kellogg, 1971; Kellogg and Lundborg, 1972). One might follow the accumulation of disappearance rates of ^{3}H-dopamine or ^{3}H-norepinephrine formed from ^{3}H-dopa after various hormonal, dietary, or environmental manipulations or after drug administration to the mother. Nevertheless, the use of dopa to label norepinephrine and dopamine pools is limited by problems in interpretation. First, ^{3}H-dopa bypasses the rate-limiting tyrosine hydroxylase step and thus may not accurately reflect alterations in synthesis rates. Second, the labeled dopamine and norepinephrine formed from dopa may not equilibrate with endogenous catecholamine stores due to formation of dopamine in serotonergic neurons or capillaries and incomplete mixing within dopamine and norepinephrine neurons. Since dopa is normally converted to dopamine immediately upon its formation from tyrosine, an artificially high proportion of the endogenous dopamine pools may be labeled unless tracer doses are employed. These problems related to nonspecificity appear to be more serious in studies of dopaminergic function; if one simply follows the rate of disappearance of ^{3}H-norepinephrine, the use of ^{3}H-dopa is less questionable.

During postnatal development, determination of conversion rates of labeled tyrosine to dopamine and norepinephrine should yield valuable information about the dynamics of norepinephrine metabolism in the developing animal. Some inferences about synthesis and control processes in the newborn can be drawn from recent studies using drugs such as 6-hydroxydopamine, α-methyltyrosine, reserpine, monoamine oxidase inhibitors, and amphetamine.

6. DRUG ACTIONS AT NORADRENERGIC AND DOPAMINERGIC SYNAPSES

A variety of drugs are available that either block or mimic and enhance noradrenergic and dopaminergic activity. To date only a few of these agents have been employed in developmental studies; their sites of action are indicated in Fig. 3 (for a review, see Moore, 1971; Cooper et al., 1970).

α-Methyltyrosine inhibits tyrosine hydroxylase and thus reduces dopamine and norepinephrine concentrations both in the periphery and in brain (Weissman et al., 1966). The reduction of catecholamine contents in nerve terminals of adult rats is dependent upon nerve impulse conduction (Andén et al., 1966). Loizou (1971a) found that administration of α-methyltyrosine to the newborn rat markedly decreased brain catecholamine-related fluorescence in both cell bodies and the few observable nerve terminals. Depletion was faster in dopaminergic than in noradrenergic neurons. Also, neuronal contents of catecholamines in the newborn were gradually repleted, but this process was slower than in 7-day or older animals. These results suggest that catecholaminergic neurons of the newborn rat brain can synthesize the amines from tyrosine and possibly release catecholamines in response to nerve conduction to the terminals. Thus, Loizou (1971a) suggested that biochemical and functional differentiation precedes complete morphological differentiation of catecholaminergic neurons.

Rat brain catecholamine contents were likewise sensitive to reserpine from the time of initial observance of catecholamine fluorescence (Loizou, 1971a). Eleven-day-old rats were more sensitive to the catecholamine-depleting effects of reserpine (0.1 mg/kg i.p.) than were adult rats (Kulkarni and Shideman, 1966), perhaps due to an immature storage mechanism as suggested by Coyle and Axelrod (1971) and Kellogg et al. (1971). Reserpine, administered into the yolk sac of 3-day-old chick embryos decreased brain stem norepinephrine in week-old chicks and also delayed and decreased hatchability (Sparber and Shideman, 1968).

6-Hydroxydopamine produces a selective and long-lasting degeneration of catecholaminergic nerve terminals (Tranzer and Thoenen, 1968; Uretsky and Iversen, 1970). In effect, 6-hydroxydopamine administration causes a chemical sympathectomy or, if given intracisternally or intraventricularly, a selective loss of norepinephrine and dopamine-containing nerve terminals in the brain (Ungerstedt, 1968; Bloom et al., 1969). Recent studies have examined both peripheral (Angeletti and Levi-Montalcini, 1970; Angeletti, 1971) and central (Breese and Traylor, 1971, 1972; Clark et al., 1972; Lytle et al., 1971; Traylor and Breese, 1971) effects of 6-hydroxydopamine in developing rats.

Intracisternal administration of 6-hydroxydopamine to early postnatal rats reduced brain contents of dopamine and norepinephrine and produced a permanent deficit in rate of body growth (Breese and Traylor, 1972; Lytle et al., 1972; Smith et al., 1973). For example, 6-hydroxydopamine, administered intracisternally on postnatal day 7 or 14, caused reductions in brain dopamine and norepinephrine contents and tyrosine hydroxylase activity of at least 75%, which persisted for at least 50 days. Administration of 6-hydroxydopamine on day 7 but not on day 14 produced a permanent retardation in rate of body growth, suggesting the existence of a short, specific period when interference with noradrenergic or dopaminergic function results in long-lasting effects (Breese and Traylor, 1972). With appropriate treatment schedules dopamine or norepinephrine can be selectively depleted. For example, by pretreating neonatal rats with demethylimipramine to prevent uptake of 6-hydroxydopamine into noradrenergic terminals, Smith et al. (1973) produced a selective, long-lasting depletion of brain dopamine. These workers found that neonatal rats with depletion of dopamine alone or both dopamine and norepinephrine exhibited marked decrements in rate of body growth, consummatory behavior, acquisition of conditioned avoidance responding, and locomotor activity. Thus, dopamine appeared critical for the integrity of these behaviors. Animals with a selective depletion of brain norepinephrine exhibited enhanced acquisition of conditioned avoidance responding and hyperactivity.

Systemic administration of 6-hydroxydopamine to rats in one or more doses during the first postnatal week caused a long-lasting and marked depletion of norepinephrine content in the forebrain but an increase in the brain stem (Clark et al., 1972; Lew and Quay, 1971; Pappas and Sobrian, 1972; Singh and de Champlain 1972). Thus, it appears that the catecholaminergic cell bodies were relatively resistant to the effects of 6-hydroxydopamine under these conditions. Lytle and co-workers (1972) observed no effect on whole brain norepinephrine contents when 6-hydroxydopamine was administered intraperitoneally to newborn rats; perhaps a decrease in forebrain was masked by an increase in brain stem content. Sachs (1973) studied the development of the blood–brain barrier to 6-hydroxydopamine in the developing rat. She observed a rapid development of the barrier in the cerebral cortex between days 7 and 9; the barrier in the hypothalamus was relatively complete by day 5 and that in the spinal cord developed more slowly and never completely. Clark et al. (1972) found that systemic 6-hydroxydopamine treatment during development decreased nocturnal locomotor activity at 10 weeks of age. Exploratory behavior upon first exposure to a Y-runway was also reduced. These initial reports emphasize that 6-hydroxydopamine can be a valuable tool for investigating the functional roles of catecholamines during development.

6-Hydroxydopamine is proving to be a valuable tool for examining the recently discovered phenomena of noradrenergic axon regeneration and collateral sprouting (Katzman *et al.*, 1971; Björklund and Stenevi, 1971; Björklund *et al.*, 1971). Use of 6-hydroxydopamine avoids the trauma and subsequent gliosis associated with mechanical or electrolytic lesions (Nygren *et al.*, 1971). These latter authors used intraspinal 6-hydroxydopamine injections to examine regeneration of spinal noradrenergic neurons in both adult and developing rats. Such studies in developing animals may be used to elucidate the factors responsible not only for the sprouting phenomenon but also the normal maturation of nerve terminals and dendrites.

6-Hydroxydopamine is generally considered specific for catecholamine-containing neurons (Breese and Traylor, 1970; Uretsky and Iversen, 1970). Nevertheless, compensatory adjustments may occur in neurons impinging upon the affected catecholaminergic neurons. Such changes might be detected only by determination of synthesis rates or turnover rates in the appropriate neuronal systems. Nevertheless, Smith *et al.* (1973) found that treatment of neonates with 6-hydroxydopamine did not alter choline acetyltransferase or tryptophan hydroxylase activities.

Black *et al.* (1972) found that in the superior cervical ganglion of the immature mouse 6-hydroxydopamine treatment reduced not only the postsynaptic tyrosine hydroxylase activity but also choline acetyltransferase activity in the presynaptic nerve terminal. Thus, the postsynaptic adrenergic neurons appeared to regulate the biochemical maturation of presynaptic cholinergic nerve terminals. Conversely, decentralization of the developing mouse superior cervical ganglion reduced not only choline acetyltransferase activity but tyrosine hydroxylase activity as well, suggesting that the presynaptic nerve terminals regulated development of the postsynaptic adrenergic neurons (Black *et al.*, 1971). Thus, disruption of a discrete group of neurons also caused a disruption of an impinging group of neurons. Similar phenomena may occur in neurons of the developing CNS.

Administration to newborn rats of the monoamine oxidase inhibitors increased the norepinephrine content and catecholamine-related fluorescence in the brain, suggesting that monoamine oxidase is functional in the newborn rat (Karki *et al.*, 1962; Kulkarni and Shideman, 1968; Loizou, 1971a).

d-Amphetamine is thought to produce behavioral arousal by releasing or blocking reuptake of norepinephrine or dopamine at presynaptic nerve terminals in brain (Carr and Moore, 1969; Stein and Wise, 1969). Thus, it is interesting that amphetamine produces hyperactivity (Campbell *et al.*, 1969; Fibiger *et al.*, 1970) and gnawing (McGeer *et al.*, 1971) in rats less than 1 week old (see Section VIII,B). Apomorphine produces similar effects (Lal and Sourkes, 1973). This and other evidence that

TABLE II. Evidence for Functional Catecholaminergic Systems in Newborn Rat Brain

Evidence	Reference
1. Amphetamine, which in the adult is thought to act by releasing brain catecholamine, elicits a grawing response and hyperactivity in rats less than 1 week old	Campbell et al. (1969); McGeer et al. (1971)
2. α-Methyltyrosine inhibits tyrosine hydroxylase and causes a nerve impulse-dependent depletion of brain catecholamines in adults; it has the same effect in the newborn rats	Loizou (1971a)
3. Uptake of norepinephrine by rat brain synaptosomes shows some adult characteristics as early as day 19 of gestation (same K_m and similar sensitivity to desipramine, an inhibitor of neuronal membrane uptake)	Coyle and Axelrod (1971)
4. Responses to norepinephrine applied to cerebellar Purkinje cells using the microiontophoretic technique at postnatal days 1–3 suggest that chemosensitivity actually precedes synaptic development	Woodward et al. (1971)

central catecholaminergic neuronal systems are at least partially functional at birth and shortly thereafter is summarized in Table II.

B. 5-Hydroxytryptamine (Serotonin)

5-Hydroxytryptamine (serotonin) is a proposed CNS transmitter, possibly involved in sleep mechanisms (Jouvet, 1968; Koella, 1969), temperature regulation (Feldberg and Myers, 1964), and hormone release (Wurtman, 1971). Like the serotonin-containing neurons, the sleep, temperature, and hormone-releasing regulatory mechanisms are immature in most newborn mammals. Thus the developing organism may serve as a useful model for correlative studies of developing serotonergic metabolism with physiological and behavioral parameters.

In invertebrates, serotonin is vital for cleavage and early cellular differentiation (Baker and Quay, 1969). Evidence for similar functions of serotonin in mammals is not definitive. Notwithstanding, the present discussion will focus only on possible neurotransmitter or synaptic modulator functions of this amine. The development of central serotonergic functions has been reviewed by Tissari (1973).

1. DISTRIBUTION AND LOCALIZATION

In the CNS, the highest concentrations of serotonin are found in the hypothalamus, limbic structures, and basal ganglia (Bodanski et al.,

1957; Maickel *et al.*, 1968) and are localized in nerve terminals (Whittaker, 1959). Most serotonergic cell bodies lie in the midbrain raphe nuclei; their axons project both rostrally via the medial forebrain bundle to various forebrain structures and caudally to the spinal cord.

The developmental pattern of serotonin contents in brain has been described for several species (see Table III) and generally parallels that of brain catecholamine contents. Relatively immature neonates such as the rat, mouse, cat, and rabbit have low brain serotonin contents at birth, whereas the precocious guinea pig and chick possess nearly adult contents of the amine (Karki *et al.*, 1962; Smith *et al.*, 1963). Karki *et al.* (1962) found that the serotonin contents of rat brain increased sharply just prior to birth to 25% of the adult value, and had attained the adult value by 30–40 days of age (when expressed as µg/gm wet weight) or by 50–60 days (when expressed as absolute amount per brain).

Loizou and Salt (1970) found that in the rat brain the pons medulla and mes-diencephalon had attained adult contents of serotonin at 32 days, at which time telencephalic serotonin was only 68% of the concentration in mature brain (Fig. 4). A similar developmental pattern has been reported for kitten brain (Pscheidt and Himwich, 1966). The caudal to rostral developmental pattern indicates that maturation of cell bodies in the midbrain raphe nuclei precedes that of nerve terminals in forebrain structures. Unfortunately, histochemical fluorescence studies on the developmental patterns of brain contents of serotonin have not been reported.

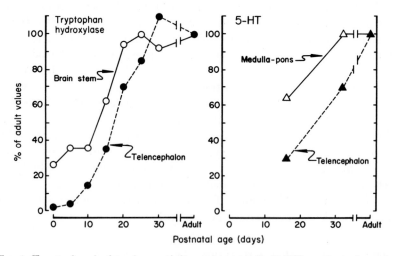

Fig. 4. Tryptophan hydroxylase activity and serotonin (5-HT) contents in various regions of the developing rat brain. (Values for tryptophan hydroxylase after Deguchi and Barchas, 1972; values for 5-HT after Loizou and Salt, 1970.)

TABLE III Summary of Developmental Studies of Central Serotonergic Neuronal Systems

Species	5-HT	Trp-OH	Trp	5-HIAA	MAO	AAD	Tissue analyzed	Reference
Rat	+						Whole brain	Pepeu and Giarman, 1962
	+				+		Whole brain	Nachmias, 1960
	+						Brain regions	Kurzepa and Bojanek, 1965
	+						Whole brain	Kato, 1960; Loizou and Salt, 1970
	+						Whole brain	Karki et al., 1962
						+	Circadian rhythm	Okada, 1971
	+						Whole brain	Smith et al., 1963
	+		+				Whole brain	Gornicki et al., 1963
			+	+			Whole brain	Tyce et al., 1964
	+			+	+	+	Whole brain	Bennett and Giarman, 1965
	+						Whole brain	Tissari and Pekkarinen, 1966
		+					Whole brain	Wapnir et al., 1971; Schmidt and Sanders-Bush, 1971
		+					Brain stem, cerebral cortex	Deguchi and Barchas, 1972
Mouse	+			+			Brain stem, cortex	Tissari, 1973
	+						Brain regions	Baker and Hoff, 1972
Chick	+				+		Whole brain	Bourne, 1965
	+						Whole brain	Pscheidt and Taimimie, 1966
	+					+	Brain regions	Eiduson, 1966

[a] + indicates that data were presented for the respective compound or enzyme activity: 5-HT, 5-hydroxytryptamine; Trp-OH, tryptophan hydroxylase; Trp, tryptophan; 5-HIAA, 5-hydroxyindoleacetic acid; MAO, monoamine oxidase; AAD, aromatic-L-amino acid decarboxylase.

2. SYNTHESIS

The biosynthetic and catabolic pathways for serotonin are depicted in Fig. 5. Tryptophan hydroxylase is generally considered to be the rate-limiting enzyme in the biosynthesis of serotonin (Grahame-Smith, 1964; Ashcroft *et al.*, 1965). Technical difficulties in the *in vitro* assay have, until recently, limited the study of this enzyme. In rat brain, the regional distribution of tryptophan hydroxylase activity parallels that of serotonin contents (Deguchi and Barchas, 1972).

In the developing rat brain, tryptophan hydroxylase activity increased sixfold between postnatal days 7 and 30 (Schmidt and Sanders-Bush, 1971). In the brain stem and telencephalon of the rat, the enzyme activity attained adult values at 3 and 4 weeks of age, respectively (Fig. 4; Deguchi and Barchas, 1972). Thus, development of brain tryptophan hydroxylase activity parallels that for serotonin contents (Loizou and Salt, 1970). Contrasting results were obtained by Wapnir *et al.* (1971) who found the major increase (four to fivefold) to occur from 2 days pre- to 2 days postpartum, reaching a value greater than adult enzyme activity. Methodological differences may account for the different results.

In the mature rat brain, the availability or uptake of tryptophan into neurons may normally control the rate of serotonin biosynthesis (Fern-

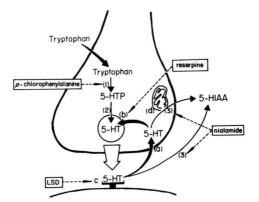

FIG. 5. A schematic representation of a serotonergic synapse depicting probable sites of action of some of the drugs discussed in the text. Numbers represent reactions catalyzed by the following enzymes: (1) tryptophan hydroxylase, (2) aromatic L-amino acid decarboxylase, (3) monoamine oxidase. The letters identify the sites of (a) 5-HT transport mechanism in the membrane of the presynaptic nerve terminal, (b) 5-HT transport mechanism in the synaptic vesicle, (c) 5-HT receptor on the postsynaptic neuronal membrane, (d) mitochondrion. 5-HT, 5-hydroxytryptamine or serotonin; 5-HTP, 5-hydroxytryptophan; 5-HIAA, 5-hydroxyindoleacetic acid; LSD, D-lysergic acid diethylamide. For additional details, see text or Moore, 1971.

strom and Wurtman, 1971; Grahame-Smith, 1971; Tagliamonte *et al.*, 1971). For example, elevation of brain tryptophan contents within normal limits by administration of small doses of tryptophan was associated with an increase in brain serotonin (Fernstrom and Wurtman, 1971). Moreover, drugs known to stimulate serotonin synthesis rates increased brain tryptophan concentrations (Tagliamonte *et al.*, 1971).

Tryptophan availability is evidently not rate limiting in the newborn rat, since the brain tryptophan concentration was threefold greater than in the adult (Gornicki *et al.*, 1963; Tyce *et al.*, 1964). Whether a similar pattern is observed in other species is not known.

In view of the high tryptophan and low serotonin contents in newborn rats, the gradual increase in tryptophan hydroxylase activity observed by Schmidt and Sanders-Bush (1971) would be the expected pattern. The relative importance of tryptophan availability versus tryptophan hydroxylase activity could be evaluated by a correlative study of tryptophan and serotonin contents and tryptophan hydroxylase activity in brain regions at various times during development and by determinations of synthesis rates of ^{14}C-serotonin from ^{14}C-tryptophan.

Bennett and Giarman (1965) reported that the developmental pattern of brain 5-hydroxytryptophan decarboxylase (aromatic L-amino acid decarboxylase) activity in the rat follows a time course similar to that of brain serotonin contents. Thus, a sharp rise in decarboxylase activity just prior to birth to 70–80% of adult activity was followed closely by a slight fall to about 60% and then a gradual increase to adult activity sometime after the fifth week.

3. Catabolism

In the brain, serotonin is oxidatively deaminated by monoamine oxidase to form 5-hydroxyindoleacetaldehyde, which is immediately converted to 5-hydroxyindoleacetic acid or 5-hydroxytryptophol by aldehyde or alcohol dehydrogenases, respectively. 5-Hydroxyindoleacetic acid, which accounts for greater than 90% of serotonin metabolized, is removed from brain by an active process blocked by probenecid (Neff and Tozer, 1968). The role of monoamine oxidase, relative to that of reuptake or diffusion, in terminating synaptic actions of serotonin is not clear. The observation that monoamine oxidase activity represents the composite of several isozymes (Eiduson, 1971) further hinders interpretation of the significance of developmental patterns of monoamine oxidase activity.

Bennett and Giarman (1965), using serotonin as substrate, found the development of monoamine oxidase activity in rat to have a pattern like that of many other brain enzymes (see Flexner, 1955). That is, monoamine oxidase increased sharply just prior to birth, fell slightly, and then gradually increased to nearly adult activity by 40 days. In the guinea pig brain, monoamine oxidase activity attained the adult value during the first postnatal week (Karki et al., 1962).

4. DYNAMICS

Turnover or synthesis rates of brain serotonin can be determined by several methods (see Costa, 1969; Costa and Neff, 1970) and provide an index of serotonergic neuronal activity. Such studies have not been done in young animals, however. Stimulation of serotonergic cell bodies in the raphe nuclei increased forebrain contents of 5-hydroxyindoleacetic acid (Sheard and Aghajanian, 1968; Kostowski and Giacolone, 1969). Thus, in the mature rat brain 5-hydroxyindoleacetic acid contents have been considered an index of ongoing serotonergic activity. It is interesting, therefore, that rat brain 5-hydroxyindoleacetic acid reportedly fluctuated little from birth to maturity (Tyce et al., 1964), although total plasma 5-hydroxyindoles increased from 10% of adult values at birth to adult concentrations by 21 days of age. The high 5-hydroxyindoleacetic acid concentrations in the newborn may result from (1) faster utilization of 5-hydroxytryptamine, (2) immature storage capacity and thus easier access to monoamine oxidase, (3) an undeveloped transport system for 5-hydroxyindoleacetic acid efflux from brain. Haber and Kamano (1964) found the percentage of total brain serotonin in the particulate fraction of a brain homogenate to be constant (75%) during postnatal life. In both newborn rabbits and rats, 5-hydroxyindoleacetic acid contents were relatively higher in brain stem than in cerebral cortex (Tissari and Pekkarinen, 1966).

Negative feedback control of serotonin biosynthesis in the CNS is not a physiologically important phenomenon, since following monoamine oxidase inhibition, serotonin contents increased two- to threefold before any demonstrable diminution in serotonin synthesis rates occurred (Tozer et al., 1966; Neff and Tozer, 1968; Macon et al., 1971). In addition to regulation by tryptophan availability, more subtle regulatory mechanisms related to neuronal firing may be operative in the control of serotonin synthesis. As suggested above, study of serotonin metabolism in developing animals may shed light not only on changes occurring during development but on the regulatory mechanism operative in the mature animal as well.

A high affinity neuronal membrane uptake system for serotonin present in cerebral tissue (Ross and Renyi, 1967; Shaskan and Snyder, 1970) most likely terminates synaptic actions of serotonin. Developmental aspects of this uptake system remain to be studied.

Study of the development of circadian rhythms in brain serotonin contents and related enzymes may lead to new insights regarding the controlling factors of serotonin metabolism. A circadian rhythm of serotonin concentrations in whole rat brain was evident at 3 weeks but it did not resemble the adult rhythm until 5 weeks postnatally (Asano, 1971; Okada, 1971). Studies examining only whole brain have little merit, however, in view of the unsynchronized circadian and ultradian rhythms in various regions of rat brain (Scapagnini et al., 1971; Friedman and Walker, 1968) and cat brain (Reis et al., 1969).

In conclusion, the developing animal offers a unique model for investigation of serotonin metabolism and function. Examples of questions which lend themselves to a developmental approach include: (1) What is the nature of the cell body–nerve terminal relationship? (2) What is the nature of the control of serotonin neuronal metabolism? (3) What is the role of serotonin in the ontogenesis of sleep patterns, temperature regulation, and certain behaviors?

5. Drug Actions at Serotonergic Synapses

The use of drugs as tools for examining possible roles of serotonin in the CNS has been generally disappointing owing primarily to lack of drug specificity. Reserpine, monoamine oxidase inhibitors, tricyclic antidepressants, and hallucinogens affect brain catecholamines as well as serotonin. Even 5-hydroxytryptophan does more than selectively increase brain serotonin contents, since it can be decarboxylated to form serotonin in catecholaminergic neurons resulting in norepinephrine and dopamine displacement with a "false transmitter." Originally p-chlorophenylalanine was reported to selectively deplete brain serotonin contents by inhibiting serotonin synthesis at the step catalyzed by tryptophan hydroxylase (Koe and Weissman, 1966). More recent studies, however, indicate the p-chlorophenylalanine causes significant initial alterations in brain norepinephrine and dopamine stores, at least in the rat (Miller et al., 1970). In general, attempts to correlate behavioral and biochemical actions of p-chlorophenylalanine have been disappointing, perhaps due to the effects of this drug on catecholamines as well as to nonspecific effects (Volicer, 1969; Thornburg and Moore, 1971).

Studies of D-lysergic acid diethylamide and methysergide on isolated smooth muscle preparations suggest that these drugs block postsynaptic receptors for serotonin. In the rat brain, D-lysergic acid diethylamide slows serotinin turnover rates, decreases raphé stimulation-induced increases in forebrain 5-hydroxyindoleacetic acid, and alters firing rates of raphé neurons upon iontophoretic application. These data are more consistent with a presynaptic or somal action than with a postsynaptic site of action in the CNS. Thus, use of D-lysergic acid diethylamide as a tool is hindered by a lack of knowledge of its mechanism of action.

By mechanisms presumably analogous to that of 6-hydroxydopamine on catecholaminergic neurons, 5,6-dihydroxytryptamine and 5,7-dihydroxytryptamine produce a long-lasting although modest depletion of the brain content of serotonin when injected into the lateral ventricles of rats (Baumgarten et al., 1971; Baumgarten and Lachenmayer, 1972). At present, the lack of specificity for serotonergic neurons and the low potency at nontoxic doses may limit the usefulness of these compounds, although appropriate combinations with monoamine oxidase inhibitors and/or tricyclic imipramine-like compounds may greatly enhance their utility. For the present, however, a deficit of serotonergic function is best achieved by lesions of the midbrain raphe nuclei.

C. γ-Aminobutyric Acid (GABA)

In the mammalian CNS, GABA may be both an inhibitory neurotransmitter and a vital intermediate in the "GABA shunt" (see Section VII,C,2). An inhibitory transmitter role for GABA has been demonstrated conclusively at the neuromuscular junction and stretch receptor neuron of crustacea (evidence reviewed by Cooper et al., 1970) but not at any one synapse in mammalian CNS. The precise metabolic function of the "GABA shunt" is not clear. With respect to possible roles of GABA in physiological functions and behavior, no clear relationships have been established. The metabolism of GABA in both adult and developing organisms has been reviewed (Roberts and Kuriyama, 1968; Baxter, 1970; Roberts, 1971).

1. Distribution and Localization

GABA is confined exclusively to the CNS in mammals. The distribution and localization of GABA lend support to the view that this compound is a CNS neurotransmitter. It has a discrete regional distribution; distinct layers of cerebellum and retina containing inhibitory neurons (Purkinje cells and amacrine cells, respectively) have the highest GABA contents of these particular structures. Exogenous GABA is preferentially concentrated in nerve-ending fractions of brain tissue although apparently not in synaptic vesicles (Iverson and Neal, 1968; Iversen and Snyder, 1968).

Nevertheless, GABA, unlike other proposed neurotransmitters, is found in glial cells as well as neurons (Utley, 1963; Wollerman and Devenyi, 1963) and occurs in relatively high concentrations in brain tissue (micromoles/gram compared to nanomoles/gram for monoamines, Fahn and Côté, 1968a). These facts, however, may merely reflect multiple functions of GABA. Lack of a specific, sensitive histochemical technique for localizing GABA has prevented anatomic identification of possible GABA-containing neuronal tracts. Autoradiographic localization of ³H-GABA following intraventricular administration may aid in delineating GABA-containing neurons (Schon and Iversen, 1972).

2. Synthesis and Metabolism

The pathways for the synthesis and metabolism of GABA are shown in Fig. 6. Glutamic acid, the immediate precursor of GABA, is formed in brain from glucose and represents an important energy source in brain via its entry into the tricarboxylic acid cycle. Glutamic acid enters the tricarboxylic acid cycle either by direct conversion to α-ketoglutarate or by entering the "GABA shunt." The metabolic significance of the "shunt" is not known, although possibly 10–40% of total brain metabolism funnels through the shunt (see Baxter, 1970).

GABA is formed only by α-decarboxylation of glutamic acid, a reaction catalyzed by glutamic acid decarboxylase. This enzyme, like GABA, is found concentrated in but not confined to a nerve-ending fraction of brain (Løvtrup, 1961; Salganicoff and DeRobertis, 1965; Fonnum, 1968).

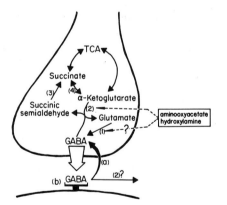

Fig. 6. A schematic representation of a GABA synapse depicting probable sites of action of some of the drugs discussed in the text. Numbers represent reactions catalyzed by the following enzymes: (1) glutamic acid decarboxylase, (2) GABA transaminase, (3) succinic semialdehyde dehydrogenase (steps 2 and 3 constitute the "GABA shunt"), (4) glutamic acid dehydrogenase. The letters represent the sites of (a) GABA transport mechanism in the presynaptic nerve terminal, (b) GABA receptor on the postsynaptic neuronal membrane. GABA, γ-aminobutyric acid; TCA, tricarboxylic acid cycle. For additional details, see text or Moore, 1971.

The developmental pattern of GABA contents of whole brain has been reported for the mouse, rat, kitten, dog, guinea pig, and chick (Table IV). Only the guinea pig has adult contents of GABA at birth. In other species, GABA concentrations increase two- to threefold postnatally, attaining adult values at various ages (see Himwich, 1962; Agrawal and Himwich, 1970). In the rabbit brain, GABA contents increase fastest at the time of a decrease in the proportional volume of dendrites. Timewise, the attainments of adult GABA levels and a mature EEG pattern correlate well (Schadé and Baxter, 1960). Nevertheless, the only value of such correlations lies in suggestions for future research. As Flexner (1955) clearly demonstrated, many unrelated events occur simultaneously during development, the challenge is in demonstrating cause and effect relationships.

GABA is one of a group of metabolically active amino acids including aspartic acid and glutamic acid that increase in concentration in brain during the period of postnatal maturation. Like GABA, glutamic acid and aspartic acid are both metabolically active and are also putative neurotransmitter substances. Concentrations of other amino acids decrease or remain constant during the postnatal period (Agrawal and Himwich, 1970; see Section III).

The developmental pattern of glutamic acid decarboxylase activity has been studied in the brain of the rabbit, rat, mouse, dog, guinea pig, and chick (Table IV). Postnatally, glutamic acid decarboxylase activity and GABA concentrations exhibit progressive, parallel increases until adult values are attained. In the embryonic chick cerebellum, the maximal increase in glutamic acid decarboxylase activity occurs at a time of maximal increase in nerve terminal proliferation but subsequent to the major rise in cerebellar weight and protein content (Roberts, 1971). Schadé and Baxter (1960), in a study of rabbit cerebral cortex morphology, found that the largest increase in glutamic acid decarboxylase activity occurs concomitantly with the major development of dendritic surface area. The above evidence suggests that glutamic acid decarboxylase is, to a large extent, localized in nerve terminals.

GABA is degraded in a transamination reaction with α-ketoglutarate catalyzed by GABA transaminase in which succinic semialdehyde and glutamate are formed. Succinic semialdehyde is then rapidly oxidized to succinic acid, a tricarboxylic acid cycle intermediate, in a reaction catalyzed by succinic semialdehyde dehydrogenase. Although the degradation of GABA is obviously important from a metabolic standpoint, its importance in terminating possible synaptic actions of GABA is less clear. Roberts (1971) proposed that in the chick cerebellum GABA is formed in

TABLE IV Summary of Developmental Studies of Central GABA-Containing Neuronal Systems

Species	Parameter measured[a]				Tissue analyzed	Reference
	GABA	GAD	GABA-T	SS-A		
Rat	+				Whole brain	Agrawal et al., 1966b
	++				Whole brain	Oja and Piha, 1966
	++	+++			Whole brain	Bayer and McMurray, 1967
		+++	+++		Whole brain	Van den Berg et al., 1965
		++	++	+	Whole brain	Sims and Pitts, 1970
					Whole brain	Van den Berg and Van Kempen, 1964
					Whole brain	Sims et al., 1968
				+	Whole brain; cerebellar layers	Pitts and Quick, 1967
Mouse	+++	++			Caudate nucleus	McGeer et al., 1971
	++				Whole brain	Roberts et al., 1951
Cat		++			Cerebral cortex	Berl, 1964; Berl and Purpura, 1963
Rabbit	+	++			Cerebral cortex	Schadé and Baxter, 1960
					Whole brain	Himwich, 1962
Guinea pig	+++				Whole brain; regions—newborn vs adult	Agrawal et al., 1968b
					Whole brain	Davis et al., 1968
Dog	+++	++			Whole brain	Himwich, 1962
					Whole brain	Dravid and Himwich, 1964
					Whole brain	Himwich, 1962
Chick	+	+++			Optic lobes cerebral cortex	Sisken et al., 1961
	+++				Whole brain	Van den Berg et al., 1965
			++		Cerebellum	Kuriyama et al., 1968
					Cerebellum	Roberts, 1971
	+++				Whole brain	Levi and Morisi, 1971

[a] + indicates that data were presented for GABA (γ-aminobutyric acid) or the respective enzyme activity: GAD, glutamic acid decarboxylase; GABA-T, GABA transaminase; SS-A, succinic semialdehyde dehydrogenase.

presynaptic structures (e.g., basket cells) and upon release is metabolized at postsynaptic sites (e.g., Purkinje cells) by GABA transaminase. Nevertheless, in a histochemical study of GABA transaminase activity in adult rat cerebellar cortex, the enzyme was present in all neural structures examined (Woodward et al., 1969a). Assuming that GABA has both metabolic and transmitter roles, however, ubiquity of the enzyme is only expected and cannot be taken as evidence that it is not involved in terminating synaptic actions of GABA. Recently Sims et al. (1972) developed a histochemical technique for localizing brain succinic semialdehyde dehydrogenase; this technique may prove valuable for delineating synapses mediated by GABA.

Nevertheless, a sodium-dependent, high affinity membrane transport system located at presynaptic nerve terminals may be the primary means of terminating transmitter actions of GABA (Iversen and Neal, 1968; Snyder et al., 1969). Demonstration of the importance of a membrane reuptake mechanism for GABA requires specific nontoxic inhibitors of the uptake mechanism, but to date none have been found (Iversen and Johnston, 1971). Exogenous GABA may be highly concentrated by non-GABA-containing neurons, thereby further complicating analysis of studies of GABA uptake (Snyder et al., 1969).

During development, changes in GABA transaminase activity parallel changes in glutamic acid decarboxylase activity in the rat (Van den Berg and Van Kempen, 1964; Sims et al., 1968) and chick (Roberts, 1971). Woodward et al. (1969a,b) demonstrated the presence of GABA transaminase histochemically in various types of neurons in the rat cerebellar cortex during the first postnatal week. Pitts and Quick (1967) determined succinic semialdehyde dehydrogenase activity during development in various layers of rat cerebellum. The ontogeny of neuronal uptake capacity for GABA in brain tissue has not been examined.

3. Dynamics

Study of the dynamics of GABA metabolism is presently subject to severe methodological limitations including (1) lack of sensitive histochemical or immunocytochemical techniques specific for GABA or glutamic acid decarboxylase, (2) lack of specific inhibitors of GABA synthesis, degradation, and uptake and possible postsynaptic actions, (3) lack of methodology for determining turnover or synthesis rates of GABA. This latter problem and the general interpretation of changes in GABA metabolism are due to the multiple pools of GABA which may serve very different functions.

Certain problems with current techniques are frequently overlooked.

For example, the GABA contents of fresh brain tissue increase 40–60% within 2 minutes after death (see Baxter, 1970). Studies of GABA contents in both adult and developing brain may be greatly affected by such postmortem alterations unless proper precautions are observed. Use of quick-freeze techniques or the microwave irradiation method of sacrifice (Schmidt et al., 1971, 1972) may eliminate this problem. The only means presently available to estimate capacity for GABA synthesis and degradation is based on in vitro assays for glutamic acid decarboxylase and GABA transaminase. In developmental studies, even relative changes in apparent enzyme activity may not represent the true in vivo situation because of differences in substrate or cofactor availability, immature regulatory mechanisms, or differences in enzyme stability.

Certain GABA-containing neuronal systems are particularly amenable to study, however. Both the adult and developing cerebellum of the rat and chick are well characterized with respect to morphology, electrophysiology, and cell localization. Importantly, specific types of neurons occur in well-defined patterns. With the development of more specific and sensitive methodology, very elegant studies of GABA metabolism and function in discrete cerebellar neuronal systems should be feasible. Woodward et al. (1969a) indicated that distinct correlations exist between electrophysiological and histochemical maturation of cerebellar Purkinje cells and the development of basic motor capabilities as described by Tilney (1933). Thus, future experiments may be able to establish the relative contribution of the cerebellar cortex, which may or may not involve GABA, to the ontogeny of motor function.

Several workers have proposed that GABA may regulate its own synthesis by end-product inhibition of glutamic acid decarboxylase (Haber et al., 1970; Sze et al., 1971; Sze, 1970; Sze and Lovell, 1970). Administration of aminooxyacetic acid, an inhibitor of GABA transaminase, to young mice resulted in an increase and subsequent decrease in brain GABA contents which were mirrored by a decrease and then an increase in glutamic acid decarboxylase activity (Sze, 1970). Glutamic acid decarboxylase of immature animals appeared to be more sensitive to GABA control than was the adult enzyme. Nevertheless, such a regulatory system would appear to be rather inefficient in rabbit cerebellum. Following aminooxyacetic acid administration, GABA contents doubled at 4 hours and then redoubled by 6 hours (Roberts and Kuriyama, 1968). No data were presented for glutamic acid decarboxylase activity after aminooxyacetic acid.

Since little is known about the dynamics of GABA metabolism in mature brain, it is not surprising that virtually nothing is known of GABA dynamics in developing brain.

4. DRUG ACTIONS AND GABA METABOLISM

A lack of specific inhibitors of glutamic acid decarboxylase and GABA transaminase has severely limited studies of GABA function (for review, see Baxter, 1970). Carbonyl trapping agents (hydroxylamine, thiosemicarbazide, and sulfhydryl reagents) are effective inhibitors *in vitro* but cause little alteration of GABA contents *in vivo*. Dietary deficiencies of pyridoxal phosphate (B_6) produce decreases in glutamic acid decarboxylase activity and GABA contents.

Certain GABA analogues and carbonyl trapping agents are effective inhibitors of GABA transaminase *in vitro*. Aminooxyacetic acid, which is active *in vivo* and appears to be surprisingly specific for GABA transaminase, has been utilized in many studies to produce elevated GABA concentrations. The functional significance of such elevated GABA contents is difficult to assess, however. For example, increased concentrations of GABA may inhibit its own synthesis (see above), possibly resulting in decreased availability of functional GABA.

D. *Acetylcholine*

Karczmar (1969) suggested that the central cholinergic nervous system may be overexploited in the sense of overinterpreting or misinterpreting data obtained by available methodology. Although perhaps overexploited in this sense, the dynamics of CNS acetylcholine metabolism and its functional roles remain relatively unknown because of methodological limitations. This is particularly true in studies of the developing central cholinergic nervous system (see Table V). Cholinergic function in the developing fetus has been reviewed by Karczmar *et al.* (1973).

1. DISTRIBUTION AND LOCALIZATION

Absolute identification of acetylcholine and other choline esters in brain tissue using a gas chromatography–mass spectrometry technique is now possible (Hammar *et al.*, 1968). This technique and other gas chromatographic procedures (see below) enable not only positive identification of acetylcholine in brain tissue and perfusates but also authentication or rejection of the presence of propionylcholine and other choline esters suggested by earlier methodology (Schmidt *et al.*, 1969; Jenden and Campbell, 1971).

Until recently acetylcholine was analyzed using often nonspecific bioassay techniques. The development of sensitive and specific gas chromatographic procedures (Stavinoha and Ryan, 1965; Hanin and Jenden,

TABLE V Summary of Developmental Studies of Central Cholinergic Neuronal Systems

Species	ACh	ChAc	AChE	ChE	Tissue analyzed	References
Rat	+				Brain regions	Westermann et al., 1970
		+	+		Caudate nucleus	McGeer et al., 1971
			+		Brain regions	Maletta et al., 1967
			+		Cerebral cortex	Gómez et al., 1970
			+	+	Brain regions	Elkes and Todrick, 1955; Maletta and Timiras, 1966
	+	+			Hypothalamohypophyseal system	Danilova, 1971
			+	+	Whole brain	Ladinsky et al., 1972
			+*		Brain regions	Nair and Bau, 1969
			+*	+*	Brain regions	Silver, 1967
		+*			Brain regions	Karczmar, 1963
		+	+		Caudate nucleus	Hattori and McGeer, 1973
Rabbit		+			Whole brain; brain regions	Hebb, 1956, 1957
		+	+			Himwich and Aprison, 1955
		+			Brain regions	Aprison and Himwich, 1954; McCaman and Aprison, 1964
Mouse		+	+	+	Whole brain	Pryor, 1968
Chick	+	+	+		Whole brain	Burdick and Strittmatter, 1965
			+		Whole brain	Iqbal and Talwar, 1971
		+*	+*	+*	Whole brain; brain regions	Filogamo and Marchisio, 1971

^{a} + indicates that data were presented for the respective substance: ACh, acetylcholine; ChAc, choline acetyltransferase; AChE, acetylcholinesterase; ChE, cholinesterase; * indicates a review discussing additional similar data.

1969; Schmidt *et al.*, 1970) and enzymatic radioassays (Feigenson and Saelens, 1969; Reid *et al.*, 1971) for acetylcholine and choline should enable specific measures of acetylcholine contents in discrete brain regions and, more importantly, permit determination of turnover rates of acetylcholine in brain tissue.

Another major problem in analysis of brain acetylcholine is that postmortem changes in the concentration of this compound result from less than instantaneous inactivation of choline acetyltransferase and acetylcholinesterase. Such changes are of critical importance in analysis of acetylcholine in discrete regions because of a time lag of up to 75 seconds in freezing deep brain structures even with liquid nitrogen (Takahashi and Aprison, 1964). Also, it is nearly impossible to accurately dissect frozen tissue. The microwave irradiation method of sacrifice first suggested by Stavinoha *et al.* (1970) and modified and extended by Schmidt *et al.* (1972) may prove best in terms of most rapid and complete enzyme inactivation and subsequent ease of dissection. At present, however, lack of quantitative comparisons of the different sacrifice techniques in combination with each of the newer assays for acetylcholine precludes a definitive statement as to the "best" combination of procedures. Possible strain differences and a diurnal rhythm in brain acetylcholine contents (Hanin *et al.*, 1970; Saito, 1971) must also be controlled. Acetylcholine concentrations are highest in the neostriatum and cerebral cortex and lowest in cerebellum and white matter (Schmidt *et al.*, 1972).

The lack of a histochemical method specific for acetylcholine has prevented mapping of cholinergic neuronal systems in the brain. Analysis of subcellular fractions after density gradient separation of brain homogenates suggests that acetylcholine is located in synaptic vesicles (De Robertis *et al.*, 1963) but that choline acetyltransferase is probably a cytoplasmic enzyme (see Potter, 1970).

Westermann *et al.* (1970) reported that, in the 5-day-old rat, whole brain concentrations of acetylcholine were 50 or 90% of adult values if expressed per unit wet weight of brain or milligram protein, respectively. Ladinsky *et al.* (1972) found the acetylcholine content of the 1-day-postpartum rat brain to be 73% of the adult value. Brain choline contents were significantly higher than in the adult from postnatal day 1 to day 20.

2. SYNTHESIS

Acetylcholine is formed in a reaction of choline with acetyl-CoA catalyzed by choline acetyltransferase (Fig. 7). The regional distribution of choline acetyltransferase parallels that of acetylcholine (Hebb, 1957;

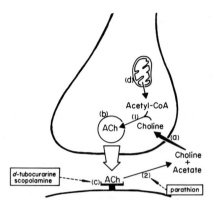

Fig. 7. A schematic representation of a cholinergic synapse depicting probable sites of action of some of the drugs discussed in the text. Numbers represent reactions catalyzed by the following enzymes: (1) choline acetyltransferase, (2) acetylcholinesterase. The letters represent the sites of (a) choline transport mechanism in the presynaptic nerve terminal, (b) synaptic vesicle, (c) ACh receptor on the postsynaptic neuronal membrane. ACh, acetylcholine. For additional details, see text or Moore, 1971.

Fahn and Côté, 1968b). The properties and methods of analysis of choline acetyltransferase have been reviewed by Schuberth (1971). Unfortunately, inhibitors of choline acetyltransferase with demonstrated specificity *in vivo* are not available.

The regulation of acetylcholine synthesis in CNS neurons is not well defined. Acetyl-CoA, a product of mitochondrial oxidative activity, is not rate limiting *in vivo*. The intraneuronal choline concentration or the membrane transport of choline could be rate limiting under some circumstances. Sharkawi and Schulman (1969) suggested that acetylcholine synthesis may be subject to negative feedback control, but more definitive evidence is required. Acetylcholine can be synthesized *in vitro* by synaptosomes or slices of brain tissue using either choline or glucose as a precursor (Marchbanks, 1969; Browning and Schulman, 1968). Such *in vitro* systems may aid in resolving the question of synthesis regulation.

Limited data (Table V) suggest that choline acetyltransferase, in a pattern similar to that of many other brain enzymes, develops most rapidly during the second and third weeks of postnatal life in the rat. For example, in the rat caudate nucleus or whole brain, choline acetyltransferase activity was less than 15% of adult activity at postnatal day 10 but then markedly increased to attain adult activity by day 24 (McGeer *et al.*, 1971; Ladinsky *et al.*, 1972). In the cerebral cortex of developing rabbit, choline acetyltransferase activity showed a similar pattern, attaining adult activity by 28 days of age (McCaman and Aprison, 1964).

3. CATABOLISM

The synaptic actions of acetylcholine can be terminated by diffusion away from receptor sites, by active reuptake by presynaptic terminals, or by acetylcholinesterase-catalyzed hydrolysis to choline and acetate. The latter process may be most important.

Much acetylcholinesterase activity is found on postsynaptic membranes at cholinergic synapses; for this reason and because it is easy to measure, acetylcholinesterase has too frequently been employed as an index of cholinergic neuronal activity, thereby contributing to the overexploitation suggested by Karczmar (1969). With this perspective, several additional findings concerning acetylcholinesterase must be considered (see Koelle, 1969): (1) in central cholinergic neurons, acetylcholinesterase is present presynaptically as well as postsynaptically, (2) acetylcholinesterase activity can be detected in noncholinergic neurons, (3) acetylcholinesterase is normally present in considerable excess so that its activity may not be a very sensitive index of cholinergic functional activity, (4) care must be taken to distinguish between acetylcholinesterase and "pseudo" or butyrylcholinesterase activity which is associated with glial cells. Thus, one may safely conclude that the significance of acetylcholinesterase activity in the CNS is not well understood.

On the other hand, some valuable information regarding cholinergic neurons may be obtained by study of acetylcholinesterase. In contrast to acetylcholine and choline acetyltransferase, acetylcholinesterase can be localized histochemically and visualized by electron microscopy. Using selective inhibitors of acetylcholinesterase and butyrylcholinesterase such as BW 62c47 [1,5-bis(4'-trimethylammoniumphenyl)-pentan-3-one-diiodide] and isoOMPA (tetraisopropylpyrophosphoramide), it is now possible to distinguish between these enzymes both chemically and histochemically (Diegenbach, 1965). In general, acetylcholine contents and choline acetyltransferase and acetylcholinesterase activities show close correlations in the various brain regions.

Whole brain acetylcholinesterase activity increased three- to fourfold from birth to attain adult activity by 4 weeks of age in the rat (Elkes and Todrick, 1955), rabbit (Himwich and Aprison, 1955), and mouse (Pryor, 1968). In the rat, acetylcholinesterase activity reached adult activity in the spinal cord at birth (Maletta et al., 1966), in the medulla and hypothalamus by 20 days, and in the cerebral cortex between 40 and 80 days of age (Nair and Bau, 1969). Thus, as with other brain enzymes, a caudal to rostral developmental progression was observed. The subcellular distribution of acetylcholinesterase activity changes during development. The proportion of acetylcholinesterase activity in the synaptosomal fraction steadily increased, whereas activity in other fractions (myelin, mitochondria) diminished to very low levels (Gómez et al., 1970). The progressive increase in synaptosomal acetylcholinesterase paralleled the increased binding of dimethyl-^{11}C-D-tubocurarine to proteolipids in the synaptosomal fraction, suggesting that acetylcholinesterase activity may be a good index of development of postsynaptic cholinergic sites. A major implication of the study of Gómez et al. (1970) is the extreme caution, coupled with strict morphological control, that must be used in applying cell fractionation methods to brain tissue during development.

Burdick and Strittmatter (1965) determined the changes in concentrations of acetylcholinesterase, choline acetyltransferase, acetylcholine, choline, and protein during the embryonic development of the chick. Interestingly, development of choline acetyltransferase activity and acetylcholine contents preceded that of acetylcholinesterase activity.

4. Dynamics

Drugs such as morphine, barbiturates, and general anesthetics (Giarman and Pepeu, 1962; Richter and Goldstein, 1970) as well as various behavioral alterations (Toru et al., 1966; Aprison et al., 1968) cause significant changes in acetylcholine contents in brain. Unless such changes can be related to alterations in rates of synthesis, release, or degradation, however, their significance will remain unknown.

Unfortunately at the present, the dynamic aspects of acetylcholine metabolism in the CNS are almost completely unknown; some inferences can be drawn based upon limited knowledge of dynamics of acetylcholine in peripheral cholinergic systems. Nevertheless, techniques are now available by which processes of synthesis, release, storage, and uptake as they relate to ongoing neuronal activity can be investigated. Schuberth et al. (1969) have developed a method for determining turnover rates for acetylcholine in mouse brain. Hanin et al. (1972) have coupled the gas chromatographic method of Hanin and Jenden (1969) for acetylcholine and choline with use of intravenous administration of ^{14}C-phosphorylcholine to permit estimation of specific activities of both choline and acetylcholine in rat salivary glands. Similarly, the enzymatic radioassay of Reid et al. (1971) could be adapted to determine turnover rates of acetylcholine in brain and other tissues.

Release of acetylcholine onto the surface of the cerebral cortex or from subcortical sites with subsequent collection by push–pull cannulae has been demonstrated; however, such release has not been related directly to stimulation of specific neuronal systems (Philis *et al.*, 1968; Jasper and Koyama, 1969; Beleslin and Myers, 1970).

The dynamic aspects of central cholinergic metabolism in the developing animals are virtually unknown.

5. DRUG ACTIONS AT CHOLINERGIC SYNAPSES

Some of the basic types of drug actions occurring at cholinergic synapses are illustrated in Fig. 7 and are thoroughly discussed elsewhere (Goodman and Gilman, 1970). Perusal of recent reviews of developmental pharmacology (Young, 1967; Kornetsky, 1970; Mirkin, 1970; Becker, 1970), however, indicates that studies of cholinergic drug effects, either biochemical or behavioral, in the CNS of developing animals are almost totally lacking. A few such studies in the developing peripheral nervous system are reviewed by Filogamo and Marchisio (1971); see Section VIII for a discussion of the role of developing cholinergic mechanisms in behavior (Campbell *et al.*, 1969; Fibiger *et al.*, 1970).

E. Histamine

Histamine participates in such diverse physiological processes as allergic and inflammatory reactions and secretion of gastric acid (Håkanson, 1970). A possible role of histamine in synaptic functions in the CNS, however, remains to be defined (Green, 1970).

Considerable recent evidence suggests that histamine may modulate growth processes in the developing brain (Pearce and Schanberg, 1969; Young *et al.*, 1971; Schwartz *et al.*, 1971). For example, Young *et al.* (1971) found that histamine concentrations of rat brain reach a peak of 250 ng/gm wet weight during the first 10 days postnatally and then gradually decline to an adult value of 50 ng/gm at 17 days. This developmental pattern is in sharp contrast to that of 5-hydroxytryptamine or norepinephrine but closely parallels that of spermidine (Pearce and Schanberg, 1969). Moreover, during this early postnatal period, 90% of the histamine content of rat brain is found in the crude nuclear fraction obtained by differential centrifugation (Young *et al.*, 1971) in contrast to the small amount in the nuclear fraction of adult brain. Development of brain histamine contents proceeds in a caudocephalic direction like the general developmental pattern of brain neurotransmitters (Young *et al.*, 1971).

Histamine synthesis in the brain may be controlled by the free histidine concentration (about 0.1 mM in rat brain) which is far below the saturating concentration (10 mM) for histidine decarboxylase (Schwartz et al., 1971). These authors speculate that in children with histidinemia, alterations in brain histamine formation may be related to observed mental disturbances. The developing animal may be an extremely useful model to examine this possibility and the general question of the CNS functions of histamine.

VII. Behavioral Effects of Drugs Administered during the Prenatal Period

A. Clinical Investigations

Little effort has been made to examine the effects of drugs administered during pregnancy or labor on the behavior of the human infant. The major reasons are obvious; well-controlled studies in humans are difficult to conduct, and poorly controlled studies are impossible to evaluate. Despite the many problems involved, however, there are some pertinent clinical studies that should be considered.

To causally relate neonatal depression to a drug action one must eliminate other possible causes of depression (e.g., prolonged or precipitous labor, maternal diseases such as preeclampsia or diabetes). When these possible causes are eliminated, it is clear that some central depressant drugs when administered to the mother before or during labor can depress the newborn infant.

In the delivery room depression is generally reported on the basis of a 10 point Apgar score which considers heart rate, reflex irritability, muscle tone, and skin color (Apgar, 1953). Ratings are generally made at 1 and 5 minutes after birth. A low 1-minute score indicates an increased chance of subsequent neurological abnormalities, and a low 5-minute score indicates some threat to survival. The Apgar score is a more reliable index of newborn depression from hospital to hospital than are general descriptions such as slightly depressed, moderately depressed, etc. A similar type of quantitative scoring system is needed to determine "CNS depression" at later times during postnatal life.

1. ACUTE DRUG ADMINISTRATION DURING LABOR

There is a remarkable lack of well-controlled, quantitative clinical reports on the effects of prenatally administered centrally active drugs on the postnatal behavior of infants. At least three factors determine the degree of neonatal depression resulting from the administration of a central depressant drug to the mother during labor: the dose of the drug, the route of administration, and the period of time between drug administration and delivery. Unfortunately, this information is not always reported. Moya and Thorndike (1963) reviewed the effects of drugs administered to the mother during labor (skeletal muscle relaxants, general anesthetics, barbiturates, tranquilizers, and other sedatives) on the fetus and the newborn infant. Emphasis was placed upon the pharmacokinetic properties of these drugs (e.g., transfer across the placenta and blood–brain barrier) rather than on their behavioral or biochemical actions. Selected reports on the behavioral effects in the newborn of many of these same drugs are summarized in the next section; most of these studies have appeared since the 1963 review.

Shnider and Moya (1964) made a retrospective study of over 1000 women who delivered full-term infants vaginally and received no general anesthesia. The women were divided into three major groups: those receiving no medication, those receiving intramuscular injections of meperidine (50, 75, or 100 mg) 10 minutes–4 hours prior to delivery, and those receiving similar doses of meperidine plus secobarbital (100 mg i.m. or 200 mg p.o.) simultaneously with the meperidine. They divided the infants into two groups depending on Apgar scores at 1 minute and the time to sustain respiration. Depressed infants had Apgar scores of less than 6 and a greater than 90 second time to sustain respiration. Irrespective of the time of drug administration there was no significant difference in the incidence of depressed infants from women who received meperidine and those who received no mediation. There was, however, a significantly higher incidence of depressed babies from mothers who received both meperidine and secobarbital prior to delivery. The highest incidence of depression occurred in infants born to mothers who received meperidine and secobarbital 2–4 hours prior to delivery. In a single-blind study Borgstedt and Rosen (1968) compared infants born to mothers who received no medication with those who received meperidine or phenobarbital 7 minutes to 10 hours prior to delivery. When examined 6 hours after birth, infants from medicated mothers were "behaviorally impaired" and exhibited an altered EEG involving an increase in the low-voltage fast wave activity recorded from the frontal cortex. The EEG effects but not the behavioral ratings were altered for 3 days in 30% of the infants. Since there were no differences in Apgar scores between infants from medicated and nonmedicated mothers the authors concluded that the Apgar rating system is not as sensitive an indicator of drug-induced depression of the newborn as is the EEG.

Benson *et al.* (1969) evaluated data from a large number of pregnancies, comparing the hazards of elective cesarean section and normal spontaneous vaginal deliveries. They concluded that cesarean section was more hazardous to the baby, as evidenced by increased neonatal mortality and morbidity, than was vaginal delivery. This appeared to be due, at least in part, to the greater depth of anesthesia required in the former procedure. When general rather than regional anesthesia was employed, significantly lower Apgar scores were noted at both 1 and 5 minutes in babies delivered by elective cesarean section; the scores were inversely related to the depth of anesthesia employed. Greater depression of the newborn infant resulted when the mother received secobarbital rather than meperidine during labor. A similar conclusion was reached by Batt (1968) who noted that administration during labor of rather large doses of vinbarbital (240–420 mg) with or without a phenothiazine resulted in infants who had lower Apgar scores and took longer before they were able to sustain respiration than did administration of meperidine (50–100 mg) alone or with a phenothiazine. The latter investigator did not attempt a long-term evaluation, but Benson et al. (1969) reviewed the results of subsequent neurological examinations of the offspring. At 4 months, abnormal or suspect neurological examinations were recorded in 16% of infants delivered by cesarean section under general anesthesia as compared with only 10% delivered vaginally; there were no differences in the two groups when examined at 1 year. The low Apgar scores and the 4-month neurological examination reported in this extensive study support the premise that general anesthesia can be a major factor in the increased morbidity of infants during the first year of life.

Brazelton (1961) studied the influence of obstetrical anesthesia on responsiveness of newborn infants to breast feeding. He found that the type of anesthesia administered during delivery was unimportant with respect to the alertness of the baby for nursing; there were no obvious differences between babies from mothers who received a local anesthetic and those who received an inhalant anesthetic (ether, nitrous oxide). On the other hand, preanesthetic administration of barbiturates caused a significant depression. Infants from mothers who received large doses of barbiturates ($>$150 mg) 1–6 hours before delivery were much less responsive than babies from mothers who received low doses of barbiturates ($<$60 mg) during the same period; barbiturate administration prior to delivery delayed by 48 hours the ability of the neonate to adapt to breast feeding. This effect was also reflected in the weight gain of the infants; babies from mothers receiving the lower doses of barbiturates began gaining weight 24 hours before those from the higher dose group. The author emphasizes that these results should be interpreted cautiously because of the many variables associated with delivery and also because the effects might have resulted, in part, from the sedative effects of the barbiturates in the mother. Nevertheless, the results do suggest that effects of maternal drug administration can alter the subsequent behavior of the neonate during the first week of life and perhaps for an even longer period. In a subsequent report Brazelton (1970) expressed concern that despite the fact that depressant drugs administered during pregnancy may adversely effect mother–infant relationships, little has been done to alter the accepted obstetrical practice of medicating the mother in labor.

In an elegant study by Kron et al. (1966), infants born to mothers given secobarbital (200 mg) for obstetrical sedation during labor 10–180 minutes prior to delivery had slightly lower Apgar scores but exhibited markedly reduced sucking rates and pressures and consumed less nutrients than did infants from nonmediated mothers. These effects lasted for at least 5 days, the time the infants remained in the nursery.

Budnick et al. (1955) reported that administration of reserpine 15 minutes—21 hours before delivery resulted in infants who exhibited nasal discharge and thoracic retraction lasting from 1 to 5 days. Lethargy and poor feeding, which appeared associated with the nasal obstruction, were also observed, but no gastrointestinal symptoms were recorded. The same symptoms plus bradycardia were observed by Desmond et al. (1957) in newborn infants who received reserpine prior to delivery. Unfortunately, neither of these investigators followed the subsequent behavioral development of the children. Chlordiazepoxide (100 mg i.m.) given on a double-blind basis during the first stage of labor did not significantly alter the following measures in newborn infants: Apgar scores at 1 and 5 minutes, temperature, pulse, respiration, and the amount of fluid intake (Decancq et al., 1965). It was noted that the approximate half-life of the drug in the newborn (61 hours) was approximately 20% longer than in the adult. Thus at this dose, chlordiazepoxide crossed the placenta but did not depress the newborn infant. It was also noted, however, that parturient women receiving chlordiazepoxide did not achieve significant benefits when compared with those receiving placebo, indicating that this dose was ineffective for the purposes for which it was administered.

From the standpoint of behavioral testing, the study reported by Stechler (1964) is particularly interesting. He measured the attentive behavior (time spent viewing a blank card or cards containing pictures of a die or a face) in 2- to 4-day-old infants from mothers who had received various drugs but no general anesthetic prior to delivery. Babies from mothers who received the highest doses of the drugs (meperidine, alphaprodine, pentobarbital, promethazine) were the least attentive; infants from mothers who received the drugs within 90 minutes of delivery were less attentive than those from mothers who received the drugs at an earlier time. Unfortunately, the small sample size and the use of multiple drug combinations did not permit examination of the effects of specific drugs. It was not possible from this study to determine if the reduction of attentive behavior was related to the persistence of the drug in the infant or if it was secondary to a drug-induced delay in the functional development of the central nervous system. Although the drugs produced significant effects 2–4 days after birth, it would have been interesting to determine if these effects could be detected at later times. This study can be severely criticized from a pharmacological standpoint, but it affords great possibilities for behavioral testing of newborn, since quantitative clinical data can be obtained. Hopefully, similar studies can be performed taking special cognizance of the dose and the time of administration before delivery of different classes of drugs.

2. Chronic Drug Administration during Pregnancy

In infants, the most obvious behavioral effects resulting from prenatal drug administration to the mother are caused by drugs that produce physical dependence in the mother and the fetus. These drugs include narcotic analgesics, barbiturates, and alcohol. To our knowledge there are no reports of behavioral alterations in children born to mothers who have chronically taken such drugs as amphetamines, hallucinogens (e.g., LSD), or marijuana. Nevertheless, adverse symptoms in infants from mothers who have taken such drugs may go unrecognized or be attributed to other etiological factors.

a. Narcotic Analgesics. It has long been recognized that most infants born to mothers who are truly physically dependent upon heroin or other narcotic analgesics exhibit adverse symptoms beginning 1–96 hours after birth (for a historical review, see Cobrinik et al., 1959). These symptoms, undoubtedly analogous to withdrawal symptoms in the adult, include hyperactivity, hyperirritability and restlessness, tremor, disturbed sleep, sneezing, vomiting and diarrhea, hyperthermia, sweating, dehydration, and high-pitched crying (Cobrinik et al., 1959; Hill and Desmond, 1963; Henley and Fisch, 1966; Kahn et al., 1969; Stone et al., 1971; Zelson et al., 1971). Schulman (1969) noted abnormal sleep patterns in infants from addicted mothers; quiet sleep did not occur, and REM periods were disorganized. As would be expected, the longer the period of abuse and the larger the maternal intake of heroin, the more frequent the incidence of withdrawal symptoms in the offspring. The differences in time of onset of symptoms obviously relate to the time and size of the last dose taken by the mother.

Goodfriend et al. (1956) reported an overall mortality rate of 34% among infants born to mothers addicted to narcotic analgesics; Hill and

Desmond (1963) calculated a 9% death rate in a summary of reports during the period of 1947 to 1962. More recently, Zelson et al. (1971) reported the incidence of neonatal death in a fairly large series of heroin addicts as only 3.6%; this was compared to a rate of 3% in the overall population. At least part of the reduction in mortality rate must be related to the better recognition and treatment of withdrawal symptoms in the infant. Treatment has generally involved the use of paregoric, barbiturates, and chlorpromazine, alone or in combination (Cobrinik et al., 1959; Hill and Desmond, 1963; Rosenthal et al., 1964; Stern, 1966; Kahn et al., 1969; Zelson et al., 1971). The length of treatment needed varied from less than 10 to more than 40 days. The slightly higher incidence of postnatal mortality of infants born to narcotic addicts may be due to a number of factors. The lack of proper prenatal care and nutrition is obviously important. Stone et al. (1971) and Perlmutter (1969) reported that approximately 75% of the addicts made no attempt to obtain prenatal care even though they suffered from a high incidence of disease (hepatitis, venereal disease). Lack of proper maternal care during the postnatal period may also be a factor; most of the infants are not raised by their natural mother but are made wards of the court and subsequently adopted. With treatment that is now currently employed, few deaths appear to be directly related to withdrawal symptoms per se, although prematurity is a complicating factor (Stern, 1966; Kahn et al., 1969). Approximately 50% of infants from addict mothers weigh less than 2.5 kg compared to only 7–17% in the overall infant population of comparable hospitals (Perlmutter, 1969; Blinick et al., 1969; Kahn et al., 1969; Stone et al., 1971; Zelson et al., 1971). Although there does appear to be an increased incidence of prematurity, most of the infants born to narcotic addicts are small full-term babies.

It is generally believed that most "heroin" addicts abuse a variety of drugs in addition to the narcotic analgesics. In the study reported by Kahn et al. (1969) heroin addicts also took drugs such as glutethimide, amphetamines, barbiturates, and alcohol and were heavy smokers of cigarettes. Accordingly, any interpretation of the relationship between prenatal heroin administration and infant behavior must be tempered by the fact that drugs other than narcotic analgesics could be responsible for altering offspring behavior.

Rajegowda et al. (1972) reported a high incidence of withdrawal symptoms in infants born to mothers receiving methadone on a maintenance program. As might be expected from the known pharmacological effects in adults, these withdrawal symptoms (tremor, irritability) were of longer duration (4–16 days) than those observed in infants born to heroin addicts (2–8 days).

b. Barbiturates. Despite the fact that barbiturates are widely used and can produce severe physical dependence in adults, there is little information on the neonatal withdrawal symptoms related to maternal use of these drugs. Desmond *et al.* (1972) recently reported on 15 infants born to mothers who had taken barbiturates during pregnancy either for illicit or therapeutic purposes (i.e., prescribed for epilepsy or anxiety). When compared with a group of 13 infants from heroin addicts who generally exhibited low birth weights and postnatal depression (40% had Apgar scores of less than 7), babies of mothers "addicted(?)" to barbiturates appeared normal at birth. Infants from heroin addicts first exhibited withdrawal symptoms 10 minutes to 48 hours after birth (median of 6 hours), whereas infants of mothers taking barbiturates did not begin to exhibit symptoms until 3–10 days after birth. The symptoms in the latter group included hyperreflexia, restlessness, disturbed sleep, tremor, shrill crying, hyperphagia, and hyperacusia. Similar but milder effects were also noted in infants of mothers receiving barbiturates during the latter part of gestation for the treatment of anxiety, hypertension, and epilepsy. The less severe behavioral symptoms in this group may be related to differences in the doses and in the types of barbiturates administered. Short-acting barbiturates (amobarbital or secobarbital) were used illicitly, whereas phenobarbital was generally prescribed therapeutically. Except for the time of onset, the symptoms in infants from barbiturate addicts were remarkably similar to those in offspring from heroin addicts. The delayed onset of withdrawal symptoms may be related to the reduced rate of metabolism of barbiturates in the newborn. The drug may remain in the tissues for several days before the concentration is reduced enough to precipitate withdrawal.

The report by Desmond *et al.* (1972) is at variance with two recent studies in which phenobarbital was administered to pregnant women for several weeks prior to delivery in order to induce hepatic enzymes capable of metabolizing bilirubin (Ramboer *et al.*, 1969; Mauer *et al.*, 1968). In these latter studies 30–130 mg of phenobarbital per day for a minimum of 2 weeks prior to delivery significantly reduced the plasma bilirubin content but did not alter behavioral characteristics of the infants. These studies were not primarily designed to evaluate behavior, and behavioral alterations may have been overlooked. Alternatively, the lack of behavioral effect may be related to a lower dose of barbiturates and to the fact that infants were observed only during the first 4–7 days of life. Desmond *et al.* (1972) noted that in many instances "withdrawal symptoms" were not observed in infants until after they were discharged from the hospital, since the median time of onset of symptoms was 7 days.

Bleyer and Marshall (1972) reported an infant born to a mother, who had consumed high doses of secobarbital during pregnancy, exhibited withdrawal symptoms soon after delivery. The symptoms appeared to be more severe than those reported by Desmond *et al.* (1972). A second episode of barbiturate withdrawal symptoms occurred again in the same infant at age 4 months. These symptoms, which included repetitive grand mal seizures, followed separation from the mother, who had administered daily doses of secobarbital to the infant. When examined at 2 years the child's EEG, growth and neurological function were considered normal.

c. Alcohol. Despite the high incidence of alcoholism there are only two reports of withdrawal symptoms in infants born to alcoholic mothers. In a case reported by Schaefer (1962) the mother was known to be continuously drunk for 2 months prior to admission to the hospital and was actually stuporous at the time of delivery. She delivered a small but full-term baby who was severely depressed at birth and developed withdrawal symptoms consisting of jerky movements, tremors of hands and feet, restlessness, sleeplessness, shrill high-pitched crying, and hyperresponsiveness to sensory stimuli 12–18 hours later. These symptoms were most pronounced 24 to 48 hours after birth and disappeared after about 1 week. In a case reported by Nichols (1967), an infant was delivered to a woman who was entering an early period of delerium tremens. The mother experienced typical symptoms (extreme agitation, tremors, hallucinations) for 4 days after delivery. The time course of symptoms in her infant (hyperactivity, tremor of extremities, twitching of eyelids) appeared to parallel those of the mother, but it was not possible to follow the course of these symptoms, because alcohol and chlorpromazine were administered to the infant during the first 4 days of life. At 7 months the infant was considered neurologically normal.

d. Other Drugs. Hill *et al.* (1966) reported that two children born to a schizophrenic mother who had taken high doses of phenothiazines during pregnancy exhibited symptoms that could be associated with an extrapyramidal disturbance (hypertonia, tremor, hand posturing) for 6–10 months. It was suggested that the motor dysfunction in the infants might have resulted from the maternal intake of the phenothiazine tranquilizers. Monson *et al.* (1973) examined the possibility that anticonvulsant drugs taken during pregnancy (diphenylhydantoin, barbiturates, benzodiazepines) adversely affect the fetus. They concluded that fetal outcome (complications of pregnancy, fetal malformations, stillbirths) was not influenced by maternal intake of anticonvulsant drugs. Unfortunately, they did not examine the behavioral characteristics of the offspring. These conclusions differ from those of Hill *et al.* (1974) who described a cluster of abnormal physical findings in the offspring of mothers receiving anticonvulsant medication during pregnancy. Bitman (1969) reported a case of an infant born to a mother who had taken 25 mg of chlordiazepoxide 4 times a day during pregnancy. Labor was induced and the infant was judged to be about 1-month premature. Apgar scores at 1, 5, and 10 minutes were 7, 8, and 9. At 3 days the infant was inactive and exhibited poor feeding, weak crying, and sluggish reflexes. These symptoms lasted for approximately 2 weeks, but thereafter the infant developed normally.

3. POSSIBLE LONG-TERM EFFECTS

An important question that needs to be answered is: Do children who exhibit signs of physical dependence to narcotic analgesics, barbiturates, or alcohol shortly after birth exhibit permanent alterations in behavioral characteristics in later life? Unfortunately, there is little specific information on this point from clinical studies. Hill and Desmond (1963) reported on a limited follow-up of infants born to heroin addicts. These infants, who were adopted, showed steady weight gain during the first year of life but exhibited a slight lag in development as determined by physical examination and psychological testing. Desmond et al. (1972) directed their attention to the possible long-term effects in infants born to mothers addicted to barbiturates or heroin. They found that although the infants appeared to improve when discharged from the hospital, "withdrawal" symptoms (tremors, flexor–extensor movements of lower limb, hyperphagia, hyperacusia, and outbursts of screaming) persisted in the home setting for several months. This same group of researchers have now noted that offspring of heroin addicts continue to exhibit behavioral and autonomic abnormalities for up to 2 years of age (G. A. Wilson, personal communication). Perhaps with more discriminating behavioral tests, effects may be discerned for an even longer period of time. It would be interesting to determine if similar results can be confirmed by other investigators.

It is obviously difficult to estimate the duration of withdrawal symptoms in humans, realizing that the environment will greatly influence infant behavior. Mother–infant interaction may be responsible for extended abnormal behavior of the infant so that, as pointed out earlier, it is extremely difficult to determine if the behavior observed in the infant is the result of a direct action of a drug. For example, mothers who receive barbiturates during pregnancy to control anxiety and apprehension may continue to exhibit these symptoms during the postnatal period and thereby adversely influence the behavior of their children. Maternal care or the lack of it may also be important factors in offspring of addict mothers. The majority of babies born to addict mothers appear to be subsequently adopted. Another obvious difficulty in evaluating the long-term effects in infants born to mothers who received drugs capable of producing physical dependence is related to the use of adequate controls of nonphysically dependent mothers who come from a similar environment, who receive similar prenatal care (or the lack of it), and who provide equivalent postnatal care to their infants. Obviously, studies which attempt to evaluate these variables are much easier to perform in experimental animals.

B. Experimental Animal Investigations

In the not too distant past it was believed that the behavior of a mother during pregnancy could "mark" her child; the birth of physical or behavioral "monsters" was explained on this basis. Gross structural defects in offspring are now generally attributed to genetic, viral, or chemical influences. Abnormal offspring behavior may result from genetic defects or from brain injury at birth, but in many instances the etiology of behavioral abnormalities is unknown. The role of prenatal drug administration cannot be dismissed. Many drugs and hormones in the maternal blood can pass the placental barrier and in some instances produce dramatic structural alterations in the developing fetus (teratogenic effects). It is not unreasonable that chemicals, in addition to producing structural defects in the central nervous system, can also produce subtle effects on neuronal systems that become manifest as alterations in behavior. The next sections (VII,B,2 and VIII,B) review some of the studies that have attempted to demonstrate drug-induced alterations in the neurochemical and behavioral development of experimental animals.

1. GENERAL PROBLEMS IN EXPERIMENTAL DESIGN

As indicated in Section VII,A, the effects of drugs administered to human mothers during the prenatal period on the subsequent behavioral development of the offspring are difficult to evaluate because of the many problems associated with conducting such investigations under adequate control conditions. Furthermore, it is not possible to conduct correlative behavioral and neurochemical studies in humans. Accordingly, animal experiments have been employed, but even here inadequate controls have often created difficulties in interpreting the experimental results. The administration of drugs during the prenatal period presents problems concerning the use of appropriate controls that are not generally encountered in pharmacological research; these types of problems, however, have been considered by researchers in the fields of psychology and nutrition. Drugs administered to the mother may influence offspring by having: (1) a direct effect on brain development during the prenatal period, (2) an indirect effect on brain development during the prenatal period as a result of maternal influence, (3) an effect on the mother during the postnatal period which, by causing inadequate or inappropriate maternal care, influences subsequent development of the offspring. In order to determine which of these factors is responsible for a neurochemical or behavioral effect observed in the offspring, it is extremely important to employ adequate control procedures.

a. Physical Environment. Changes in the physical environment of the pregnant female may alter the psychological state and thereby alter the chemical composition of the maternal blood. This in turn may influence the normal maturation of the CNS in the fetus in such a manner that subsequent postnatal behavior may be affected. A variety of psychological stresses encountered by the human mother during pregnancy have been reported to cause alterations in such offspring behavior as crying, reading ability, and temperament (Archer and Blackman, 1971). Results of such studies are difficult to assess because of the problems of conducting this type of research in human subjects under adequate control conditions.

The effects of a number of prenatal physical factors have been examined on the survival rate, morphology, and behavior of animal offspring. With a few exceptions (e.g., X-ray), most physical factors affecting the fetus appear to act through indirect mechanisms. Since there are no neural connections between mother and fetus, these factors obviously must involve alterations in the composition of maternal blood which could include changes in the concentration of oxygen, intermediary metabolites, and various hormones. Possible hormonal changes include the release of catecholamines from sympathetic nerve endings and the adrenal medulla and the release of corticosteroids from the adrenal cortex. Other endocrines may also be involved (Mason, 1968). An increased concentration of these hormones in the maternal blood may influence fetal development directly or indirectly by inducing changes in concentrations of critical intermediary metabolites.

Experimental studies in animals suggest that the severity and duration of stress are more important than the type of stress in producing hormonal changes, as reflected by quantitative measurements of plasma corticosterone or blood glucose concentrations. For example, Carr and Moore (1968) reported that a supposedly "mild stress," such as removing an animal from its home cage and placing it in a new environment, produced adrenocortical responses equivalent to those seen in animals following the presentation of prolonged and obviously painful electric shocks. Similar results have been reported by Friedman and Ader (1967). Hutchings and Gibbon (1970) suggested that disrupting normal ongoing behavior of an animal by removing it from its home cage may be a more stressful experimental manipulation than the presentation of some additional "stressful procedures." Accordingly, the various procedures that have been used to induce prenatal stress, including conditioned avoidance responding, handling, injections of water, saline, or caustic agents by various routes, crowding, swimming, and open-field testing, are probably not different from one another in terms of their effects on the fetus.

Of critical importance, however, are the duration of the stress and the time during gestation at which the stress is presented. Effects of prenatal drug administration on postnatal behavior may reflect both a specific pharmacological action of the drug and a nonspecific stressful effect associated with drug administration. Moreover, the relative contributions of the drug and stress may differ depending upon the stage of gestation during which the drug is administered. Although nonspecific stress might produce different effects on offspring behavior depending on the trimester of pregnancy in which it was presented, not enough studies have been performed to formulate general conclusions, nor has there been any trend linking the duration of stress presentation during pregnancy to the effects on offspring behavior (Archer and Blackman, 1971). Prenatal stress may also cause long-lasting neurochemical changes in the offspring. Huttunen (1971) found that offspring of female rats receiving a foot-shock stress from the fifteenth to the nineteenth day of gestation exhibited an apparent increase in turnover of brain norepinephrine when compared to offspring of nonshocked mothers. Thus, both behavioral and neurochemical effects may result from environmental factors or manipulative procedures rather than from the action of the drug per se (also see Section VIII,A).

In order to identify true drug effects adequate controls must be used. Drug-treated and control mothers must be housed under the same conditions (lighting, cage size, etc.) and handled and injected in the same manner. The route of injection and the volume of injected material should be the same in control and experimental groups. Havlena and Werboff (1963) demonstrated that offspring behavior is affected differently by drugs depending upon the route of injection. The drug vehicle rather than water or saline (unless these solvents are the vehicle) should be injected into the control group. If the drug is insoluble and must be injected as a suspension, an inert material with similar physical properties might be suspended and injected into the control animals. For example, suspensions of tyrosine have been used as controls for the injections of insoluble suspensions of α-methyltyrosine (Moore, 1966). Administration of drugs in the diet or in the drinking water has been used to circumvent problems inherent in handling and injections. Care must be taken, however, to ensure that the presence of the drug does not disrupt the normal food or water intake.

b. Maternal Behavior. Drugs administered during the prenatal period may alter subsequent maternal behavior during the postnatal period and thereby influence the neurochemistry or behavior of the offspring. For example, prenatal drug or hormone administration may result in inadequate lactation or cause maternal neglect. Residual drug may remain in the mother and be transferred to the offspring during nursing. To avoid this influence cross-fostering procedures are used. Cross fostering can be carried out in a number of ways but generally offspring from experimental mothers (those injected with the drug) are divided so that some remain with the natural (experimental) mother and others are fostered to control mothers (those injected with the drug vehicle). In addition, offspring from control mothers are divided so that some remain with the natural (control) mother and others are fostered to experimental mothers. In this way the influence of prenatal treatments which may be transferred to offspring can be determined by removing the postnatal influences of the mother. Joffe (1965) showed that postnatal maternal behavior can influence offspring behavior. He demonstrated that rats weaned by mothers that were stressed during the prenatal period were significantly inferior to rats weaned by nonstressed mothers when tested in a conditioned-avoidance learning procedure. Offspring from the stressed mothers but fostered to nonstressed mothers were not affected. This indicates that although stress was presented prenatally, the factors that altered offspring behavior resulted from the postnatal maternal behavior of the prenatally stressed mother. Even cross-fostering techniques will not always provide a complete control. As pointed out by Kornetsky (1970), if the experimental newborn is affected by the direct placental transfer of the drug at birth and if this drug causes an immediate postnatal depression, it is possible that the experimental animal will have difficulty competing with its foster siblings for nursing. In addition, the foster mother might reject the experimental offspring if it exhibits some drug-induced abnormal behavior. During the first week of life of rat pups, the mother spends very little time away from the nest. After the first week the mother spends progressively less time in close proximity to the pups (Schaefer, 1968). The close contact of the pups and mother during the first week of life may be very important for providing "stimulation" to the pups which is essential for normal behavioral development. Any prenatal drug treatment that causes a reduction in the amount of time that the mother spends with the pups may alter their subsequent behavior.

c. Behavioral Testing. The method by which offspring behavior is tested is an important variable to consider. Since a variety of different tests have been employed, it is impossible to discuss them all, but some comments about the more commonly used tests are warranted.

The open-field test is frequently employed. In this test, exploratory activity (ambulation) and latency to move, both of which are believed to measure the readiness of an animal to explore a novel environment, and the number of fecal pellets, which is represented as an index of "emotionality," are generally recorded. The usefulness of this test as a measure of functional behavior is limited. There is no standard open-field test; the size of the field, the duration of the test, and the number of times an animal is tested vary from study to study. It is clear, however, that repeated testing of an animal reduces the measured responses. As summarized in the following sections, prenatal drug administration does alter the performance of offspring in this test. It must be noted, however, that "stress" resulting from drug administration may also influence performance. In general, prenatal stress causes the following effects in the behavior of offspring in open-field tests: (1) a reduction in exploratory activity, (2) an increase in defecation (increased number of fecal pellets), (3) equivocal responses in latency to explore (both increases and decreases have been reported).

Other types of tests and instruments are also used to measure spontaneous locomotor or exploratory activities. Some of these involve the use of various mazes that also permit the measurement of learning. For example, maze performance can be determined after the animal has learned the procedure; in this situation the drug may alter the number of errors made or the time to run the maze correctly. Learning can be determined by recording the number of trials required to reach a certain criterion of performance. The Hebb–Williams open-field maze is widely used for these types of testing. This apparatus consists of a square maze with a start box in one corner and a goal box containing food or some other reward in the diagonally opposite corner. After the animal learns to cross from the start box to the goal box, barriers are placed to form detours to the goal box. One can measure the latency to leave the goal box, crouching, defecating, or number of errors made in reaching the goal box. In general, offspring from stressed mothers exhibit increased latency and error scores in maze learning experiments.

Conditioned avoidance tests are commonly employed. An animal is trained to avoid a noxious stimulus which is cued to a nonnoxious stimulus (e.g., avoiding a painful grid shock in a shuttle box in response to a tone or a light). Other types of tests measure operant conditioning, aggressive behavior, sexual behavior, and social behavior (mouse city). Because of the variations in the way these tests are performed, it is not possible to discuss them in general terms. Specific behavioral tests, however, are discussed in the context of individual studies in Section VII,B,2.

Why a particular test is employed or what the actual test purports to measure is not always fully described. Furthermore, researchers will attempt to equate performance of animals in behavioral tests with human behavioral characteristics. Such attempts to relate experimental observations in animals to human situations are generally unwarranted and inappropriate. A more realistic approach is merely to describe the behavioral repertoire of animals in test situations and then observe how these behaviors can be altered by drugs.

d. Miscellaneous. It is frustrating that many researchers attempt to compare drug effects in their own studies with those from other laboratories with little consideration of the duration of drug administration, the trimester of pregnancy in which drug was administered, and the dose and route of administration of the drug. Furthermore, dose–response relationships are seldom considered; in many studies only a single dose of a drug is employed.

If a drug increases mortality at birth or reduces survival of offspring after birth, the effects of the drug on behavioral or biochemical measurements may actually be much greater than reported. That is, the animals most severely affected by the drug are lost from the study and thus not included in the overall evaluation of the results.

2. EXPERIMENTAL STUDIES

The past decade has seen the first attempts by several investigators to examine the effects of prenatal administration of centrally active drugs on behavior of the offspring. Although, owing to their pioneering nature, most of these studies have severe shortcomings in experimental design, they have set the stage for further, more sophisticated investigations in this important area.

In a series of similarly designed experiments, Werboff and Havlena (1962), Werboff and Dembicki (1962), and Werboff and Kesner (1963) treated gravid rats subcutaneously with water or with reasonable pharmacological doses of reserpine (0.033 mg/kg), chlorpromazine (2 mg/kg), and meprobamate (20 mg/kg) every 8 hours for 4 days during one of the three trimesters. The most obvious result was that all three drugs caused a higher total mortality of offspring than did water treatment. Treatment with meprobamate or reserpine caused decreases in body weights of offspring surviving the weaning period; chlorpromazine caused increases in body weights. Disconcertingly, the reported reduction in activity of offspring from reserpine-treated animals was directly opposite to a previous report from the same laboratory (Werboff *et al.*, 1961). Offspring from reserpine- and meprobamate-treated mothers exhibited reduced motor activity when tested on an inclined plane at 25 days or in an open-field at 55 days. Offspring from meprobamate-treated mothers required more trials to reach a criterion of learning when tested in a Lashley III maze for 8 days starting 82 days after birth. When tested for susceptibility to audiogenic seizures at 120–121 days of age, rats from drug-treated mothers tended to show a greater resistance to seizures, but variable results with respect to incidence, severity, and duration of the seizures precluded definite conclusions.

Kletzkin *et al.* (1964) were unable to duplicate some of the results reported by Werboff and co-workers; they failed to find any significant effects on body weight, activity on the inclined plane or in open-field tests, or in learning ability in a Lashley III maze in offspring of mothers injected with meprobamate (same dosage regimen employed by Werboff).

Hoffeld and co-workers (Hoffeld and Webster, 1965; Hoffeld *et al.*, 1967, 1968) attempted to duplicate the experiments of Werboff and co-workers, paying special attention to the trimester of pregnancy during which the drugs were administered and using identical doses and injection schedules. Body weights of 80-day-old offspring from water-, reserpine-, chlorpromazine-, and meprobamate-treated mothers were different depending on the trimester in which drugs were administered. For example, when meprobamate or chlorpromazine was administered during the second but not during the first or third trimesters, offspring weights were significantly less than those of water controls (Hoffeld and Webster, 1965). In a later study of identical design, Hoffeld *et al.* (1967) reported quite different results. Reserpine treatment during the first trimester resulted in offspring of low body weight, whereas drug treatment during the second trimester did not affect offspring weight. The lack of consistency in data from experiment to experiment weakened the credibility of the experimental conclusions.

Hoffeld and co-workers also found marked differences in behavioral responses of the offspring depending upon the drug administered, the trimester of drug exposure, and the behavioral test employed. For example, administration of chlorpromazine during the first trimester or reserpine during the second trimester resulted in pups that were significantly slower in learning a Lashley III maze than were those from control mothers. Administration of any of the drugs during the third trimester did not affect maze learning ability of the offspring. Acquisition of a conditioned avoidance response in 84-day-old offspring was impaired if chlorpromazine had been administered prenatally during the second or third trimester or if meprobamate had been given during the second trimester. Offspring of drug-treated mothers also extinguished the response more rapidly than did the controls.

Jewett and Norton (1966) compared the effects of prenatal administration of water, reserpine, and chlorpromazine (days 4–7 of gestation, same doses as Werboff and co-workers) on postnatal growth and behavioral responses. Neither drug affected the body weight of the mother, litter size, or body weights of offspring surviving the weaning period. Nevertheless, chlorpromazine treatment resulted in a significant increase in the number of offspring born dead or dying during the weaning period. Likewise, prenatal administration of chlorpromazine, but not of reserpine, caused reduced motor activity of the offspring on day 30 and increased susceptibility to audiogenic seizures on days 58–59. Jewett and Norton obtained pregnant rats from a commercial supplier. Stress associated with transporting the pregnant animals to a new environment may have influenced their results. Nevertheless, their results are in contrast with those of Werboff and co-workers.

Although the overall results of the experiments of these groups of investigators suggest that prenatal administration of tranquilizers influences the behavior of offspring, the nonuniformity of effects and lack of an overall trend of changes in behavioral characteristics make it extremely difficult to evaluate the significance of the results. Major flaws in experimental design of these studies included failure to use cross-fostering procedures and to determine dose–response relationships. Other sources of variation in particular studies such as transportation-induced stress of pregnant rats or variable routes or volumes of injection may have contributed to the inconsistent results obtained. These studies, however, represent the first systematic and concerted efforts to examine the effects of centrally active drugs which are administered to the mother on subsequent behavior of her offspring. Credit must be given to Werboff's group for initiating such studies and to Hoffeld and co-workers for emphasizing the importance of the trimester in which the drugs are administered. (The trimester, however, is an arbitrary division of the gestational period; reference to a specific day or days of gestation would be preferable.)

A subsequent investigation by Ordy et al. (1966) considered both the necessity for cross-fostering procedures and for determining dose–response relationships; their carefully controlled experiments should serve as a model for other investigators. Murphree et al. (1962) had previously observed an increased mortality of offspring from mothers treated during pregnancy with chlorpromazine, promazine, or thioridazine (5 mg/kg daily). Ordy et al. (1963) also noted that daily oral doses of chlorpromazine (4–16 mg/kg) to mice throughout pregnancy caused a dose-related increase in the length of time between mating and birth and a reduction in litter size and weight. Ordy and co-workers (1966) followed this toxicological study with a more intensive investigation on the prenatal effects of chloropromazine on offspring of mice. When administered orally beginning on the sixth day of pregnancy and continuing until term, chlorpromazine produced a dose-related increase in the duration of gestation and a reduction of weight gain of the mother during pregnancy. The mean litter size and weight of offspring were also reduced. At 60 days there was a significantly lower percentage of survival in the drug offspring than in the controls; this effect was independent of cross fostering. When tested at 20 and 60 days of age, offspring from chlorpromazine-treated mothers made fewer avoidances in a shock-elicited escape-avoidance learning situation and exhibited less exploratory behavior and longer latencies to move in an open-field test. Although modified slightly by maternal influences, these drug effects were not eliminated by cross fostering. For example, drug offspring raised by drug mothers made significantly fewer avoidances than drug offspring raised by placebo mothers, suggesting that postnatal effects of the drug remaining in the mother after birth influenced the avoidance behavior of the offspring. Correspondingly, control offspring raised by drug mothers had significantly longer latencies in an open-field test than control offspring raised by placebo mothers. The overall design of these experiments was much improved compared to earlier investigations and, unfortunately, was better than some subsequent experiments.

In a study by Clark et al. (1970), pregnant rats received daily subcutaneous injections of d-amphetamine (2 mg/kg), chlorpromazine (5 mg/kg), or saline on days 12–16 of gestation. At birth each litter was reduced to three male and three female pups and, at various times thereafter, the pups were tested in an open-field, a T-maze, and an operant conditioning procedure. Again, there was no consistent or logical pattern in the behavior of the offspring. These authors also ignored the use of cross-fostering procedures and dose–response relationships.

Davis and Lin (1972) examined the effects of prenatal administration of morphine on perinatal mortality and postnatal growth and behavior of rats. Beginning on the fifth day of pregnancy, rats received daily subcutaneous injections of saline or morphine. The dose of morphine sulfate was increased every second day in a stepwise fashion starting with 15 mg/kg and reaching a maximum of 45 mg/kg on days 17 and 18, at which time the morphine injections were stopped. Parturition occurred on day 21. Morphine treatment caused no maternal deaths, no evidence of fetal resorption, and no alteration in litter size at birth. Nevertheless, at birth and during the first postnatal week, the offspring from morphine-treated mothers weighed less and had a higher perinatal rate of mortality. Body weights of morphine-treated mothers were also reduced during gestation.

When subjected to an open-field testing situation at 30 or 70 days of age, offspring from morphine-treated mothers were more active and exhibited increased rearing compared to offspring from saline-treated controls. Also morphine offspring showed increased exploratory activity in a circular actophotometer and were more susceptible to audiogenic convulsive seizures. Thus, prenatal administration of morphine caused significant, long-lasting behavioral alterations in offspring. Unfortunately, no cross-fostered experimental groups were included in the study (see below, Friedler and Cochin, 1972). Also, the authors did not comment on possible withdrawal symptoms in both the mother and newborn. In view of the all too common case of the infant born to a narcotic addict (Section VII,A), further studies of the type conducted by Davis and Lin are necessary.

It is becoming increasingly apparent that pesticides and other environmental toxicants can cause acute and chronic toxicity as well as possible teratogenic effects. Al-Hachim and Fink (1967, 1968) found that administration of the insecticides, DDT (2.5 mg/kg) and parathion (3 mg/kg), orally every 2 days during a trimester of gestation in mice caused alterations in behavioral responses of offspring. These doses of DDT and parathion produced no acute toxicity in nonpregnant adult rats and had no effect on liter size. Regardless of the trimester of DDT or parathion administration, the onset of high incidence (>70%) of audiogenic seizures was delayed 2 days in offspring tested repeatedly. Prenatal administration of DDT increased the latency for seizures but only when administered during the third trimester. DDT, administered during the second or third trimester but not during the first trimester, caused a delay in acquisition of a conditioned avoidance response. Parathion did not affect acquisition regardless of the trimester administered. Although Al-Hachim and Fink suggested the possibility of transfer of DDT to the offspring in the mother's milk (Kartashova and Kartashova, 1963), they did not use cross-fostering procedures.

At the present time, official recognition of a case of methylmercury poisoning requires an overt neurological deficit. A report by Spyker et al. (1972) demonstrated, however, that exposure to methylmercury on day 7 or 9 of gestation resulted in mouse offspring which had no neurological deficits or altered growth patterns yet were significantly different from control offspring in open-field and swimming tests. The possibility that subtle behavioral alterations might also occur in humans after exposure to methylmercury and other environmental contaminants needs to be explored.

Studies of Gauron and Rowley (1969, 1971a) suggested that chronic drug exposure in female rats during their postnatal development can cause altered behavioral responses in untreated first, second, and third generation offspring. In the original study, female rat pups, from day 5 to day 55 of age, received daily subcutaneous injections of prochlorperazine (0.4 mg/kg), chlorpromazine (2 mg/kg), trifluoperazine (16 mg/kg), or an equivalent volume of saline. At 75 days of age, drugtreated animals showed impaired acquisition of a conditioned avoidance response compared to saline-treated controls. At 120 days, the females were bred. Again starting at 75 days of age, offspring of trifluoperazine- or prochlorperazine-treated females were inferior to saline offspring in acquisition of the conditioned avoidance response. Performance of offspring of chlorpromazine-treated mothers was not different from that of controls. Also, chlorpromazine treatment decreased the percentage of successful matings. In a subsequent study, Gauron and Rowley (1971a) demonstrated that second and third generation offspring of not only trifluorperazine- and prochlorpromazine-treated females but also of chlorpromazine-treated females exhibited impaired acquisition of a conditioned avoidance response compared to the saline group. Successful mating in the chlorpromazine group was not affected in the first- and second-generation females. Learning of a Hebb–Williams food maze was not impaired in second- and third-generation offspring. The drug-treated mothers, however, were not tested in the maze, so it is not clear whether or not the drug-treatment schedules altered maze learning in drug-treated animals. In subsequent studies with trifluoperazine, the cross-generational learning deficit was not a particular function of dosage or duration of drug administration (Gauron and Rowley, 1971b), and was not affected by cross fostering (Gauron and Rowley, 1973). The mechanism for these changes, possibly a genetic mutation or biochemical alteration, is unknown. Importantly, these studies are the first to suggest that behavioral effects of drugs can extend across several generations of animals.

Friedler and Cochin (1972) reported that treatment of female rats with morphine prior to conception alters the growth rate and analgesic response to morphine in their offspring. Female rats received increasing subcutaneous doses of morphine sulfate (10 mg/kg initially, then 15 mg/kg twice daily on days 2–5, and 22 mg/kg on the final day) or similar administrations of saline for $5\frac{1}{2}$ days. Five days later, when withdrawal symptoms were no longer discernible, the females were mated with untreated males. Litters from morphine- and saline-treated rats weighed the same at birth. Despite the fact that they were not exposed to morphine *in utero* or after birth, offspring from morphine-treated rats exhibited a reduced rate of growth when compared to the saline-treated controls. Although there were no differences in the number of deaths prior to weaning at 21 days, the incidence of death in litters from morphine-treated mothers (29%) was significantly higher than that of the control group (3%) during the 4- to 7-week period after birth. The effects on mortality and growth were not due to postnatal influences, since cross fostering of offspring did not alter the results significantly. When tested for an analgesic response to morphine on a hot plate at 8 weeks of age, offspring from morphine-treated mothers were less sensitive or more tolerant to a test dose of morphine than were offspring from saline-treated controls (Cochin, 1970).

As in the studies of Gauron and Rowley (1969, 1971a), premating drug experience in female rats resulted in significant effects on behavioral responses and growth of their offspring. As Friedler and Cochin suggested, a possible mutagenic effect or selection of certain clones of gametes by morphine could account for the effects observed. Alternatively, some factor present in the blood of the morphine-tolerant females may be transferred across the placenta to the fetus.

VIII. Biochemical and Behavioral Effects of Drugs Administered during the Postnatal Period

During early postnatal development, a child may encounter a variety of drugs and environmental contaminants which, in sufficient doses, may produce overt toxicity. Analogous to the situation of prenatal drug exposure, these same agents may also cause subtle yet perhaps permanent functional or behavioral effects dissociated from gross structural abnormalities. In the case of centrally active drugs, the latter possibility seems very likely considering that (1) these drugs, without exception, alter the metabolism of at least one putative neurotransmitter substance in adult brain, (2) the neurotransmitter systems of the neonatal CNS are developing rapidly. Thus, even slight interference with normal function at key points of neonatal development may disrupt the establishment of final, correct synaptic relationships.

Therefore, one objective of administration of drugs to neonates would be to screen for possible long-lasting alterations in behavior. Such studies may help avert tragedies of a mental or psychological nature but of previously unknown etiology. At present, little information is available with respect to either the human infant or the experimental animal. Obviously, ethical considerations in humans will restrict most studies to experimental animals.

The developing animal may also be a useful model system in which to examine the mechanisms of action of centrally active drugs and the neurochemical bases for various behaviors. Similarly, components of behaviors and the factors controlling maturation of normal adult metabolism of neurotransmitter substances may be studied advantageously in the developing organism. Drugs may be useful tools in such studies. For example, 6-hydroxydopamine may prove valuable for studying: (1) the long-term behavioral effects resulting from interruption of noradrenergic transmission in the neonatal CNS, (2) the role of noradrenergic systems in the development of various behaviors such as locomotor activity, temperature regulation, feeding and drinking, and conditioned avoidance responding, (3) the factors important in the maturation of noradrenergic systems, (4) the phenomena of axonal regeneration and sprouting following nerve damage (see Section VI,A,6).

A. General Problems in Experimental Design

1. ENVIRONMENTAL FACTORS

During the early postnatal period, animal behavior and biochemistry are particularly susceptible to influence by environmental factors. One must be cognizant of and attempt to control for these various factors in order to minimize any confounding effects they may have on interpretation of drug-induced effects. The presence or absence of environmental stimuli during critical periods of neonatal development may alter subsequent physiology and behavior in rodents. For example, Bell et al. (1961) found that in adult rats the blood glucose concentration determined 1 day after electroconvulsive shock varied as a function of neonatal handling. Previously unhandled animals and those handled daily beginning on postnatal day 5 had significantly elevated blood glucose concentrations; rats handled only on days 2–5 did not. Levine and Lewis (1959) demonstrated that by handling rats during the first week of life they could shorten the time it takes for the animal to respond to a cold stress with a reduction in adrenal ascorbic acid concentration; handled rats responded on postnatal day 12, whereas nonhandled rats did not respond until day 16. When exposed to an unfamiliar open-field test as adults, early handled rats generally respond with higher activity, lower defecation scores, and lower plasma adrenocorticoid concentrations than nonhandled controls (Levine and Lewis, 1959; Levine et al., 1967). The composite effect of early handling on later open-field behavior is frequently referred to as a reduced "emotionality." In a Hebb–Williams maze test, early handling was associated with increased activity although error scores were unchanged (Levine and Lewis, 1959). Denenberg (1968) demonstrated that handling during the first days of life increased the ability of the rat to learn conditioned avoidance responding procedures. It should be noted, however, that other workers using somewhat different experimental procedures reported just the opposite effects.

Hudgens *et al.* (1971) studied open-field behaviors of mother rats as a function of early handling of offspring. Their results suggest that early manipulation can have direct effects on both the mother and her offspring and thereby result in altered mother–pup interactions, which appear to be exceedingly complex.

Unless presented in the diet, administration of drugs to the neonate will necessarily involve handling. Moreover, the acute effect of the drug may alter: (1) the normal response to handling, (2) the normal feeding pattern, (3) the perception of maternal stimuli, (4) the mother's attention to the pups. Noxious effects of the drug per se such as peritoneal irritation-induced stress also could contribute to differences between treated and control groups. Thus, even though handling procedures may be kept constant between experimental groups, drug treatments may alter the responses of the neonate to handling. Possible influences of stress on postnatal behavioral development are also discussed in Section VII,B,1.

The type of housing will influence animal behavior. For example, animals raised in isolation are less active in open-field tests and more resistant to handling stress than are group-housed animals.

In summary, a number of environmental variables must be recognized and controlled in order to determine the effects of drug administration during the early postnatal period on subsequent behavioral performance. These include the degree of social stimulation, group or isolation housing, amount of handling, and previous test experiences. In some situations, however, recognition and control of all possible interacting variables may not be possible.

2. MISCELLANEOUS FACTORS

The exact experimental design of any study depends primarily upon the hypothesis to be tested and the most suitable methodological approaches. Nevertheless, in studies of effects of neonatal drug exposure on later postnatal behavior, certain factors should always be considered in the experimental design.

Possible effects of handling or nonhandling and related interactions with drug treatment were discussed in the last section. In this regard, one additional consideration is necessary if behavioral tests are to be repeated several times and if the initial tests are conducted during the period of drug administration. Association of drug administration with a behavioral test, particularly if the drug or test entails presentation of noxious stimuli, may result in "state-dependent" learning (Overton, 1966) or a drug-test interaction (Kayan *et al.*, 1969). That is, when a behavioral test is conducted immediately before or after drug administration, a resulting learned association between drug and test may alter the behavioral response in subsequent tests. Thus, if behavioral responses are to be determined both during and after drug treatment, a proper control might be to include an experimental group that is tested only after disappearance of any acute drug effect. In any case, acute and long-lasting effects of the drug should be clearly differentiated if possible.

Interpretation of long-term behavioral alterations resulting from early drug exposure may be facilitated by knowledge of possible drug effects during the preweaning period. During the first 2 postnatal weeks in rodents, however, most behaviors are not yet distinct and thus very difficult to measure. Fox (1965, 1970) has developed a battery of simple reflex tests for the mouse, kitten, and puppy which may be used to assess the degree of neural maturation and which appears to be a reliable indicator of normal development. Thus, comparison of the patterns of appearance or disappearance of the various reflexes in control and drug-treated animals may aid interpretation of behavioral alterations observed in later life. Such reflex tests are simpler to perform and may yield equally or more reliable data than examination of the EEG patterns or sleep–wakefulness patterns in neonates (Ellingson and Rose, 1970; Gramsbergen *et al.*, 1970; Jouvet-Mounier *et al.*, 1970). Other possible experimental considerations are discussed where applicable to particular studies in Section VIII,B.

B. Experimental Studies

In a study examining the effects of early postnatal drug treatment on later behavior, Meier and Huff (1962) administered reserpine (2.5 mg/kg) or saline subcutaneously to rats from postnatal day 4 to 43, and then exposed the subjects to an open-field test, a discrimination test, and a Lashley III water maze at subsequent times. Reserpine treatment did not alter the time of eye opening, onset of locomotion, body weight gain, or mortality. In the open-field test, reserpine treatment had no effect on ambulation but decreased defecation and urination. Learning performance in the Lashley III maze was not affected by reserpine. Reserpine significantly reduced the percentage of correct responses in a discrimination test, in which food-deprived rats were presented with three geometric figures, only one of which was associated with a food reward. In contrast to control animals, reserpine-treated rats showed little improvement in the number of correct responses over the course of a 9-day testing period. Thus rats administered reserpine during postnatal development showed selective alterations in later behavior, although the significance of the observed changes is equivocal.

Doty *et al.* (1964) attempted to determine if chronic treatment with chlorpromazine during infancy affected the ability of rats to utilize home cage environmental cues in subsequent problem solving requiring the use of these cues. Rats received daily intraperitoneal injections of chlorpromazine (2 mg/kg) or saline from 3 to 60 days of age, and were visually exposed to geometric forms (circle or triangle) in their home cage from 10 to 60 days. A third group of rats received no treatment and no experience with cues during this period. At 90 days of age, all rats were required to learn a discriminated avoidance problem using the geometric figures as cues. Avoidance performance was significantly and equally impaired in both chlorpromazine-treated and naive rats as compared to saline controls. Thus in this experiment, chronic chlorpromazine administration during the postnatal period of development impaired later ability to utilize cues present in the early environment. It is rather distressing that so few studies comprise the present literature concerning long-term behavioral effects of early postnatal administration of clinically used psychoactive drugs.

Prenatal exposure of rats to the insecticides, DDT or parathion, resulted in altered postnatal behavioral responses (Section VII,B,2; Al-Hachim and Fink, 1967, 1968). More recently, Sobotka et al., (1972) found that neonatal exposure of rats to maneb (ethylenebisdithiocarbamate manganese), a commonly used fungicide, produced long-lasting behavioral and neurochemical effects. Rats received diets containing 0, 0.5, 1.0, or 10 parts per million (ppm) of maneb during (1) the 28-day neonatal period, (2) the 5-month postweaning period, (3) both the neonatal and postweaning periods of life. The concentrations of maneb were well below those previously shown to affect reproductive function and physical development (Shtenberg et al., 1969), and approximated residues in agricultural products. Maneb treatment, irrespective of duration or dose, had no effect on adult body weight, thyroid or brain weights, or body weights of 30-day-old males. Neonatal exposure to 0.5 or 10 ppm of maneb resulted in reduced open-field activity and increased preshock stepout latencies in a passive avoidance test in 30-day-old rats, both results suggesting reduced exploratory activity in a novel environment. Neonatal or long-term exposure (10 ppm) to maneb caused higher avoidance scores (improved learning) in an operant conditioning test at 3–6 months of age. In contrast, postweaning exposure to maneb did not alter avoidance scores when compared to controls, suggesting that neonatal exposure is necessary for the long-lasting effect on learning.

At the termination of operant conditioning procedures at 6 months of age, plasma corticosterone concentrations were significantly elevated exclusively in rats receiving maneb postweaning only. Sobotka et al. (1972) determined cholinesterase in brain regions of 6-month-old rats since dithiocarbamate derivatives have previously been shown to inhibit brain cholinesterase activity. Cholinesterase activity of the telencephalon was significantly reduced by a 1.0 or 10 ppm maneb diet regardless of its duration. Enzyme activity in the midbrain–diencephalon or pons–medulla was significantly reduced only after preweaning or postweaning exposure to 10 ppm of maneb. In all brain regions, postweaning exposure to maneb effected the greatest reductions in cholinesterase activity. Thus neonatal exposure to maneb caused altered behavioral responses both immediately postweaning and 5 months after cessation of treatment. The neurochemical changes induced by maneb, however, did not appear to be related to the altered behavioral responses. Hopefully, this study will set a precedent for similar studies in the future with respect to (1) an attempt to correlate behavioral and neurochemical effects, (2) the use of several concentrations (doses) and durations of drug treatment. Most importantly, the study of Sobotka and co-workers indicates the immediate need for an intensive effort to examine the possibility of significant, long-lasting behavioral and neurochemical alterations resulting from exposure to environmental toxicants during early development.

Several investigators have administered p-chlorophenylalanine to rats during early development in attempts to produce an acceptable animal model of phenylketonuria in humans (Watt and Martin, 1969; Pryor and Mitoma, 1970; Kilbey and Harris, 1971; Vorhees et al., 1972; Hole, 1972b). Earlier studies (see Perry et al., 1965; Hole, 1972a) had employed large amounts of L-phenylalanine administered chronically to developing rats in attempts to obtain a model for phenylketonuria. Such phenylalanine treatment mimicked phenylketonuria to the extent that high serum phenylalanine concentrations, urinary excretion of phenylpyruvic acid, and decreased contents of brain serotonin were observed. Such rats were also deficient in learning various behavioral tasks, although the effects were generally transient. In contrast to the human condition however, phenylalanine administration to animals caused a marked elevation in serum tyrosine concentration. Woolley and van der Hoeven (1965) had proposed that the learning deficits in rats with experimental phenylketonuria were directly related to the reduced contents of brain serotonin in these animals. Thus, the report that p-chlorophenylalanine produced a specific depletion of serotonin in brain of rats (Koe and Weissman, 1966) led investigators to employ this drug in attempts to produce experimental phenylketonuria in rats. Although later biochemical studies (see Section VI,B,5) indicated that p-chlorophenylalanine is not specific for serotonergic neurons, the studies using this drug are valuable from the standpoint of demonstrating long-term behavioral changes in response to early postnatal drug exposure.

Watt and Martin (1969) found that rats receiving daily subcutaneous injections of p-chlorophenylalanine (50 mg/kg for 5 days, then 100 mg/kg for 5 days, then 200 mg/kg for the duration) from birth to postnatal day 34 made significantly more errors in learning a water maze (similar to a Lashley III maze) on day 35 than did control rats. The learning deficit was slowly reversible when treatment was withdrawn. Unfortunately since the animals were tested on the day following the last drug treatment, the observed response was at least partially due to an acute or residual drug effect. Their procedure of treating one-half of each litter with drug and one-half with vehicle is also questionable, because of possible altered pup–pup and mother–pup interactions.

Pryor and Mitoma (1970) fed rats a diet containing 0.01% p-chlorophenylalanine from birth to 6 weeks of age and subsequently determined their performance in several behavioral tasks. Brain serotonin was reduced to nondetectable concentrations during treatment and only slowly returned to control concentrations. Open-field activity of drug-treated animals was reduced during drug treatment and up to 86 days after cessation of the test diet. Nevertheless, no differences in learned responses between treatment and control groups that persisted longer than 20 days posttreatment were observed in a pole-climb avoidance test, an underwater T-maze, or a modified Lashley III maze surface swimming test, The observed differences in open-field activity tended to disappear if the test diet was presented for 8 weeks. The lack of effect of p-chlorophenylalanine on maze learning observed in this experiment contrasts with decreased learning of a similar maze observed by Watt and Martin (1969) but may be accounted for by several procedural differences. Pryor and Mitoma conducted the maze tests at least 20 days after drug treatment; also administration of the drug in the diet eliminated handling effects and also minimized noxious effects of the drug associated with intraperitoneal administration (Volicer, 1969; Thornburg and Moore, 1971). Pryor and Mitoma, however, used smaller drug litters (8–9 pups) than control litters (10–11 pups).

Kilbey and Harris (1971) administered p-chlorophenylalanine (100 mg/kg i.p.) to rats from birth to 30 days of age. Maturation of grooming and righting reflexes was slightly retarded, and activity levels were lower up to 121 days in drug-treated animals. At 180 days of age, drug-treated rats exhibited a decreased total number of responses in a pole-climb avoidance task. Brain serotonin contents were reduced by 80% during treatment but attained normal concentrations shortly after treatment was stopped.

Vorhees et al. (1972) reported that rats fed a diet of 3% excess L-phenylalanine and 0.12% p-chlorophenylalanine between 21 and 51 days of age exhibited decreased open-field activity when tested 4 or 11 days after treatment when compared to either pair-fed controls or controls fed *ad libitum*. Both pair-fed control and *p*-chlorophenylalanine-treated rats weighed significantly less than controls allowed free access to food. Thus, the results indicated that hypoactivity was not due to differences in food consumption or weight at the time of testing. By 11 days after the test diet, brain serotonin contents had returned to 80% of normal, suggesting that the decreased open-field activity was not directly related to the deficit of serotonin. These results support the findings of earlier studies that chronic administration of *p*-chlorophenylalanine during postnatal development causes a general deficit in arousal.

Hole (1972a) treated rats with *p*-chlorophenylalanine (200 mg/kg i.p.) on days 3, 7, 11, and 14 and then every second day up to 50 days of age; various behavioral tests were conducted at subsequent times. The major and consistent deficit observed in *p*-chlorophenylalanine-treated rats was reduced arousal: reduced activity in an open-field test, longer latencies in leaving start boxes in both spontaneous alternation and Lashley III maze situations, less grooming, decreased responses to shocks in a passive avoidance test, and decreased responses to auditory stimuli in a habituation test. Tendencies for more rapid habituation and slower speed in the Lashley III maze were also observed. There was no evidence of a learning deficit. Although serotonin was reduced to less than 20% of normal during treatment, its concentration was normal at the times of behavioral testing. There was a permanent decrease in brain weight but only a transient decrease in body weight followed by a significant increase in body weight at about 4 weeks.

The consistent finding in these studies is that chronic administration of *p*-chlorophenylalanine during development causes a reduced state of arousal persisting after drug treatment but not any long-lasting deficits in learned behavior. In sharp contrast, *p*-chlorophenylalanine administration to adult rats causes effects suggestive of increased arousal: locomotor hyperactivity, decreased sleep, slow habituation, and increased sensitivity to foot shock. Lesions of the serotonergic midbrain raphe nuclei also cause behavioral and electroencephalographic indications of arousal (for references, see Hole, 1972a). Accordingly, the decreased state of arousal after chronic *p*-chlorophenylalanine treatment is probably not related to a lack of brain serotonin. Nevertheless, the considerable differences in experimental procedures between studies and the nonspecific effects of *p*-chlorophenylalanine, both biochemically and behaviorally, hinder interpretation of the significance of these studies.

Campbell *et al.* (1969) hypothesized that maturation of an adrenergic arousal system precedes that of the opposing cholinergic system; hence, during an early period of development, the animals should be responsive to adrenergic stimulation but unresponsive to cholinergic stimulation. Using d-amphetamine sulfate, an adrenergic stimulant, and scopolamine, a cholinergic blocking agent, dose-locomotor activity relationships were determined in 10-, 15-, 20-, and 25-day-old and adult rats. Locomotor activity (behavioral arousal) was determined in stabilimeter cages scaled to the size of the animals. Amphetamine caused a dose-related increase in activity at all ages tested; in contrast, scopolamine increased activity only in 20-day and older rats. Also, 15-day-old rats were most sensitive to amphetamine in that the maximum increase in activity was obtained at a lower dose compared to adult animals. Correspondingly, spontaneous activity in control animals was greatest at 15 days of age (Moorcroft, 1971). Similar patterns of effects on locomotor activity for amphetamine and scopolamine have recently been demonstrated in the mouse (Thornburg and Moore, 1973). These authors also utilized the differential development of the dopaminergic and cholinergic systems to demonstrate that benztropine-induced stimulation primarily through an anticholinergic mechanism. These data suggest that an excitatory adrenergic system mediating arousal matures prior to an opposing cholinergic system. Fibiger et al. (1970) presented further evidence for this hypothesis. In adult rats amphetamine-induced locomotor activity is effectively potentiated or antagonized by simultaneous administration of scopolamine or pilocarpine, respectively. In the developing rat, however, similar effects were not significant until 20 to 25 days of age. These studies provide behavioral evidence that an excitatory adrenergic system mediating behavioral arousal is functional at birth or shortly thereafter, but that an opposing cholinergic mechanism is not functional until 20–25 days postnatally in the rat. The results also suggest that the developing brain can be studied advantageously both chemically and behaviorally to better understand the nature of two reciprocally interacting neuronal systems.

The work of Campbell and co-workers points out several important procedural considerations in activity studies in developing animals. During the first two postnatal weeks, rats and mice are poikilothermic; that is, they assume the temperature of the nest. Extended periods alone in a testing chamber at 22° to 25°C may have deleterious effects on the animal's performance and subsequent development. Therefore, these workers maintained the testing room at 29°C for the 10- to 25-day-old rats compared to 22°C for adult rats.

Activity measurements obtained using circular actophotometer cages or open-field apparatus may not be independent of the size of the animals. Thus one must be careful in equating measures of activity or locomotion with the degree of behavioral arousal or stimulation. Campbell and co-workers have used stabilimeter cages scaled to the size of the animal so that proportionately equivalent movements would be recorded as similar activity. In very young rats and mice, locomotion may consist only of turning or pivoting.

IX. Summary

The results of studies in developmental behavioral pharmacology in animals suggest that pre- or early postnatal administration of a variety of centrally acting drugs cause subtle, long-lasting biochemical and behavioral effects in the offspring. There are many difficulties in relating the results of animal experimentation to the human situation, but the results of recent clinical studies have demonstrated that chronic exposure of the mother to narcotic analgesics, tranquilizers, and barbiturates during gestation, or the acute administration of these drugs to the mother during delivery have short-term effects on the behavior of the infant. There is, however, no unequivocal evidence that perinatal drug administration causes long-term behavioral alterations in children. Perhaps studies of developmental behavioral pharmacology in animals can serve to alert the clinician to potential problems of drug use during gestation and the perinatal period. Furthermore, animal studies may suggest important studies that should be performed in humans, although many ethical and procedural problems will continue to hamper such clinical investigations.

Studies of developmental behavioral pharmacology should also be useful in examining the mechanisms of drug action. All neuronal systems do not become operational at the same time during the development of the CNS. By examining the effects of drugs at various times during the developmental period it may be possible to establish relationships between the onset of drug action and the onset of functional activity of specific neuronal systems, as evaluated by electrophysiological or biochemical measurements. This approach of correlating neurophysiology or biochemistry with behavior may be less prone to artifacts than studies that involve chemical or surgical ablation techniques to disrupt neuronal activity.

A recent interest in the developmental pharmacology of drugs acting in the CNS is evidenced by the increase in research communications dealing with this subject since 1970. This is perhaps indicative of a growing interest in closing the gaps in our knowledge about this important but heretofore largely neglected area of research.

REFERENCES

Agranoff, B. W. (1967). *In* "The Neurosciences: A Study Program" (G. C. Quarton, T. Melnechuk, and F. O. Schmitt, eds.), Vol. 1, pp. 756–764. Rockefeller Univ. Press, New York.

Agrawal, H. C., and Himwich, W. A. (1970). *In* "Developmental Neurobiology" (W. A. Himwich, ed.), pp. 287–310. Thomas, Springfield, Illinois.

Agrawal, H. C., Glisson, S. N., and Himwich, W. A. (1966a). *Biochim. Biophys. Acta* **130**, 511–513.

Agrawal, H. C., Davis, J. M., and Himwich, W. A. (1966b). *J. Neurochem.* **13**, 607–615.

Agrawal, H. C, Glisson, S. N., and Himwich, W. A. (1968a). *Neuropharmacology* **7**, 97–101.

Agrawal, H. C., Davis, J. M., and Himwich, W. A. (1968b). *J. Neurochem.* **15**, 529–531.

Al-Hachim, G. M., and Fink, G. B. (1967). *Psychol. Rep.* **20**, 1183–1187.

Al-Hachim, G. M., and Fink, G. B. (1968). *Psychopharmacologia* **12**, 424–427.

Altman, J. (1967). *In* "The Neurosciences: A Study Program" (G. C. Quarton, T. Melnechuk, and F. O. Schmitt, eds.), Vol. 1, pp. 723–743. Rockefeller Univ. Press, New York.

Altman, J. (1970). *In* "Developmental Neurobiology" (W. A. Himwich, ed.), pp. 197–240. Thomas, Springfield, Illinois.

Andén, N.-E., Corrodi, H., Dahlström, A., Fuxe, K., and Hökfelt, T. (1966). *Life Sci.* **5**, 561–568.

Angeletti, P. U. (1971). *Neuropharmacology* **10**, 55–59.

Angeletti, P. U., and Levi-Montalcini, R. (1970). *Proc. Nat. Acad. Sci. U.S.* **65**, 114–121.

Apgar, V. (1953). *Curr. Res. Anesth. Analg.* **32**, 260–267.

Aprison, M. H., and Himwich, H. E. (1954). *Amer. J. Physiol.* **179**, 502–506.

Aprison, M. H., Kariya, T., Hingtgen, J. N., and Toru, M. (1968). *J. Neurochem.* **15**, 1111–1139.

Archer, J. E., and Blackman, D. E. (1971). *Develop. Psychobiol.* **4**, 193–248.

Asano, Y. (1971). *Life Sci.* **10**, 883–894.

Ashcroft, G. W., Eccleston, D., and Crawford, T. B. B. (1965). *J. Neurochem.* **12**, 483–492.

Baker, P. C., and Hoff, K. M. (1972). *J. Neurochem.* **19**, 2011–2015.

Baker, P. C., and Quay, W. B. (1969). *Brain Res.* **12**, 273–295.

Balazs, R., Cocks, W. A., Earys, J. T., and Kovacs, S. (1971). *In* "Hormones in Development" (M. Hamberg and E. J. W. Barrington, eds.), pp. 357–379. Appleton, New York.

Batt, B. L. (1968). *Amer. J. Obstet. Gynecol.* **102**, 591–596.

Baumgarten, H. G., and Lachenmayer, L. (1972). *Z. Zellforsch. Mikrosk. Anat.* **135**, 399–414.

Baumgarten, H. G., Björklund, A., Lachenmayer, L. Nobin, A., and Stenevi, U. (1971). *Acta Physiol. Scand., Suppl.* **373**, 1–15.

Baxter, C. F. (1970). *In* "Handbook of Neurochemistry" (A. Lajtha, ed.), Vol. III, pp. 289–353. Plenum, New York.

Bayer, S. M., and McMurray, W. C. (1967). *J. Neurochem.* **14**, 695–706.

Becker, B. A. (1970). *In* "Developmental Neurobiology" (W. A. Himwich, ed.), pp. 613–651. Thomas, Springfield, Illinois.

Beleslin, D. B., and Myers, R. D. (1970). *Brain Res.* **23**, 437–442.

Bell, R. W., Reisner, G., and Linn, T. (1961). *Science* **133**, 1428–1429.

Bennett, D. S., and Giarman, N. J. (1965). *J. Neurochem.* **12**, 911–918.
Benson, R. C., Berendes, H., and Weiss, W. (1969). *Amer. J. Obstet. Gynecol.* **105**, 579–588.
Berl, S. (1964). *Progr. Brain Res.* **9**, 178–182.
Berl, S., and Purpura, D. P. (1963). *J. Neurochem.* **10**, 237–240.
Bitnum, S. (1969). *Can. Med. Ass. J.* **100**, 351 (Letter).
Björklund, A., and Stenevi, U. (1971). *Brain Res.* **31**, 1–20.
Björklund, A., Enemar, A., and Falck, B. (1968). *Z. Zellforsch. Mikrosk. Anat.* **89**, 590–607.
Björklund, A., Katzman, R., Stenevi, U., and West, K. A. (1971). *Brain Res.* **31**, 21–33.
Black, I. B., Hendry, I. A., and Iversen, L. L. (1971). *Brain Res.* **34**, 229–240.
Black, I. B., Hendry, I. A., and Iversen, L. L. (1972). *J. Physiol. (London)* **221**, 149–159.
Bleyer, W. A., and Marshall, R. E. (1972). *J. Amer. Med. Ass.* **221**, 185–186.
Blinick, G., Wallach, R. C., and Jerez, E. (1969). *Amer. J. Obstet. Gynecol.* **105**, 997–1003.
Bloom, F. E., Algeri, S., Groppetti, A., Revuelta, A., and Costa, E. (1969). *Science* **166**, 1284–1286.
Bogdanski, D. F., Weissbach, H., and Udenfriend, S. (1957). *J. Neurochem.* **1**, 272–278.
Borgstedt, A. D., and Rosen, M. G. (1968). *Amer. J. Dis. Child.* **115**, 21–24.
Bourne, B. B. (1965). *Life Sci.* **4**, 583–591.
Brazelton, T. B. (1961). *J. Pediat.* **58**, 513–518.
Brazelton, T. B. (1970). *Amer. J. Psychiat.* **126**, 1261–1266.
Breese, G. R., and Traylor, T. D. (1970). *J. Pharmacol. Exp. Ther.* **174**, 413–420.
Breese, G. R., and Traylor, T. D. (1971). *Brit. J. Pharmacol.* **42**, 88–99.
Breese, G. R., and Traylor, T. D. (1972). *Brit. J. Pharmacol.* **44**, 210–222.
Browning, E. T., and Schulman, M. P. (1968). *J. Neurochem.* **15**, 1391–1405.
Budnick, I. S., Leikin, S., and Hoeck, L. E. (1955). *Amer. J. Dis. Child.* **90**, 286–289.
Burdick, C. J., and Strittmatter, C. F. (1965). *Arch. Biochem. Biophys.* **109**, 293–301.
Caley, D. W., and Maxwell, D. S. (1971). *In* "Brain Development and Behavior" (M. B. Sterman, D. J. McGinty, and A. M. Adinolfi, eds.), pp. 89–106. Academic Press, New York.
Campbell, B. A., Lytle, L. D., and Fibiger, H. C. (1969). *Science* **166**, 635–637.
Carr, L. A., and Moore, K. E. (1968). *Neuroendocrinology* **3**, 285–302.
Carr, L. A., and Moore, K. E. (1969). *Science* **164**, 322–323.
Clark, C. V., Gorman, D., and Vernadakis, A. (1970). *Develop. Psychobiol.* **3**, 225–235.
Clark, D. W. J., Laverty, R., and Phelan, E. L. (1972). *Brit. J. Pharmacol.* **44**, 233–243.
Cobrinik, R. W., Hood, R. T., and Chusid, E. (1959). *Pediatrics* **24**, 288–304.
Cochin, J. (1970). *Fed. Proc., Fed. Amer. Soc. Exp. Biol.* **29**, 19–27.
Connor, J. D., and Neff, N. H. (1970). *Life Sci.* **9**, 1165–1168.
Cooper, J. R., Bloom, F. E., and Roth, R. H. (1970). "The Biochemical Basis of Neuropharmacology." Oxford Univ. Press, London and New York.
Costa, E. (1969). *In* "The Present Status of Psychotropic Drugs" (A. Gerletti and F. J. Bove, eds.), pp. 11–35. Excerpta Med. Found., Amsterdam.
Costa, E., and Neff, N. H. (1970). *In* "Handbook of Neurochemistry" (A. Lajtha, ed.), Vol. IV, pp. 45–90. Plenum, New York.
Coyle, J. T., and Axelrod, J. (1971). *J. Neurochem.* **18**, 2061–2075.
Coyle, J. T., and Axelrod, J. (1972a). *J. Neurochem.* **19**, 449–459.
Coyle, J. T., and Axelrod, J. (1972b). *J. Neurochem.* **19**, 1117–1123.

Coyle, J. T., and Henry, D. (1973). *J. Neurochem.* **21**, 61–67.

Dahlström, A., and Fuxe, K. (1965). *Acta Physiol. Scand., Suppl.* **232**, 1–55.

Danilova, O. A. (1971). *Histochemie* **28**, 255–264.

Davis, J. M., Himwich, W. A., and Agrawal, H. C. (1968). *Develop. Psychobiol.* **1**, 24–29.

Davis, W. M., and Lin, C. H. (1972). *Res. Commun. Chem. Pathol. Pharmacol.* **3**, 205–214.

Davison, A. N., and Dobbing, J. (1968). *In* "Applied Neurochemistry" (A. N. Davison and J. Dobbing, eds.), pp. 253–286. Davis, Philadelphia, Pennsylvania.

Decancq, H. G., Bosco, J. R., and Townsend, E. H. (1965). *J. Pediat.* **67**, 836–840.

Deguchi, T., and Barchas, J. (1972). *J. Neurochem.* **19**, 927–929.

Denenberg, V. H. (1968). *In* "Early Experiences and Behavior" (G. Newton and S. Levine, eds.), pp. 142–167. Thomas, Springfield, Illinois.

De Robertis, E., Rodriguez de Lores Arnaiz, G. R., Salganicoff, L., Pellegrino de Iraldi, A. P., and Zieher, L. M. (1963). *J. Neurochem.* **10**, 225–235.

Desmond, M. M., Rogers, S. F., Lindley, J. E., and Mayer, J. H. (1957). *Obstet. Gynecol.* **10**, 140–145.

Desmond, M. M., Schwanecke, R. P., Wilson, G. S., Yasunaga, S., and Burgdorff, I. (1972). *J. Pediat.* **80**, 190–197.

Diegenbach, P. C. (1965). *Nature (London)* **207**, 308.

Doty, L. A., Doty, B. A., Wise, M. A., and Senn, R. K. (1964). *Percep. Mot. Skills* **18**, 329–332.

Dravid, A. R., and Himwich, W. A. (1964). *Progr. Brain Res.* **9**, 170–173.

Eayrs, J. T. (1971). *In* "Hormones in Development" (M. Hamberg and E. J. W. Barrington, eds.), pp. 345–355. Appleton, New York.

Eiduson, S. (1966). *J. Neurochem.* **13**, 923–932.

Eiduson, S. (1971). *UCLA (Univ. Calif. Los Angeles) Forum Med. Sci.* **14**, 391–414.

Elkes, J., and Todrick, A. (1955). *In* "Biochemistry of the Developing Nervous System" (H. Waelsch, ed.), pp. 309–314. Academic Press, New York.

Ellingson, R. J., and Rose, G. H. (1970). *In* "Developmental Neurobiology" (W. A. Himwich, ed.), pp. 441–474. Thomas, Springfiell, Illinois.

Enemar, A., and Falck, B. (1968). *Z. Zellforsch. Mikrosk. Anat.* **89**, 590–607.

Fahn, S., and Côté, L. J. (1968a). *J. Neurochem.* **15**, 209–213.

Fahn, S., and Côté, L. J. (1968b). *Brain Res.* **7**, 323–325.

Feigenson, M. E., and Saelens, J. K. (1969). *Biochem. Pharmacol.* **18**, 1479–1486.

Feldberg, W., and Myers, R. D. (1964). *J. Physiol. (London)* **173**, 226–237.

Fernstrom, J. D., and Wurtman, R. J. (1971). *Science* **173**, 149–152.

Fibiger, H. C., Lytle, L. D., and Campbell, B. A. (1970). *J. Comp. Physiol. Psychol.* **72**, 384–389.

Filogamo, G., and Marchisio, P. C. (1971). *Neurosci. Res.* **4**, 29–64.

Filogamo, G., Giacobini, E., Giacobini, G., and Moré, B. (1971). *J. Neurochem.* **18**, 1589–1591.

Flexner, L. B. (1955). *In* "Biochemistry of the Developing Nervous System" (H. Waelsch, ed.), pp. 281–300. Academic Press, New York.

Fonnum, F. (1968). *Biochem. J.* **106**, 401–412.

Fox, M. W. (1965). *Anim. Behav.* **13**, 234–241.

Fox, M. W. (1970). *In* "Developmental Neurobiology" (W. A. Himwich, ed.), pp. 553–580. Thomas, Springfield, Illinois.

Friedler, G., and Cochin, J. (1972). *Science* **175**, 654–656.

Friedman, A. H., and Walker, C. A. (1968). *J. Physiol. (London)* **197**, 77–85.

Friedman, S. B., and Ader, R. (1967). *Neuroendocrinology* **2**, 209–219.

Gauron, E. F., and Rowley, V. N. (1969). *Psychopharmacologia* **16**, 5–15.

Gauron, E. F., and Rowley, V. N. (1971a). *Eur. J. Pharmacol.* **15**, 171–175.

Gauron, E. F., and Rowley, V. N. (1971b). *Psychol. Rep.* **29**, 497–498.

Gauron, E. F., and Rowley, V. N. (1973). *Psychopharmacologia* **30**, 269–274.

Geller, E. (1971). *In* "Brain Development and Behavior" (M. B. Sterman, D. J. McGinty, and A. M. Adinolfi, eds.), pp. 277–300. Academic Press, New York.

Ghosh, S. K., and Guha, S. R. (1972). *J. Neurochem.* **19**, 229–231.

Giarman, N. J., and Pepeu, G. (1962). *Brit. J. Pharmacol. Chemother.* **19**, 226–234.

Glowinski, J. (1970). *In* "Handbook of Neurochemistry" (A. Lajtha, ed.), Vol. IV, pp. 91–114. Plenum, New York.

Golden, G. S. (1972). *Brain Res.* **44**, 278–282.

Gómez, C. J., Pasquini, J. M., Soto, E. F., and De Robertis, E. (1970). *J. Neurochem.* **17**, 1485–1492.

Goodfriend, M. J., Shey, I. A., and Klein, M. D. (1956). *Amer. J. Obstet. Gynecol.* **71**, 29–36.

Goodman, L. S., and Gilman, A., eds. (1970). "The Pharmacological Basis of Therapeutics," 4th ed. Macmillan, New York.

Gornicki, B., Bozkowa, K., Kurzepa, K., Cabalska, B., Rutkowska, A., Lambert, I., Grodzka, Z., Duczynska, N., Padzik, H., Czupryna, A., and Suslow, I. (1963). *Pol. Med. Sci. Hist. Bull.* **6**, 18–20.

Grahame-Smith, D. G. (1964). *Biochem. Biophys. Res. Commun.* **16**, 586–592.

Grahame-Smith, D. G. (1971). *J. Neurochem.* **18**, 1053–1066.

Gramsbergen, A., Schwartze, P., and Prechtl, H. F. R. (1970). *Develop. Psychobiol.* **3**, 267–280.

Green, J. P. (1970). *In* "Handbook of Neurochemistry" (A. Lajtha, ed.), Vol. IV, pp. 221–250. Plenum, New York.

Haber, B., and Kamano, A. (1964). *Nature (London)* **209**, 404.

Haber, B., Sze, P., Kuriyama, K., and Roberts, E. (1970). *Brain Res.* **18**, 545–547.

Hammar, C. G., Hanin, I., Holmstedt, B., Kitz, R. J., Jenden, D. J., and Kárlen, B. (1968). *Nature (Lonon)* **220**, 915–917.

Hanin, I., and Jenden, D. J. (1969). *Biochem. Pharmacol.* **18**, 837–845.

Hanin, I., Massarelli, R., and Costa, E. (1970). *Science* **170**, 341–342.

Hanin, I., Massarelli, R., and Costa, E. (1972). *J. Pharmacol. Exp. Ther.* **181**, 10–18.

Håkanson, R. (1970). *Acta Physiol. Scand., Suppl.* **340**, 1–134.

Hattori, T., and McGeer, P. L. (1973). *Exp. Neurol.* **38**, 70–79.

Havlena, J., and Werboff, J. (1963). *Psychol. Rep.* **12**, 127–131.

Hebb, C. O. (1956). *J. Physiol. (London)* **133**, 566–570.

Hebb, C. O. (1957). *Physiol. Rev.* **37**, 196–220.

Henley, W. L., and Fisch, G. R. (1966). *N.Y. State J. Med.* **66**, 2565–2567.

Hill, R. M., and Desmond, M. M. (1963). *Pediat. Clin. N. Amer.* **10**, 67–87.

Hill, R. M., Desmond, M. M., and Kay, J. L. (1966). *J. Pediat.* **69**, 589–595.

Hillarp, N.-Å., Fuxe, K., and Dahlström, A. (1966). *Pharmacol. Rev.* **18**, 727–741.

Himwich, H. E., and Aprison, M. H. (1955). *In* "Biochemistry of the Developing Nervous System" (H. Waelsch, ed.), pp. 301–307. Academic Press, New York.

Himwich, H. E., Pscheidt, G. R., and Schwiegerdt, A. K. (1967). *In* "Regional Development of the Brain in Early Life" (A. Minkowski, ed.), pp. 273–296. Davis, Philadelphia, Pennsylvania.

Himwich, W. A. (1962). *Int. Rev. Neurobiol.* **4**, 117–158.

Hoffeld, D. R., and Webster, R. L. (1965). *Nature (London)* **205**, 1070–1072.

Hoffeld, D. R., Webster, R. L., and McNew, J. (1967). *Nature (London)* **215**, 182–183.

Hoffeld, D. R., McNew, J., and Webster, R. L. (1968). *Nature (London)* **218**, 357–358.

Hole, K. (1972a). *Develop. Psychobiol.* **5**, 149–156.

Hole, K. (1972b). *Develop. Psychobiol.* **5**, 157–174.

Hudgens, G. A., Chilgren, J. D., and Palardy, D. D. (1971). *Develop. Psychobiol.* **5**, 61–70.

Hutchings, D. E., and Gibbon, J. (1970). *Psychol. Rep.* **26**, 239–246.

Huttunen, M. O. (1971). *Nature (London)* **230**, 53–55.

Hyyppä, M. (1969). *Z. Zellforsch. Mikrosk. Anat.* **98**, 550–560.

Hyyppä, M. (1971). *Experientia* **27**, 336–337.

Ignarro, L., and Shideman, F. E. (1968). *J. Pharmacol. Exp. Ther.* **159**, 38–48.

Iqbal, Z., and Talwar, G. P. (1971). *J. Neurochem.* **18**, 1261–1267.

Iversen, L. L., and Johnston, G. A. R. (1971). *J. Neurochem.* **18**, 1939–1950.

Iversen, L. L., and Neal, M. J. (1968). *J. Neurochem.* **15**, 1141–1149.

Iversen, L. L., and Snyder, S. H. (1968). *Nature (London)* **220**, 796–798.

Jasper, H. H., and Koyama, I. (1969). *Can. J. Physiol. Pharmacol.* **47**, 889–905.

Jenden, D. J., and Campbell, L. B. (1971). *Methods Biochem. Anal., Suppl.* **1**, 183–216.

Jewett, R. E., and Norton, S. (1966). *Exp. Neurol.* **14**, 33–43.

Joffe, J. M. (1965). *Nature (London)* **208**, 815–816.

Jouvet, M. (1968). *Advan. Pharmacol.* **6B**, 265–279.

Jouvet-Mounier, D., Astic, L., and Lacote, D. (1970). *Develop. Psychobiol.* **2**, 216–239.

Kahn, E. J., Newmann, L. L., and Polk, D. A. (1969). *J. Pediat.* **75**, 495–500.

Karczmar, A. G. (1963). *In* "Handbuch der experimentellen Pharmackologie" (G. B. Koelle, ed.), Vol. 15, pp. 129–186. Springer-Verlag, Berlin and New York.

Karczmar, A. G. (1969). *Fed. Proc., Fed. Amer. Soc. Exp. Biol.* **28**, 147–157.

Karczmar, A. G., Srinivasan, R., and Bernsohn, J. (1973). *In* "Fetal Pharmacology" (L. O. Boréus, ed.), pp. 127–177. Raven, New York.

Karki, N., Kuntzman, R., and Brodie, B. B. (1962). *J. Neurochem.* **9**, 53–58.

Kartashova, V. M., and Kartashova, P. M. (1963). *Vestn. Sel'skokhoz Nauki (Moscow)* **8**, 88–91.

Kato, R. (1960). *J. Neurochem.* **5**, 202.

Katzman, R., Björklund, A., Owman, C., and West, K. A. (1971). *Brain Res.* **25**, 579–596.

Kayan, S., Woods, L. A., and Mitchell, C. L. (1969). *Eur. J. Pharmacol.* **6**, 333–339.

Kellogg, C., and Lundborg, P. (1972). *Brain Res.* **36**, 333–342.

Kellogg, C., Vernadakis, A., and Rutledge, C. O. (1971). *J. Neurochem.* **18**, 1931–1938.

Kellogg, C., Lundborg, P., and Ramstedt, L. (1973). *Brain Res.* **50**, 369–378.

Kilbey, M. M., and Harris, R. T. (1971). *Psychopharmacologia* **19**, 334–346.

Kletzkin, M., Wojciechowski, H., and Margolin, S. (1964). *Nature (London)* **204**, 1206.

Kobayashi, K., and Eiduson, S. (1970). *Develop. Psychobiol.* **3**, 13–34.

Koe, K. B., and Weissman, A. (1966). *J. Pharmacol. Exp. Ther.* **154**, 499–516.

Koella, W. P. (1969). *Neurosci. Res.* **2**, 229–251.

Koelle, G. B. (1969). *Fed. Proc., Fed. Amer. Soc. Exp. Biol.* **28**, 95–100.

Kornetsky, C. (1970). *Psychopharmacologia* **17**, 105–136.

Kostowski, W., and Giacolone, E. (1969). *Eur. J. Pharmacol.* **7**, 176–179.

Kron, R. E., Stein, M., and Goddard, K. E. (1966). *Pediatrics* **37**, 1012–1016.

Kulkarni, A. S., and Shideman, F. E. (1966). *J. Pharmacol. Exp. Ther.* **153**, 428–433.

Kulkarni, A. S., and Shideman, F. E. (1968). *Eur. J. Pharmacol.* **3**, 269–271.

Kuriyama, K., Sisken, B., Ito, J., Simonsen, D. G., Haber, B., and Roberts, E. (1968). *Brain Res.* **11**, 412–430.

Kurzepa, S., and Bojanek, S. (1965). *Biol. Neonatorum* **8**, 216–221.

Ladinsky, H., Consolo, S., Peri, G., and Garattini, S. (1972). *J. Neurochem.* **19**, 1947–1952.

Lal, S., and Sourkes, T. L. (1973). *Arch. Int. Pharmacodyn. Ther.* **202**, 171–182.

Lamprecht, F., and Coyle, J. T. (1972). *Brain Res.* **41**, 503–506.

Levi, J., and Morisi, G. (1971). *Brain Res.* **26**, 131–140.

Levine, S., and Lewis, G. W. (1959). *Science* **129**, 42–43.

Levine, S., and Mullins, R. F. (1968). *In* "Early Experiences and Behavior" (G. Newton and S. Levine, eds.), pp. 168–197. Thomas, Springfield, Illinois.

Levine, S., Haltmeyer, G. C., Karas, G. G., and Denenberg, V. H. (1967). *Psychol. Behav.* **2**, 55–59.

Lew, G. M., and Quay, W. B. (1971). *Res. Commun. Chem. Pathol. Pharmacol.* **2**, 807–812.

Loizou, L. A. (1971a). *Brit. J. Pharmacol.* **41**, 41–48.

Loizou, L. A. (1971b). *Z. Zellforsch. Mikrosk. Anat.* **114**, 234–252.

Loizou, L. A. (1972). *Brain Res.* **40**, 395–418.

Loizou, L. A., and Salt, P. (1970). *Brain Res.* **20**, 467–470.

Løvtrup, S. (1961). *J. Neurochem.* **8**, 243–245.

Lundbourg, P., and Kellogg, C. (1971). *Brain Res.* **29**, 387–389.

Lytle, L. D., Shoemaker, W. J., Cotman, K. E., and Wurtman, R. J. (1971). *Pharmacologist* **13**, 275.

Lytle, L. D., Shoemaker, W. J., Cotman, K., and Wurtman, R. J. (1972). *J. Pharmacol. Exp. Ther.* **183**, 56–64.

McGaman, R. E., and Aprison, M. H. (1964). *Progr. Brain Res.* **9**, 220–233.

McGeer, E. G., Gibson, S., Wada, J. A., and McGeer, P. L. (1967). *Can. J. Biochem.* **45**, 1943–1952.

McGeer, E. G., Fibiger, H. C., and Wickson, V. (1971). *Brain Res.* **32**, 433–440.

Macon, J. B., Sokoloff, L., and Glowinski, J. (1971). *J. Neurochem.* **18**, 323–331.

Maickel, R. P., Cox, R. H., Saillant, J., and Miller, F. P. (1968). *Neuropharmacology* **7**, 275–281.

Maletta, G. J., and Timiras, P. S. (1966). *J. Neurochem.* **13**, 75–84.

Maletta, G. J., Vernadakis, A., and Timiras, P. S. (1966). *Proc. Soc. Exp. Biol. Med.* **121**, 1210.

Maletta, G. J., Vernadakis, A., and Timiras, P. S. (1967). *J. Neurochem.* **14**, 647–652.

Manshardt, J., and Wurtman, R. J. (1968). *Nature (London)* **217**, 574–575.

Marchbanks, R. M. (1969). *Biochem. Pharmacol.* **18**, 1763–1766.

Mason, J. W. (1968). *Psychosom. Med.* **30**, 774–790.

Mauer, H. M., Wolff, J. A., Finster, M., Poppers, P. J., Pantuck, E., Kuntzman, R., and Conney, A. H. (1968). *Lancet* **2**, 122–124.

Meier, G. W., and Huff, F. W. (1962). *J. Comp. Physiol. Psychol.* **55**, 469–471.

Miller, F. P., Cox, R. H., Snodgrass, W. R., and Maickel, R. P. (1970). *Biochem. Pharmacol.* **19**, 435–442.

Mirkin, B. L. (1970). *Annu. Rev. Pharmcol.* **10**, 255–272.

Mirkin, B. L. (1972). *Fed. Proc., Fed. Amer. Soc. Exp. Biol.* **31**, 65–73.

Mirkin, B. L. (1974). *In* "Drugs and the Developing Brain" (A. Vernadakis and N. Weiner, eds.), p. 199. Plenum, New York.

Molinoff, P., Weinshilboum, R., and Axelrod, J. (1971). *J. Pharmacol. Exp. Ther.* **178**, 425–431.

Monson, R. R., Rosenberg, L., Hartz, S. C., Shapiro, S., Heinonen, O. P., and Slone, D. (1973). *N. Engl. J. Med.* **289,** 1049–1052.

Moorcroft, W. H. (1971). *Brain Res.* **35,** 513–522.

Moore, K. E. (1966). *Life Sci.* **5,** 55–65.

Moore, K. E. (1971). *In* "An Introduction to Psychopharmacology" (R. H. Rech and K. E. Moore, eds.), pp. 79–136. Raven, New York.

Moore, K. E., and Dominic, J. A. (1971). *Fed. Proc., Fed. Amer. Soc. Exp. Biol.* **30,** 859–870.

Moya, F., and Thorndike, V. (1963). *Clin. Pharmacol. Ther.* **4,** 628–653.

Murphee, O. D., Monroe, R. L., and Seager, L. D. (1962). *J. Neuropsychiat.* **3,** 295–297,

Nachmais, V. T. (1960). *J. Neurochem.* **6,** 99–104.

Nair, V., and Bau, D. (1969). *Brain Res.* **16,** 383–394.

Neff, N. H., and Tozer, T. N. (1968). *Advan. Pharmacol.* **6A,** 97–109.

Nelson, P. G. (1967). *In* "The Neurosciences: A Study Program" (G. C. Quarton, T. Melnechuk, and F. O. Schmitt, eds.), Vol. 1, pp. 772–775. Rockefeller Univ. Press, New York.

Nichols, M. M. (1967). *Amer. J. Dis. Child.* **113,** 714–715.

Nygren, L.-G., Olson, L., and Seiger, A. (1971). *Histochemie* **28,** 1–15.

Oja, S. S., and Piha, R. S. (1966). *Life Sci.* **5,** 865–870.

Okada, F. (1971). *Life Sci.* **10,** 77–86.

Olson, L., Seiger, A., and Fuxe, K. (1972). *Brain Res.* **44,** 283–288.

Ordy, J. M., Latanick, A., Johnson, R., and Massopust, L. C. (1963). *Proc. Soc. Exp. Biol. Med.* **113,** 833–836.

Ordy, J. M., Samorajski, T., Collins, R. L., and Rolsten, C. (1966). *J. Pharmacol. Exp. Ther.* **151,** 110–125.

Overton, D. A. (1966). *Psychopharmacologia* **10,** 6–31.

Pappas, B. A., and Sobrian, S. K. (1972). *Life Sci.* **11,** 653–659.

Pearce, L. A., and Schanberg, S. M. (1969). *Science* **166,** 1301–1303.

Pepeu, G., and Giarman, N. J. (1962). *J. Gen. Physiol.* **45,** 575–583.

Perlmutter, J. H. (1969). *Amer. J. Obstet. Gynecol.* **99,** 569–572.

Perry, T. L., Ling, G. M., Hansen, S., and MacDougall, L. (1965). *Proc. Soc. Exp. Biol. Med.* **119,** 282–287.

Philis, J. W., Tebecis, A. K., and York, D. H. (1968). *J. Pharm. Pharmacol.* **20,** 476–478.

Pitts, F. N., and Quick, C. (1967). *J. Neurochem.* **14,** 561–570.

Porcher, W., and Heller, A. (1972). *J. Neurochem.* **19,** 1917–1930.

Potter, L. T. (1970). *In* "Handbook of Neurochemistry" (A. Lajtha, ed.), Vol. IV, pp. 263–284. Plenum, New York.

Pryor, G. T. (1968). *Life Sci.* **7,** 867–874.

Pryor, G. T., and Mitoma, C. (1970). *Neuropharmacology* **9,** 269–275.

Pscheidt, G. R., and Himwich, H. E. (1966). *Brain Res.* **1,** 363–368.

Pschedit, G. R., and Taimimie, H. S. (1966). *Biochem. Pharmcol.* **15,** 1629–1632.

Rajegowda, B. K., Glass, L., Evans, H. E., Maso, G., Swartz, D. P., and Leblanc, W. (1972). *J. Pediat.* **81,** 532–534.

Ramboer, C., Thompson, R. P. H., and Williams, R. (1969). *Lancet* **1,** 966–968.

Reid, W. D., Haubrich, D. R., and Krishna, G. (1971). *Anal. Biochem.* **42,** 390–397.

Reis, D. J., and Wurtman, R. J. (1968). *Life Sci.* **7,** 91–98.

Reis, D. J., Weinbren, M., and Corvelli, A. (1968). *J. Pharmacol. Exp. Ther.* **164,** 135–145.

Reis, D. J., Corvelli, A., and Connors, J. (1969). *J. Pharmacol. Exp. Ther.* **167,** 328–333.

Richter, J. A., and Goldstein, A. (1970). *J. Pharmcol. Exp. Ther.* **175,** 685–691.

Roberts, E. (1971). *Advan. Exp. Med. Biol.* **13,** 207–214.

Roberts, E., and Kuriyama, K. (1968). *Brain Res.* **8,** 1–35.

Roberts, E., Harman, P. J., and Frankel, S. (1951). *Proc. Soc. Exp. Biol. Med.* **78,** 799–803.

Robinson, N. (1968). *J. Neurochem.* **15,** 1151–1158.

Rosenthal, T., Patrick, S. W., and Krug, D. C. (1964). *Amer. J. Pub. Health* **54,** 1252–1262.

Rosenzweig, M. B., Krech, D., Bennett, E. L., and Diamond, M. C. (1968). *In* "Early Experience and Behavior" (G. Newton and S. Levine, eds.), pp. 258–298. Thomas, Springfield, Illinois.

Ross, S. B., and Renyi, A. L. (1967). *Life Sci.* **6,** 1407–1415.

Sachs, C. (1973). *J. Neurochem.* **20,** 1753–1760.

Saito, Y. (1971). *Life Sci.* **10,** 735–744.

Salganicoff, L., and De Robertis, E. (1965). *J. Neurochem.* **12,** 287–309.

Scapagini, U., Moberg, G. P., Van Loon, G. R., de Groot, J., and Ganong, W. F. (1971). *Neuroendocrinology* **7,** 90–96.

Schadé, J. P., and Baxter, C. F. (1960). *Exp. Neurol.* **2,** 158–178.

Schaefer, O. (1962). *Can. Med. Ass. J.* **87,** 1333–1334.

Schaefer, T. (1968). *In* "Early Experiences and Behavior" (G. Newton and S. Levine, eds.), pp. 102–141. Thomas, Springfield, Illinois.

Schapiro, S. (1971). *In* "Brain Development and Behavior" (M. B. Sterman, D. J. McGinty, and A. M. Adinolfi, eds.), pp. 307–334. Academic Press, New York.

Scheibel, M. E., and Scheibel, A. B. (1971). *In* "Brain Development and Behavior" (M. A. Sterman, D. J. McGinty, and A. M. Adinolfi, eds.), pp. 1–21. Academic Press, New York.

Scheving, L. E., Harrison, W. H., Gordon, P., and Pauly, J. E. (1968). *Amer. J. Physiol.* **214,** 166–173.

Schmidt, D. E., Szilagyi, P. I. A., Alkon, D. L., and Green, J. P. (1969). *Science* **165,** 1370–1371.

Schmidt, D. E., Szilagyi, P. I. A., Alkon, D. L., and Green, J. P. (1970). *J. Pharmacol. Exp. Ther.* **174,** 337–345.

Schmidt, D. E., Speth, R. C., Welsch, F., and Schmidt, M. J. (1972). *Brain Res.* **38,** 377–389.

Schmidt, M. J., and Sanders-Bush, E. (1971). *J. Neurochem.* **18,** 2549–2552.

Schmidt, M. J., Schmidt, D. E., and Robison, G. A. (1971). *Science* **173,** 1142–1143.

Schon, F., and Iversen, L. L. (1972). *Brain Res.* **42,** 503–507.

Schuberth, J. (1971). *Methods Biochem. Anal., Suppl.* **1,** 275–296.

Schuberth, J., Sparf, B., and Sundwall, A. (1969). *J. Neurochem.* **16,** 695–700.

Schulman, C. (1969). *Neuropediatrie* **1,** 89–94.

Schwartz, J.-C., Lampart, C., Rose, C., Rehault, M. C., Bischoff, S., and Pollard, H. (1971). *J. Neurochem.* **18,** 1787–1789.

Sharkawi, M., and Schulman, M. P. (1969). *Brit. J. Pharmacol.* **36,** 373–379.

Shaskan, E. G., and Snyder, S. H. (1970). *J. Pharmacol. Exp. Ther.* **175,** 404–418.

Sheard, M. H., and Aghajanian, G. K. (1968). *J. Pharmacol. Exp. Ther.* **163,** 425–430.

Shih, J.-H. C., and Eiduson, S. (1969). *Nature (London)* **224,** 1309–1310.

Shih, J.-H. C., and Eiduson, S. (1971). *J. Neurochem.* **18,** 1221–1227.

Shnider, S. M., and Moya, F. (1964). *Amer. J. Obstet. Gynecol.* **89,** 1009–1015.

Shtenberg, A., Kirlich, A., and Orlova, N. (1969). *Vop. Pitan.* **28,** 66–72.

Silver, A. (1967). *Int. Rev. Neurobiol.* **10,** 57–109.

Sims, K. L., and Pitts, F. N. (1970). *J. Neurochem.* **7**, 1607–1612.

Sims, K. L., Witztum, J., Quick, C., and Pitts, F. N. (1968). *J. Neurochem.* **15**, 667–672.

Sims, K. L., Weitsen, H. A., and Bloom, F. E. (1972). *Science* **175**, 1479–1480.

Singh, B., and de Champlain, J. (1972). *Brain Res.* **48**, 432–437.

Sisken, B., Sano, K., and Roberts, E. (1961). *J. Biol. Chem.* **236**, 503–507.

Smith, G. C., and Simpson, R. W. (1970). *Z. Zellforsch. Mikrosk, Anat.* **104**, 541–556.

Smith, R. D., Cooper, B. R., and Breese, G. R. (1973). *J. Pharmacol. Exp. Ther.* **185**, 609–619.

Smith, S. E., Stacey, R. S., and Young, I. M. (1963). *Proc. Int. Pharmacol. Meet., 1st, 1961* **8**, 101–105.

Snyder, S. H., Hendley, E. D., and Gfeller, E. (1969). *Brain Res.* **16**, 469–477.

Sobotka, T. J., Brodie, R. E., and Cook, M. P. (1972). *Develop. Psychobiol.* **5**, 137–148.

Sparber, S. B., and Shideman, F. E. (1968). *Develop. Psychobiol.* **1**, 236–244.

Spyker, J. M., Sparber, S. B., and Goldberg, A. M. (1972). *Science* **177**, 621–623.

Stavinoha, W. B., and Ryan, L. C. (1965). *J. Pharmacol. Exp. Ther.* **150**, 231–235.

Stavinoha, W. B., Pepelho, B., and Smith, P. W. (1970). *Pharmacologist* **12**, 257.

Stechler, G. (1964). *Science* **144**, 315–317.

Stein, L., and Wise, C. D. (1969). *J. Comp. Physiol. Psychol.* **67**, 189–198.

Stern, R. (1966). *Amer. J. Obstet. Gynecol.* **94**, 253–257.

Stone, M. L., Salerno, L. J., Green, M., and Zelson, C. (1971). *Amer. J. Obstet. Gynecol.* **109**, 716–723.

Sze, P. Y. (1970). *Brain Res.* **19**, 322–325.

Sze, P. Y., and Lovell, R. A. (1970). *J. Neurochem.* **17**, 1657–1664.

Sze, P. Y., Kuriyama, K., Haber, B., and Roberts, E. (1971). *Brain Res.* **26**, 121–130.

Tagliamonte, A., Tagliamonte, P., Perez-Cruet, J., Stern, S., and Gessa, G. L. (1971). *J. Pharmacol. Exp. Ther.* **177**, 475–480.

Takahashi, R., and Aprison, M. H. (1964). *J. Neurochem.* **11**, 887–898.

Tennyson, V. M. (1970). *In* "Developmental Neurobiology" (W. A. Himwich, ed.), pp. 47–116. Thomas, Springfield, Illinois.

Tennyson, V. M., Barrett, R. E., Cohen, G., Cote, L., Heikkila, R., and Mytilineou, C. (1972). *Brain Res.* **46**, 251–285.

Tennyson, V. M., Mytilineou, C., and Barrett, R. E. (1973). *J. Comp. Neurol.* **149**, 233–258.

Thornburg, J. E., and Moore, K. E. (1971). *Arch. Int. Pharmacodyn. Ther.* **194**, 158–167.

Thornburg, J. E., and Moore, K. E. (1973). *Res. Commun. Chem. Pathol. Pharmacol.* **6**, 313–320.

Tilney, F. (1933). *Bull. Neurol. Inst. New York* **3**, 252–358.

Timiras, P. S., Vernadakis, A., and Sherwood, N. M. (1968). *In* "Biology of Gestation" (N. S. Assali, ed.), Vol. 2, pp. 261–319. Academic Press, New York.

Tissari, A., and Pekkarinen, E. M. (1966). *Acta Physiol. Scand., Suppl.* **277**, 201.

Tissari, A. H. (1973). *In* "Fetal Pharmacology" (L. O. Boréus, ed.), pp. 237–257. Raven, New York.

Toru, M., Hingtgen, J. N., and Aprison, M. H. (1966). *Life Sci.* **5**, 181–189.

Tozer, T. N., Neff, N. H., and Brodie. B. B. (1966). *J. Pharmacol. Exp. Ther.* **153**, 177–182.

Tranzer, J. P., and Thoenen, H. (1968). *Experientia* **24**, 155–156.

Traylor, T. D., and Breese, G. R. (1971). *Fed. Proc., Fed. Amer. Soc. Exp. Biol.* **30**, 334.

Tyce, G., Flock, E. V., and Owen, G. A. (1964). *Progr. Brain Res.* **9**, 198–203.

Udenfriend, S. (1966). *Pharmacol. Rev.* **18**, 43–51.

Ungerstedt, U. (1968). *Eur. J. Pharmacol.* **5**, 107–110.

Ungerstedt, U. (1971a). *Acta Physiol. Scand., Suppl.* **367**, 1–48.

Uretsky, N. J., and Iversen, L. L. (1970). *J. Neurochem.* **17**, 269–278.

Uteley, J. D. (1963). *Biochem. Pharmacol.* **12**, 1228–1230.

Van den Berg, C. J., and Van Kempen, G. M. J. (1964). *Experientia* **20**, 375–376.

Van den Berg, C. J., Van Kempen, G. M. J., Schade, J. P., and Veldstra, H. (1965). *J. Neurochem.* **12**, 863–869.

Volicer, L. (1969). *Neuropharmacology* **8**, 361–364.

Vorhees, C. V., Butcher, R. E., and Berry, H. K. (1972). *Develop. Psychobiol.* **5**, 175–180.

Wapnir, R. A., Hawkins, R. L., and Stevenson, J. H. (1971). *Biol. Neonatorium* **18**, 85–93.

Watt, D. D., and Martin, P. R. (1969). *Life Sci.* **8**, 1211–1222.

Watts, J. S., Mendez, H. C., Reilly, J. F., and Krop, S. (1969). *Arch. Int. Pharmacodyn. Ther.* **178**, 130–136.

Weiner, N., and Rabadjija, M. (1968). *J. Pharmacol. Exp. Ther.* **164**, 103–114.

Weiner, R. I., and Ganong, W. F. (1972). *Neuroendocrinology* **9**, 65–71.

Weissman, A., Koe, K. B, and Tenen, S. S. (1966). *J. Pharmacol. Exp. Ther.* **151**, 339–352.

Werboff, J. (1970). *In* "Principles of Psychopharmacology" (W. G. Clark and J. del Giudice, eds.), pp. 343–353. Academic Press, New York.

Werboff, J., and Dembicki, E. L. (1962). *J. Neuropsychiat.* **4**, 87–91.

Werboff, J., and Havlena, J. (1962). *Exp. Neurol.* **6**, 263–269.

Werboff, J., and Kesner, R. (1963). *Nature (London)* **197**, 106–107.

Werboff, J., Gottlieb, J. S., Havlena, J., and Word, T. J. (1961). *Pediatrics* **27**, 318–324.

Westermann, K. H., Fischer, H.-D., and Oelssner, W. (1970). *Acta Biol. Med. Gem.* **25**, 855–861.

Whittaker, V. P. (1959). *Biochem. J.* **72**, 694–706.

Wollerman, M., and Devenyi, T. (1963). *J. Neurochem.* **10**, 83–88.

Woodward, D. J., Hoffer, B. J., and Lapham, L. L. (1969a). *Exp. Neurol.* **23**, 120–139.

Woodward, D. J., Hoffer, B. J., and Lapham, L. L. (1969b). *In* "Neurobiology of Cerebellar Evolution and Development" (R. Llinas, ed.), pp. 725–741. Amer. Med. Ass. Educ. Res. Found., Chicago, Illinois.

Woodward, D. J., Hoffer, B. J., Siggins, G. R., and Bloom, F. E. (1971). *Brain Res.* **34**, 73–97.

Woolley, D. W., and van der Hoeven, T. (1965). *Int. J. Neuropsychiat.* **1**, 529–544.

Wurtman, R. J. (1971). *Neurosci. Res. Program, Bull.* **9**, 172–297.

Young, A. B., Pert, C. D., Brown, Taylor, K. M., and Snyder, S. H. (1971). *Science* **173**, 247–249.

Young, R. D. (1967). *Psychol. Bull.* **67**, 73–86.

Yuwiler, A. (1971). *In* "Brain Development and Behavior" (M. B. Sterman, D. J. McGinty, and A. M. Adinolfi, eds.), pp. 43–57. Academic Press, New York.

Zelson, C., Rubio, E., and Wasserman, E. (1971). *Pediatrics* **48**, 178–189.

5
Clinical Implications
of Perinatal Pharmacology

Sumner J. Yaffe
Leo Stern

I. Introduction

Consideration of the total perinatal environment encompasses the entire span from conception, through pregnancy and the gestational period, labor and delivery, and often through the neonatal period. Accordingly, the clinical implications of perinatal pharmacology begin appropriately with consideration of teratogenic effects which may either terminate the pregnancy or cripple it even prior to birth—through effects of drugs on the fetus either directly or by maternal administration. The situation *vis-à-vis* the newborn infant is reflected in the problem of hepatic immaturity which illustrates many of the problems faced by the newly born, developing organism. We have, therefore, chosen to examine in detail the question of bilirubin metabolism to serve as an *in vivo* marker of this immaturity whose occurrence is not only frequent (up to 30% of all newborns are visibly jaundiced), but of extreme clinical importance (cf. kernicterus). Finally, as an example of the opposite effect to the exogenous administration of pharmacological agents, we have chosen to explore the pharmacological and physiological role of an endogenous class of agents (catecholamines) which may have profound effects on the organism, independent of any exogenous administration or use.

II. Teratogenic Effects

A. Historical Perspectives

The recognition of congenital malformations is as old as mankind. The malformations were almost invariably attributed to witchcraft, and the only contributions of environmental conditions were confined to some action or slight of the mother. From about 1900 on it was, however, shown in a number of laboratories by embryologists, initially in avian embryos and later in mammals, that a multiplicity of environmental factors, e.g., nutritional, mechanical, and physical in addition to chemical substances and drugs, were able to alter normal development. Though occasional cases of drug-adverse effect on fetuses following maternal treatment had been reported, rubella virus was the first teratogen to be incriminated beyond a doubt in humans (Gregg, 1941). In the early 1960's thalidomide, considered to be an ideal drug because of its apparent virtual lack of toxicity, was shown to result in severe limb defects (phocomelia) when given to pregnant women during the first trimester (McBride, 1961; Lenz and Knapp, 1962). This brought with it a sudden and increased interest in teratology, not only among embryologists but also among clinicians, pharmacologists, and toxicologists.

Classically, teratology refers to the study of congenital malformations observed grossly at birth and induced by exogenous agents during the organogenetic period. Today, however, the concepts of teratology have widened more and more to include any adverse effects, morphological, biochemical, behavioral, etc., induced during fetal life, detected at birth or later (World Health Organization, 1966). This evolution has brought teratology and developmental pharmacology closer to each other.

The causes of congenital malformations are usually multifactorial and comprise an interaction between genetic and environmental factors. It has been estimated that 25% of human malformations can be attributed to genetic factors, 3% to chromosomal aberrations, and 3% to environmental factors such as maternal infections, radiation, and drugs. The etiology of the remaining 69% is still essentially unknown (Cohlan, 1969).

The following discussion will cover basic principles of teratology and their application to man with special reference to preventive measures.

B. Teratogenic Principles

The possible occurrence of a congenital malformation is dependent upon the interplay of the following four teratogenic principles: timing, the nature of agent and its accessibility to the fetus, genetic makeup, and level and duration of dosage. The discussion refers to human conditions whenever such are known. It should, however, be remembered that these basic principles have been acquired from animal experimentation.

1. TIMING

The timing of intervention determines the type of expected malformation. Very little is known about the damage that can be produced to the gametes before fertilization. Chromosomal breakages have been found after high doses of LSD in mice (Skakkebaek et al., 1968). In nine children exposed in utero to LSD, a significant increase in breakages was found in somatic cells but there were, however, no associated abnormalities (Cohen et al., 1968). In a prospective study of 972 children, a significantly greater number of trisomic children were found after maternal abdominal radiation exposure (Uchida et al., 1968). On the whole, however, there is an interest, especially among geneticists, for possible mutagenic effects of environmental factors.

During the preimplantation period, the embryo is generally said to be relatively resistant to adverse effects from the environment. In animal experiments, however, it is possible to interfere with blastocyst formation in rabbits both in vitro and in vivo (Lutwak-Mann and Hay, 1962). An effect during this period most probably results in severe damage and death of the embryo with subsequent abortion. There is an increased incidence of abnormalities in aborted fetuses (Nishimura et al., 1968). A number of chemicals and drugs have been shown to penetrate into tubular fluid and even into the preimplantation blastocyst when administered to pregnant rabbits in doses comparable to those encountered in the human (Fabro and Sieber, 1969).

During the organogenetic period (in the human approximately 15 to 56 days) the type of malformation will relate closely to the stage of development at which the intervention took place. In humans, for example, the period of sensitivity for the nervous system is days 15 to 25, for the heart days 20 to 40, and for the limbs days 24 to 46 (Smith, 1970). Similar tables have been developed for the most commonly used laboratory animals to facilitate comparison. Since many organs are developing at the same time, the outcome often represents a combination of different abnormalities. As a corollary of this, it is often possible for a specific cluster of malformations to predict when the adverse effect took place. In the case of thalidomide, it was almost always possible to date the exposure from the constellation of defects (Lenz and Knapp, 1962). Rubella is most harmful when contracted during the seventh week when the sensitive targets, eyes and heart, are undergoing their most rapid development (Katz et al., 1968). In animal experiments this period has been defined as the period of maximum sensitivity for most substances with a high rate of fetal death as well as a high rate of malformations (Wilson, 1965).

After the first trimester, most organs are already formed with certain important exceptions such as the genital apparatus, the teeth, and the further maturation of the central nervous system. During this so-called fetal period, the fetus will be at risk for the same drug-adverse effect as can be induced in adults. Only a few examples will be mentioned here; for further information see Section III. Hemorrhages have occurred following dicoumarol treatment of the mother (Bloomfield, 1970).

Some effects might not appear until later in postnatal life and even in adulthood although induced prenatally. Behavioral changes of various types have been noticed following treatment with tranquilizing drugs and sex hormones (Brazelton, 1970). Most information has until now been derived from animal experiments but this is an exciting new field which needs further attention. A recently observed increased incidence of vaginal adenocarcinoma in young girls whose mothers had been treated with high doses of stilbestrol for vaginal bleeding during pregnancy, underlines the fact that the teratogenic effect may appear in the next generation (Herbst et al., 1971).

2. Nature of the Agent

Several agents can induce the same types of malformations, and one agent can induce more than one type. A wide variety of teratogens and teratogenic conditions have been identified in animals and no structural activity relationships have yet been found. In humans, however, only a few teratogens have been proved beyond a doubt. Hearing loss can follow exposure to rubella (Anderson et al., 1970) and in a few cases following streptomycin medication (Robinson and Cambon, 1964). On the other hand, rubella can give rise to heart defects and cataracts, depending on the timing. Certain agents, however, seem to have a preferential type of damage, for example, thalidomide with mainly limb defects, and irradiation with microcephalia (Plummer, 1952). In this connection it should be mentioned that the final and most recognizable defect can be a secondary effect, such as renal agenesis following failure of development of the ureteric bud or microcephalia following underdevelopment of the brain.

3. GENETIC MAKEUP

The genetic makeup modifies the environmental influence so that the final response differs among species, strains, and individuals. In animal experiments, this has been shown several times relative to cleft palate in mice (Kalter, 1954), which (see below) has been a valuable tool for studying the basic mechanism. In humans, this is apparent in the fact that not all mothers who took thalidomide during the calculated critical period gave birth to damaged children (Lenz and Knapp, 1962). Another example is the higher incidence of rubella-induced deafness in children with a genetic disposition for hearing impairment (Anderson et al., 1970).

It is also well known (see below) that no final conclusion can be drawn from experiments in animals to the situation in man. This is of the utmost importance for drug testing. Unfortunately, adverse effects on the embryo and fetus can only be evaluated conclusively in man.

4. DOSAGE

The teratogenic dose is said to be between the dose for temporary impairment and the dose for fetal death. As in most toxicological considerations, teratogenicity follows a dose–effect relationship. In most cases the teratogenic zone is narrow and the dose–effect curve has a steep slope. The glaring exception, however, is thalidomide where a large increase in dose means only a slight increase in fetal morbidity.

The two most well-known human teratogens, thalidomide and rubella, usually leave the mother with no ill effect. For most animal teratogens, however, the dose is rather close to the maternal LD_{50}, even though the relationship can vary considerably within, for example, such a relatively homogeneous group as tumor-inhibiting drugs (Murphy, 1965).

The duration of the total dosage is also of great importance. Chronic administration of a drug may give rise to enzyme induction with consequent lowering of the dose at the sensitive moment. On the other hand, increased teratogenic activity may also be seen following repeated dosage which may be due to pathological damage resulting in reduced metabolic activity or accumulation of toxic substances.

Table I lists those drugs which have been incriminated in the production of congenital malformations in man. Drugs have been grouped in descending order with respect to their estimated potential for adverse effect. The small number of drugs is further testimony for the need for more prospective and fundamental research in man.

C. Application to Man

It has long been known that drugs and other environmental influences may induce adverse effects in the human fetus. The adverse effects could be expected from adverse effects known to occur in adults. The reported cases were, however, few and their significance not seriously considered. With the thalidomide disaster in the early 1960's attention was drawn to the possibilities of inducing congenital malformations with a drug that was considered almost nontoxic in man. This also meant an increasing interest in teratology and the possibilities of fetal damage through environmental influences. Numerous reviews were written which urged great caution in the treatment of pregnant or any woman of childbearing age. Unfortunately, this in many instances led to therapeutic nihilism. However, when treatment is necessary, it should be instituted since untreated maternal illness can be harmful to the developing fetus.

Other more constructive measures for preventing a new thalidomide tragedy include drug testing, central registration of birth defects, and further teratological research. Some areas of interest in teratological research today are mechanisms of normal and faulty development, mechanisms behind strain differences and development, and improvement of different methods of drug testing as discussed above.

In early recommendations, reproduction studies were included as a possible part of a chronic toxicity test (Barnes and Denz, 1954). Since 1961, when thalidomide was first suspected of being teratogenic in humans, discussions have been focused on the design of a teratogenic test for the safety evaluation of drugs for human use. In 1966, a WHO group reviewed the scientific bases then available for testing drugs for teratogenicity. Suggestions were made with full awareness of the limitations involved and many countries have developed their own recommendations. Usually a drug is required to be tested during all stages of pregnancy including the perinatal and lactation period. It should also be stressed that no absolute conclusions can be drawn from results in animals to man. In this connection it should be mentioned that many drugs which we today consider almost safe and irreplaceable, such as salicylate, antihistamines, and several antibiotics, have been shown to induce malformations in several animal species under the conditions outlined for teratogenic tests.

TABLE I   Human Teratogens[a]

Drug	Adverse effect	Reference
Group I: Teratogens with high potential		
Aminopterin	Gross malformations	Thiersch, 1952; Emerson, 1962
Thalidomide	Gross malformations	Lenz and Knapp, 1962; McBride, 1961
Group 2: Teratogens with low potential		
Androgens	Masculinization	Wilkins, 1960
Busulfan, chlorambucil, cyclo-phosphamide	Gross malformations and fetal death	Stutzman and Sokal, 1968
Progesterone	Masculinization	Wilkins, 1960; Jacobson, 1962
Salicylate	Minor malformations	Richards, 1969; Nelson and Forfar, 1971
Streptomycin	VIII Nerve damage	Robinson and Cambon, 1964; Conway and Birt, 1965
Group 3: Suspected teratogens		
Cortisone	Abortion, fetal death	Warrell and Taylor, 1968
Coumarin	Hemorrhage, fetal death	Bloomfield, 1970; Fillmore and McDevitt, 1970
Diphenylhydantoin	Cleft lip	Mirkin, 1971
LSD (lysergic acid diethylamide)	Chromcsomal breakage, skeletal malformations	Smart and Bateman, 1968; McGlothlin et al., 1970
Quinine	VIII Nerve damage, skeletal malformations	Matz and Naunton, 1968; Uhlig, 1957
Tetracycline	Cataracts	Harley et al., 1964
Tolbutamide	Gross malformations	Larsson and Sterky, 1960; Schiff et al., 1970

[a] Drugs which may affect the human fetus during the first trimester.

It is generally believed that a good system of central registration of birth defects could have detected the relationship between thalidomide and abnormalities earlier and prevented hundreds of children from being born with defects. Many countries now have a central register for birth defects. It is also possible to calculate how many new cases are needed for statistical recognition of a new syndrome on a monthly basis in a given population (Kallen and Winberg, 1969).

Investigation of the etiology of congenital malformations in man may be either prospective in which intense surveillance of drug intake is maintained during pregnancy, or retrospective in which exposure to environmental factors is ascertained in infants with birth defects (Nora et al., 1967; Richards, 1969).

The study of the underlying mechanisms for development of congenital malformation has been made possible through their induction in high percentages by teratogenic agents and the application of biochemical methods and isotope techniques. Cleft palate, for example, has been used as a model where its appearance has been related to the inhibition of the synthesis of sulfomucopolysaccharides, RNA, and/or DNA (Larsson, 1962; Zimmerman et al., 1970). Some of the achievements in this field have come about by the introduction of new methods, such as tissue culture for the study of limb buds (Shepard et al., 1971) or growing blastocysts in vitro for the study of early development (Fabro and Sieber, 1969).

Differences between strains have also been used as a tool for studying underlying mechanisms, e.g., for salicylate-induced damage, both early and late in pregnancy (Larsson and Boström, 1965; Eriksson, 1971). Even here progress has been facilitated by the introduction of new techniques, such as blastocyst transfer (Marsk et al., 1971).

III. Pharmacology of the Fetus

For many years the therapeutic use of drugs during pregnancy has been directed toward maternal disease. It is evident that under these circumstances the fetus will also function as a drug recipient. Appreciation of this concept has been greatly stimulated as a result of the thalidomide tragedy of the early 1960's. More recently, the increasing ability to diagnose and treat fetal disease in utero has been associated with the prescription of drugs to the pregnant woman in order to affect directly the intrauterine host. Knowledge concerning fetal pharmacology is a prerequisite in helping the obstetrician and pediatrician understand how certain pharmacological agents may produce deleterious effects while others may be employed for their therapeutic benefit to either the mother or the fetus.

A. General Principles

Numerous factors govern the action of the drug within the organism. These include mechanisms that determine the duration of action of a chemical agent and factors which control the concentration of the substance at the receptor site. Irrespective of the route of administration which in the case of the fetus is usually to the pregnant woman, a drug must traverse one or several semipermeable membranes before the required receptor is reached. On both sides of each membrane the net effects of storage, excretion, and inactivation tend to modify the effective concentration of the drug. In administering a drug to a pregnant woman, either for her benefit or to treat the fetus, the physician must consider: (1) maternal pharmacological mechanisms; (2) effects on the placenta, including its pharmacodynamic capability; and (3) effects on the fetus as an additional recipient of the drug. Fetal pharmacology must, therefore, examine the interplay between the fetus and the mother with the placenta mediating this dual relationship.

1. THE ROLE OF THE PLACENTA

The transfer of drugs occurs across the placenta from the maternal arterial supply by way of the intervillous spaces into the fetal capillaries in the villi and into the umbilical venous blood. (Placental transfer is discussed in Chapter 1.) Maternal factors, such as distribution and metabolism, can affect the amount of drug delivered to the placenta through the uterine arteries. Little is known about these factors relative to the supply of drugs to the placenta except that during active labor, uterine arterial blood flow decreases during contractions, thus affecting the supply of drug to the placenta and to the fetus. Since pregnancy is associated with dramatic and profound physiological and biochemical changes in the maternal organism, it would not be surprising if the drug-metabolizing capability of the mother was also altered. Data on this point are nonexistent in the human, but evidence in animals suggests that drug metabolism by maternal hepatic microsomes is markedly reduced during pregnancy (Guarino et al., 1969). This decrease would result in the delivery of more lipid-soluble, nonmetabolized drug to the placenta for transport to the fetus.

Discussion of the passage of drugs between the pregnant woman and the fetus must emphasize at the outset the inadequacy of our present knowledge, specifically with regard to quantitative kinetic data which would permit calculation of transfer rates. This is particularly true for detailed systematic measurements made at various times throughout pregnancy as it is known that the tissue layers interposed between fetal capillaries and maternal blood become progressively thinner during gestation. What happens to placental transmission of drugs during toxemia and other abnormalities of pregnancy is also not clear. Alterations in maternal and fetal blood flow through the placenta induced by contractions, position of the mother or fetus, anesthesia, or cord compression may also effect transmission of drugs. Difficulties in obtaining data regarding actual rate of transfer are compounded because of the circumstances under which investigations must be conducted. Because of marked species differences in placental structure, reliable data can be collected only from humans rather than by extrapolation from animal experiments. And in this instance, obviously, fetal concentration of drugs can be measured only once: at the moment the fetus is delivered. Thus the typical study in man entails the administration of a drug to the mother just before delivery and determination of drug concentrations in cord blood at the time of birth. Information about rates of equilibrium has to be pieced together from a great many separate experiments in different individuals. The recent introduction of techniques in which fetal scalp blood is sampled during labor may help to provide meaningful data from which equilibrium rates can be determined. The deficiency in sampling cord blood without distinguishing umbilical venous and umbilical arterial blood is another negative factor in the present collection of data.

In addition to and synchronous with its role as an organ of transport, the placenta contains numerous active enzyme systems which function in the biosynthesis and degradation of chemical compounds and drugs. Recent investigations have demonstrated that hydrolytic and reductive reactions are most active in homogenates of term placentas (Juchau and Dyer, 1972). Conjugating activity is very low in placental tissue and is likely to be overwhelmed by hydrolytic enzymes whose activity probably serves to facilitate the bidirectional transfer of drug substrates between mother and fetus. Exceptions with respect to conjugation reactions appear to be acetylation and glycine coupling. Recently, it has been shown that environmental agents can modify the metabolic capabilities of the placenta. Benzpyrene hydroxylase activity cannot be measured in homogenates of term placenta, but becomes detectable in the placenta of women who have smoked 10 to 30 cigarettes a day (Welch et al., 1968). While these studies were carried out at the end of pregnancy, it is likely that other reactions may be mediated by the placenta during early gestation. The role of interactions of this type in the general well being of the mother and particularly of the fetus is not only interesting to contemplate but may be of considerable functional significance. It has been hypothesized that the placenta supplements the fetal liver and should thus be able to metabolize drugs maximally early in gestation when the developing fetal liver is metabolically most incompetent (see Section III,A,3). While the significance of drug biotransformation by the placenta has not been fully clarified, it should be pointed out that these metabolic conversions could influence the developing fetus in a number of ways: Metabolites could act directly upon fetal tissues to produce abnormal effects; drug substrates could compete for enzyme systems within the placenta normally used for the metabolism of endogenous substances such as hormones, thus disturbing the internal environment of the fetus; or drug metabolites could inhibit the biochemical functions of the placenta which are important in the energy-requiring transport mechanisms of this unique organ. While biotransformation reactions in the placenta are discussed in detail in Chapter 2, their potential importance for the successful outcome of pregnancy needs to be mentioned when discussing the role of the placenta.

2. FETAL RECEPTOR FUNCTION

The exposure of fetal tissue to maternally administered drugs is dependent upon the kinetics of equilibration between maternal and fetal blood as well as upon special features of distribution within the fetus. These are discussed in detail in Chapter 3. A few points deserve mention here even though the dynamics of the fetal circulation *in vivo* are not completely understood because of the technical difficulties involved in this type of investigation, particularly in humans. The fetal brain receives a much greater proportion of the cardiac output than does the brain of the newborn infant or older child. Since perfusion of the brain increases with either fetal hypoxia or hypercapnia, interference with placental fetal circulation (such as occurs during labor) may affect cerebral blood flow and thereby the delivery of drugs to that tissue. The ultimate effect of these differences in fetal circulation on drug distribution within the fetus is not clear. However, it should also be mentioned that compared to the adult organism, little is known about rates of membrane transport and permeability in the fetus.

The initiation of the pharmacological response usually results from the interaction between the drug molecules and active sites (receptors) in the tissues. Boréus (1967) and McMurphy and Boréus (1968) have recently examined receptor function within the human fetus by means of *in vitro* experiments utilizing segments of fetal ilium. They demonstrated that autonomic receptors are present during early human ontogenesis (at the beginning of the second trimester) and furthermore, that the responsiveness of these receptors to chemical stimulation does not appear to change with increasing fetal age. Cholinergic agents produced contraction of the ilium whereas adrenergic agents resulted in relaxation. Administration of adrenergic antagonists prevented relaxation. Since all of the antagonists where β blocking agents, this indicated that adrenergic relaxation was mediated through a sensitive β receptor. Inihibition could not be achieved with α blocking agents suggesting that adrenergic relaxation in the human fetal intestine is due to β receptor function exclusively. These results differ considerably from studies in adult humans and animals where both α and β adrenergic receptors are considered by most investigators to participate in relaxation of the intestinal musculature. The development of receptor function early in gestation is an indication that the fetus is capable of responding to pharmacological agents. This must be considered when drugs are prescribed to the mother.

3. FETAL DRUG METABOLISM

Drug action in the intact organism is usually terminated by chemical change with urinary excretion of the native drug being of little quantitative importance. The biochemical mechanisms for drug transformation are accomplished by enzymes which are found to be minimal at or near term in experimental animals except for enzyme systems involved in the transfer or hydrolysis of sulfate. There are exceptions to this rule as, for example, glucuronide conjugating activity in the gastrointestinal mucosa of newborn rats is higher than at other stages of life. While the general view exists that fetal tissues are unable to metabolize foreign compounds, it should be emphasized that the investigations have been carried out using nonprimate fetal tissues. Endocrinologists have provided ample evidence that human fetal tissues (especially liver and adrenal) obtained in early and midgestation are able to carry out a number of metabolic functions with steroid substrates, including oxidation, reduction, demethylation, sulfation, and glucuronidation. In fact cell suspensions of human trophoblast grown in tissue culture are capable of acetylating sulfonamides and hydroxylating other drug substrates. While these studies have been concerned with hormones as substrates, recent data have shown many similarities between the enzyme systems which hydroxylate steroids and those which hydroxylate drugs. The inability to detect drug-metabolizing activity *in vitro* may be due to the endogenous substrates, e.g., hormones, preventing drug substrates from gaining access to the active site of the microsomal enzyme molecule. Experimental evidence has recently been obtained which has demonstrated the presence of the cytochrome pigment P-450 in human fetal tissues during the second trimester in amounts comparable to that found in adult rat liver (Yaffe *et al.*, 1970). Human fetal liver microsomes also contain the electron transport components necessary for drug hydroxylation reactions. These investigators demonstrated significant rates of mixed-function oxidation of an endogenous substrate such as testosterone or laurate but variable results were obtained with drug substrates (aminopyrine, benzpyrene). Positive results were later obtained for the oxidative N-demethylation of demethylimipramine and ethylmorphine and the p-hydroxylation of aniline in human fetal liver preparations *in vitro* by Rane and Ackermann (1972). These findings were somewhat surprising in view of the inability of a large number of investigators to detect significant quantities of cytochrome P-450- or P-450-dependent drug hydroxylation reactions in liver microsomes from fetuses of a wide variety of animal species, even at comparatively late stages of gestation.

During the studies with human fetal liver it was noted that the microsomal 105,000 g pellets were small compared to pellets from adult rat liver when the same amount of liver had been used for the preparation of the homogenate. Rane subsequently utilized marker enzymes to investigate the centrifugal distribution of the endoplasmic reticulum and other subcellular elements from human fetal liver. With the conventional technique for isolation of microsomes (centrifugation at 9000 g followed by 105,000 g) about 63% of the total microsomal enzyme activity was recovered in the 105,000 g pellet in human adult liver. The corresponding percentage in human fetal liver was only 14% and almost all of the remainder was recovered in the 9000 g pellet. In order to elucidate a possible interference with the microsomal sedimentation by intact hepatic and hematopoietic cells and hepatic cell nuclei, initial centrifugations at 900 and 200 g were employed. It was found that 79 and 64% of the total microsomal enzyme activity remained in the 900 and 200 g pellets, respectively. A partial explanation was afforded by electron microscopic studies of the various pellets. The low-spin pellets were dominated by two structures, mitochondria and rough endoplasmic reticulum. The high-speed pellet was composed of vesicles of varying size some of which were studded with ribosomes. The loss of microsomal enzymes into the low-speed pellets thus seems to be due in part to insufficient fragmentation of the endoplasmic reticulum during the homogenization of the fetal liver. In contrast specific activities for the various enzymes were highest in the high-speed pellet. This was also true for the *in vitro* oxidation of ethylmorphine and aniline.

Juchau and Pedersen (1973) have recently shown that microsomal fractions of human fetal adrenal gland homogenates contain large quantities of carbon monoxide-binding pigment which exhibits an absorption maximum between 446 and 448 nm. Human fetal liver microsomes exhibited similar spectral properties but the concentration of the pigment in the adrenal microsomes appeared to be at least one order of magnitude higher then that observed in fetal liver microsomes. Arylhydrocarbon hydroxylase specific activities in fetal adrenal microsomes approached those observed in analogous preparations of adult rat livers. These investigations have shown the cytochrome P-450 concentration in human fetal liver microsomes to average 0.22 nmoles/mg of protein which is similar to those reported for human adult liver microsomes. Recently the presence of cytochrome P-450 has been demonstrated in human placental tissue obtained at term.

This is in contrast to previously reported negative results and may be explained by the relative instability of the placental 450 form. In addition, contamination with hemoglobin which is extremely difficult to remove from placental particulate fractions may also have been a factor in the reporting of negative findings. The carboxyhemoglobin spectrum overlaps that of the degraded form of cytochrome P-450. Consequently, the rate of conversion of the 450 form to the 428 form could be retarded markedly if buffered solutions containing 10^{-4} M dithiothreitol and 20% glycerol were utilized for the resuspension of placental particulate fractions. These results would appear to reinforce the hypothesis of affinity differences between natural and external substrates and the enzyme molecule. Final assessment of the drug metabolic capability of the human fetus must await investigations with human tissue, employing conditions which take into consideration the role of hormones as natural substrates.

Studies during the last 10 years have shown that the chronic administration of many drugs to the intact organism causes a nonspecific increase in the metabolism of drugs by microsomal enzymes. As a consequence the duration and intensity of drug action *in vivo* is decreased. This phenomenon of induction has been applied to the fetus, and it has been demonstrated that agents such as phenobarbital, administered to pregnant animals late in gestation, can stimulate the activities not only of the mixed-function oxidase system in fetal liver microsomes but also of several other drug-metabolizing systems including that of glucuronidation. These findings have led to the clinical application in the human infant for the treatment of the unconjugated hyperbilirubinemia of the newborn. (See Section III,B.) The apparent lack of effect of these inducers earlier in gestation may indicate the insensitivity of a biochemical system which has yet to make its evolutionary appearance or it may be due to the inhibitory effect of high concentrations of endogenous substrates, particularly steroid hormones.

While the placenta and fetus have been discussed up to this point separately for the sake of clarity, it is obvious that these two organs do not function separately but rather are integrated into a single unit. The concept of fetal–placental unit evolved from studies of steroid metabolism where one or more key enzymes were found to be absent in either fetal liver or placenta. Since the enzymes lacking in one tissue were present in the other, the fetus and placenta together could carry out biochemical transformations which neither could accomplish alone. The interdependence of the fetus and placenta appears to be a natural phenomenon when one considers the physiology of the developing embryo and fetus. This functional concept has not as yet been applied to studies in fetal pharmacology but will undoubtedly prove to be a fruitful area for future investigation.

B. Therapy of the Fetus

Appreciation of the fact that the fetus serves as a recipient of maternally administered drugs has been repeatedly mentioned in this chapter. It is surprising, therefore, that so few attempts have been made to administer drugs using either the maternal route or directly into the fetus for the treatment of fetal disease itself. The administration of penicillin to the pregnant female infected with *Treponema pallidum* is a striking example of this concept. The treatment of syphilis resulted in a cure of fetal infection which after all was of far greater consequence and produced a greater toll than the maternal disease itself. Another historical example has been the use of γ-globulin in mothers who have been exposed to rubella during early pregnancy. γ-Globulin, although administered to the mother, was given in a prophylactic manner to prevent serious fetal disease from rubella virus. More recently, the energetic management of the fetus severely at risk from erythroblastosis fetalis by means of intrauterine transfusion becomes the first example of a direct therapeutic approach to the fetus. In this instance, blood is injected directly into the peritoneal cavity of the fetus, usually during the third trimester of pregnancy. The dose of the drug (in this case blood) is calculated in a manner similar to calculation of dosage in the adult organism and the following factors are taken into consideration in arriving at a calculation of the volume of blood to be infused: (1) 70% of red cells given intraperitoneally are absorbed and circulate in the peripheral circulation; (2) the blood volume of the fetus is approximately 80 mg/kg; (3) the hematocrit of the donor red blood cells is approximately 95%; and (4) the desired concentration of blood in the fetus is a hematocrit of 40–50%. Using these four factors, Duhring found a 48% survival rate in over a 5-year period in 25 fetuses who were subjected to intrauterine fetal transfusion (Duhring and Zwirek, 1971). Duhring actually went further and calculated the dosage interval by dividing the volume of red cells needed for transfusion into three equal aliquots and giving each of these 2 weeks apart.

Bowman in Manitoba, Canada has a much greater experience, having given 437 intrauterine transfusions to 193 fetuses (J. D. Bowman, personal communication, 1971). The survival rate was approximately 60%. The risk appears to be greater if the fetus is less than 26 weeks of age when the first intrauterine transfusion is given. It is of interest that as with all new therapeutic endeavors with a high risk, the risk is greater during the initial period of use of the procedure. This was true in the Manitoba series where the survival rate during the first 2 years was only about 25%.

Another example of drug administration to the fetus arises from analysis of their approach to the management of severe erythroblastosis fetalis. A major therapeutic problem in erythroblastosis fetalis occurs when the fetus develops severe heart failure because of anemia secondary to massive hemolysis. In these patients digitalis has been added to the therapeutic regimen. This is undertaken when the diagnosis of severe fluid retention or hydrops can be established in utero on the basis of gross ascites present at the time of intrauterine transfusion. Digoxin is instilled into the peritoneal cavity of the fetus in a dosage of 0.035 mg per estimated kg of body weight of the fetus. It should be emphasized that at present such therapy is highly empiric, its effectivenes has not been adequately assessed, and that no measurements of concentrations of the drug in the fetus have been obtained. As the need for direct fetal drug therapy increases, more scientific data will be required upon which to base the rational selection and dosage of drugs.

Another example of fetal therapeutics is the application of the concept of pharmacological induction of drug metabolic enzyme activity. This approach has been employed primarily to treat the unconjugated hyperbilirubinemia of the newborn and premature infant. The administration of phenobarbital orally (30 to 120 mg/day) to the mother for 2 weeks prior to delivery has been shown to produce a marked decrease in neonatal serum bilirubin concentrations when contrasted to a control group of infants born to untreated mothers. Retrospectively it has been noted that infants born to mothers receiving phenobarbital as therapy for epilepsy were less jaundiced than control infants. The mechanism by which phenobarbital caused a decrease in serum bilirubin concentration is not entirely clear, although induction of the activity of glucuronyltransferase plays a significant role. The risks of using phenobarbital are unknown and may outweigh its benefits since the phenobarbital inductive effect is nonspecific and activities of other liver microsomal enzymes are also increased after its administration. For example, a number of steroid hydroxylases are increased in activity by administration of phenobarbital. Alterations in steroid concentrations at such a critical period of development as the perinatal period may have long-lasting consequences which may not become apparent until much later in postnatal life. The use of phenobarbital is probably justifiable in treating a fetus known to be sensitized with hemolytic disease. In this case, benefits from induction may be greater than the risks mentioned above. Of greater significance is the concept of pharmacological induction as an example of fetal therapeutics, which may hold great promise for the future management of fetal growth and development.

C. Therapy of the Mother

As discussed above, all pharmacological agents (with rare exceptions), when administered to the mother, will be transported across the placenta to the fetus although in varying degree depending upon the characteristics of the transport process for the particular drug. In the following paragraphs, several classes of drugs commonly administered to the pregnant woman in mid and late gestation are reviewed. The purpose is not to present a complete list for the physician to memorize what to avoid but rather to exemplify principles of fetal pharmacology. (See Chapter 1 for detailed discussion.)

1. GENERAL ANESTHETICS

Except for patients who receive local anesthetics, pregnant women are usually given a general anesthetic in the latter part of the first stage and the second stage of labor. Gaseous volatile agents are commonly used and anesthesia is usually maintained at the level of analgesia to minimize the severe pain as the head of the fetus passes through the vulva. With forceps delivery and for repair of lacerations or an episiotomy, anesthesia is deepened to stage three (surgical anesthesia). All of the agents used in inhalation anesthesia rapidly and easily diffuse across the placenta and the effect upon the infant will depend upon the amount of drug present and the rate of equilibration between mother and fetus. Since the gases, with the exception of trichloroethylene, are primarily excreted by exhalation without prior metabolism, the duration of anesthetic effect in the newborn infant after delivery will depend upon the infants ventilatory capacity as well as the amount of drug present. The most frequently used anesthetic gases during the second stage of labor are cyclopropane and nitrous oxide. Moderate analgesia can be achieved with a concentration of nitrous oxide of 40 to 60% which will not produce visible depression of the newborn infant. In order to produce anesthesia with nitrous oxide, a mixture containing 75% or more of this gas must be administered for several minutes. Infants born following such anesthetic management of the mother in labor are generally asphyxiated at birth and are slow to breathe spontaneously. Three to 5% cyclopropane administered to the mother for brief periods of time produces satisfactory analgesia without adverse effect upon the infant. However, if the same agent is used to produce maternal anesthesia, the infant may be seriously depressed.

Ultrashort-acting barbiturates are used intravenously either to induce or to maintain general anesthesia. These compounds are not very effective analgesics and, except during deep anesthesia, are used in combination with other agents which possess pain-relieving properties. Thus, other agents may be given to the mother and be present in the infant at birth to interact with the barbiturate. The ultrashort-acting barbiturates must be metabolized via hepatic microsomal enzymes prior to excretion. Their effect on the brain is short lived because of the rapid redistribution within the organism. These two factors, however, may combine to produce deep depression in the newborn infant. Redistribution from sites in maternal brain may lead to a high concentration in the newborn infant whose ability to oxidize the barbiturate is much less than the older, more mature organism. Clinically, significant neonatal depression has been seen when thiobarbiturates are used to produce anesthesia for delivery by cesarean section but is not usually seen when infants are delivered vaginally following intravenous barbiturate anesthesia.

Finally, it should be mentioned that a certain number of women undergo general anesthesia for surgical reasons during earlier stages of gestation. No adverse effects upon the fetus have been noted but it should be emphasized that no prospective study specifically aimed at this point has been undertaken.

2. LOCAL ANESTHETICS

Local anesthetics given either by regional infiltration or by the intrathecal, epidural, or caudal route have been used extensively during delivery without obvious harmful effect on the fetus or infant unless maternal hypotension has occurred. This hazard to both the mother and fetus occurs when these drugs are used for spinal anesthesia. The reduction in uteroplacental blood flow can result in severe fetal asphyxia. Local anesthetics in general use are either of the ester or the amide type. The esters include procaine and are usually characterized by a fairly long latent period between administration and action, a relatively short duration of action, and a relatively poor ability to penetrate tissues. They have given way in clinical usage to the amides which act more rapidly and longer and can penetrate tissues better. This type (lidocaine, prilocaine, mepivacaine) undergoes metabolic degradation by amidases in the liver in contrast to the ester group which is hydrolyzed by both plasma esterases as well as by hepatic enzymes. The young organism is unable to metabolize the amide group as efficiently as he can hydrolyze esters. Consequently, as many as 30% of infants whose mothers received amide type of regional anesthetics via either the epidural or paracervical routes have recognizable adverse effects at birth. These vary from central nervous system depression to bradycardia from the direct effect of the anesthetic into the fetal circulation.

3. ANALGESICS

The goal of obstetric analgesia is to provide pain relief for the mother without affecting the fetus or the delivery process. Opiates and their synthetic substitutes, such as meperidine, easily reach the fetus when given to the mother during delivery. Respiratory depression in the newborn infant is frequently seen since glucuronidation, the major conjugating mechanism for morphine, functions at a low level in the fetus and newborn infant. All of the narcotic analgesics are competitively antagonized by nalorphine and levallorphan, congeners of morphine, which have been used effectively to combat the depressant effects seen in the newborn infant. Antagonism can only be obtained when the drug is injected into the mother immediately prior to delivery because of the rapidity of placental transport of these agents. The use of morphine in obstetric anesthesia today is a rare event because of the widespread publicity which neonatal respiratory depression from this agent received. Meperidine, however, continues to result in depressed infants, particularly when it is administered to the mother more than 1 hour prior to actual delivery.

Morphine and heroin addiction can occur *in utero* but the diagnosis may be missed because of the late appearance, several days after birth, of withdrawal signs in the newborn infant. So characteristic is the withdrawal picture, however, that it can be the clue to the diagnosis of addiction in the mother. The heroin abstinence syndrome in the neonate can be quite severe although reliable figures as to the exact mortality and morbidity rate in untreated cases are either not available or are controversial. As mentioned above, while considerable attention has been paid to the quantitation of respiratory depression in the newborns of mothers who receive small acute analgesic doses of morphine or meperidine during active labor, little attention has been paid to the study of infants exposed chronically during gestation to narcotics. This is particularly true with respect to the long-term assessment of these infants. This lack of reliable data regarding outcome in the passively addicted newborn is further compounded by the marked variations which exist in drug intake in addicted mothers. Early recognition and treatment of the withdrawal syndrome in the newborn infant is mandatory in order to prevent death which can occur from severe withdrawal.

The nonnarcotic analgesics, of which salicylate is the major prototype, are used in a free and uncontrolled manner throughout pregnancy. In a study of 272 consecutive deliveries Palmisano found that 10% of all newborns had a measurable salicylate level in cord blood (Palmisano and Cassady, 1969). Mechanisms for conjugation of salicylate via either glucuronide formation or coupling with glycine are limited in the immediate newborn period. Nevertheless, overt toxic effects in the newborn from maternal administration of salicylate have been only rarely noted until recently when effects on platelet function and on synthesis of factor XII (Hageman) have been found (Bleyer and Breckenridge, 1970). Of significance was the fact that in their series hemorrhagic phenomena occurred in three of the 14 aspirin-exposed infants. The effects of salicylate administration to the mothers have been shown to be due to an action on platelet aggregation (Corby and Schulman, 1971). Salicylate appears to inhibit the release of adenosine diphosphate (ADP) from platelets, and thus aggregation to form a platelet plug, which results from ADP release, is impaired. Impairment of platelet function occurred even though mothers had last taken the aspirin in usual dosage as long as a week prior to delivery. Furthermore, newborn platelets appeared to be strikingly sensitive to the effects of salicylate *in vitro*. The study by Corby and Schulman also demonstrated that another compound used for analgesic purposes during labor, promethazine, was also capable of markedly impairing platelet aggregation in the newborn infant. In this case (in contrast to salicylate) no effect was demonstrable on the maternal platelets *in vitro*.

4. ANTIHYPERTENSIVE AGENTS

Aggressive pharmacological management of toxemia of pregnancy and its associated hypertension has led to a profound decrease in maternal and fetal mortality. Antihypertensive drugs have played a major role in the treatment program but they have been associated on occasion with adverse effects in the offspring. Thrombocytopenia has been reported in infants born to mothers receiving thiazide diuretics. This is apparently a rare event and is most likely due to a direct toxic effect on fetal megakaryocyte production since maternal platelet counts are normal. Reserpine, the most commonly prescribed of the *Rauwolfia* alkaloids, is associated with a significant incidence (10%) of morbidity in infants born to mothers who have been treated with therapeutic doses during the last trimester of pregnancy. These infants exhibit a clinical syndrome which is characterized by severe noninfective nasal discharge, lethargy, anorexia, and respiratory depression. The syndrome is self-limiting and symptoms usually subside spontaneously within the first week of life, although on rare occasions local therapy with nasal decongestants is necessary because of the interference with oral feeding in the affected infant. Despite the common occurrence of this syndrome, no pharmacological investigations have been undertaken to explain the symptomatology, which more than likely is due to prolonged blockage of norepinephrine uptake at neurotransmitter storage sites in the infant.

Magnesium sulfate is frequently used in the management of toxemia of pregnancy. The form of therapy employing the intravenous route is extremely safe for the mother and has a solid foundation in the practice of obstetrics. With frequent and repetitive administration of the drug to the mother, a steady increase in intracellular concentration of magnesium in the fetus ensues. This causes central depression and peripheral neuromuscular block by a curarelike action on the motor end plate. In the newborn, magnesium is excreted rather slowly in the urine with plasma concentrations requiring as long as 72–96 hours postpartum to become normal. As a consequence, infants born after magnesium therapy in the mother may be flaccid and lethargic and may have a delay in onset of spontaneous respirations. Vigorous supportive therapy must be instituted once the diagnosis can be established. In extreme cases exchange transfusion may be life saving. Such exchange transfusion should always be carried out with citrated blood because of the added beneficial effect of the citrate–magnesium binding. This also requires an awareness of the potential hazards of magnesium therapy in the mother and communication of the fact that this therapy has been given to the physician caring for the infant. Although calcium ion has been shown to be an effective antagonist in the adult, no such efficacy has been demonstrated in the newborn infant.

5. ANTITHYROID DRUGS

The fetal thyroid gland begins to function during the fourth month of gestation. Any antithyroid agent administered to the mother thereafter may affect the function and subsequent development of the infant's thyroid–pituitary axis, since antithyroid drugs readily cross the placenta while thyroid hormones do not. Thiouracil derivatives inhibit thyroxine synthesis in the fetus in the independently functioning fetal thyroid gland. It is this effect which is probably responsible for many congenital goiters. In most instances the enlargement of the thyroid gland regresses spontaneously in the postnatal period when the infant is separated from the maternal medication. No therapy is needed unless there is mechanical obstruction of the airway due to compression from the enlarged thyroid gland. Transient hyperthyroidism may occur (the syndrome is similar to heroin or methadone withdrawal) and may require rigorous supportive measures with intravenous fluids and sedatives.

The use of radioactive iodine during pregnancy can produce severe hypothyroidism in the fetus because of the local destructive effects on the fetal thyroid. These findings have been varified in animal experiments and noted in human stillborn infants. The potential for initiation of malignant change in the infant thyroid at some later date should also serve to preclude the use of radioactive iodine during pregnancy.

6. Psychopharmacological Agents

Phenothiazines (chlorpromazine, promethazine, promazine) are frequently prescribed during pregnancy both for their antiemetic effect during early pregnancy and as adjuncts to anesthesia at the time of labor and delivery. While there has been considerable controversy regarding their potential for teratogenesis, no clear-cut causal relationship has been established. When these compounds are used in labor they appear to be efficacious. However, they have been variously indicted as being responsible for depression in the newborn infant. While it is, of course, possible that use of these compounds during labor and their transmission to the newborn infant may be associated with long-term effects on behavior, no such observations have been made. It should also be emphasized that phenothiazines produce α adrenergic receptor blockade with hypotension in the mother and diminished uteroplacental blood flow. Since these receptors are operative in the newborn infant, it is conceivable that blockage may have deleterious effects on such important homeostatic mechanisms as norepinephrine-mediated thermogenesis. Here again, no prospective detailed investigation regarding temperature regulation in infants born to mothers receiving phenothiazines has been reported. Although this family of drugs is known to be associated frequently with liver toxicity in adults, there is no evidence that it potentiates neonatal hyperbilirubinemia. In fact there is a body of clinical evidence which suggests that it may actually induce fetal liver enzyme systems. Recently concern has been expressed that chronic treatment with chlorpromazine during pregnancy might possibly produce retinopathy in the fetus because of the affinity of the compound to melanin-containing tissues (Herxheimer, 1971). Thus the clinical recommendation has been put forth that the eyes of all infants whose mothers received large doses of chlorpromazine during pregnancy be examined carefully. Similar eye lesions have been reported in human neonates after pregnant women had received chloroquine for discoid lupus (Hart and Naunton, 1964).

7. STEROIDS HORMONES

Steroid hormones are widely used in clinical obstetrics to prevent abortion, sustain placentation, and decrease uterine tone. Discussion of pharmacological effects must begin with consideration of the physiological role of these hormones during fetal development. There is ample experimental evidence to indicate that in contrast to extrauterine existence, no fetal endocrine gland is indispensable for survival of the fetus, perhaps because of the presence of placental or maternal hormone. Homeostasis in the fetus can thus be regulated by the maternal environment mediated through the placenta. Fetal hormones evidently have their major role in the determination of physiological and morphological development of their own target organs.

Permanent structural changes are a conspicuous effect of gonadal hormones and fetal female masculinization may follow the use of testosterone or 17-substituted steroid hormones in certain pregnant women. The mechanism for this pharmacological effect has been clearly elucidated by Jost, who demonstrated a critical period during development when masculinization of the female fetus can occur (end of first trimester) with resultant fusion of the urethral folds and development of a penislike phallus (Jost, 1961). Administration of the hormone after this critical period may only lead to an enlarged clitoris. The drug effect, in this case androgenic action, is exerted at the time during normal development when sex differentiation is taking place. The function of fetally produced androgen is to prevent the genital tract of males from differentiating along the female line; feminine differentiation is non-hormone-dependent. Thus it follows that excess androgen in the external environment (maternal) finds a sensitive receptor organ when it is present at the time of differentiation of the female genital tract. A variety of exogenous progestational compounds can, if administered to the mother, result in masculinization of the female fetus. It should be noted that diethylstilbestrol has also produced this effect, probably indicating that estrogen may either stimulate the fetal adrenals to increase androgen secretion or become metabolized to compounds with androgenic activity. There are undoubtedly many instances of fertilization occurring prior to the subsequent institution of oral contraceptive therapy; yet there is no reliable clinical evidence that the small amounts of progestins in these compounds can masculinize the human fetus. Androgens may also be derived from virilizing ovarian tumors in the mother or from congenital adrenal hyperplastic glands of the infant itself. Masculinization results, similar to that seen when the androgens are administered to the pregnant woman. Psychological evaluation of girls exposed *in utero* to excess fetal androgens either via the adrenogenital system or because of progestin treatment of the mothers have exhibited a tomboyish behavior (Ehrhardt and Money, 1967). Of added interest was the higher mean IQ measured in these patients in contrast to a control population. On the other hand, studies by the same investigators of patients with Turner's syndrome who have either no gonads or only vestigial streaks and who differentiate morphologically as females, showed that they had the same degree of femininity as their controls (Ehrhardt *et al.*, 1970). Thus the fetal ovary does not appear essential for the subsequent differentiation of normal female gender identity.

The report of the appearance of seven young patients with adenocarcinoma of the vagina tragically illustrates one of the most important concepts in pediatric pharmacology, namely, that exposure to drugs or chemicals may have latent, unforeseen effects on development (Herbst *et al.*, 1971). Patients ranging in age from 14 to 22 sought medical advice because of vaginal bleeding. Subsequent examination confirmed that all had adenocarcinoma of the vagina, an extremely rare tumor at this age. Epidemiologic study of the seven patients revealed that the mothers had received stilbestrol during pregnancy and that administration had begun during the first trimester and was continued throughout pregnancy. Other cases have now been reported and the causal relationship between malignancy and prenatal exposure to stilbestrol appears strong although by no means proved. The phenomenon appears to be rare in that many women have been given stilbestrol for vaginal bleeding in early pregnancy without untoward effects on their fetuses.

Adrenal steroid hormones are frequently used for the treatment of a variety of chronic diseases in pregnant women. As previously mentioned, cortisone and related steroids may be responsible for some cases of cleft palate but the data do not at all support a cause and effect relationship, despite the fact that ample evidence in animal species has proved that cortisone administered in large doses early in pregnancy may produce cleft palate. In addition to concern for direct toxic effects on the fetus, there is a possibility that the infant's pituitary–adrenal function might be suppressed by adrenal steroids administered to the mother. A review of the world literature in 1960, however, revealed only one possible case occurring in 260 pregnancies (Bongiovanni and McPadden, 1960). More recently, direct measurement of cortisol secretion in eight newborns whose mothers had been treated with steroids demonstrated normal production and none of the infants showed symptoms of relative hypoadrenocorticism (Kenny *et al.*, 1966). There have been occasional cases reported, however, in which hypoglycemia developed shortly after birth. It would, therefore, seem prudent to follow such an infant clinically but not to administer routine prophylactic steroid therapy.

8. ANTIMICROBIAL AGENTS

This class of pharmacological agents is used frequently during pregnancy for maternal infections and obviously have a role in the prevention of intrauterine fetal infection. As previously indicated, the administration of penicillin to the mother has proved to be effective in the treatment of congenital syphilis. Generally, therapeutic concentrations of a great number of antimicrobial substances are achieved in the fetus and amniotic fluid. Most of the available data in man have been obtained during labor and delivery or at the time of cesarean section. In such studies, single doses of drug are given to mothers at varying times before delivery and paired samples of maternal and cord plasma are obtained at birth for assay. All antibacterial agents studied cross the placenta at varying rates. Cephalothicin, studied at term, reaches peak levels in the infant 30 to 50 minutes after maternal peak concentrations but the concentrations achieved are much lower than those obtained in normal newborns treated directly. The transplacental passage of methicillin, dicloxacillin, and ampicillin has been studied and correlated to their degree of protein binding. Dicloxacillin (96% protein bound) achieves low levels in fetal serum and insignificant concentrations in amniotic fluid. Methicillin (40% protein bound) is rapidly cleared from maternal serum and reaches high concentrations in the fetus and amniotic fluid. Ampicillin (20% protein bound) shows further reduction in maternal serum levels and even higher concentrations on the other side of the placenta. Therapeutic approaches to the pregnant woman can take advantage of these different rates of transfer. For dichloxacillin, reducing the total dose and injecting it intramuscularly will lower the maximum concentration in the mother and at the same time the amount crossing the placenta will be minimal. Therefore, maternal infections could be treated with no effects on the fetus (MacAulay *et al.*, 1968). Conversely, the treatment of fetal disease could take advantage of the reverse situation and use ampicillin to achieve maximal drug concentrations in the fetus.

There are no data indicating that sulfonamides have an adverse effect on the fetus *in utero*. Their competition with bilirubin for albumin-binding sites in the fetus is probably unimportant clinically since the placenta is well able to clear unconjugated bilirubin from the fetus to the mother. This pharmacological effect is hazardous near term because once the umbilical cord is clamped the neonate must depend upon his own metabolic capbilities for clearance of bilirubin and the sulfonamides can then compete with bilirubin for albumin binding, displace bilirubin, and enable the pigment to enter the brain at lower serum levels. Long-acting sulfonamides in particular should therefore not be administered near term.

Several of the aminoglycoside antibiotics cross the placenta and there are isolated reports that chronic treatment of the mother with streptomycin during pregnancy can lead to permanent otic damage. There are sporadic reports of similar toxicity occurring with kanamycin administration. In the first half of pregnancy streptomycin administered to the mother is not detected in amniotic fluid but later on high concentrations can be found. This would indicate that the fetal kidneys eventually acquire the capacity to excrete the drug. Similar results have been found with cephalothicin near term.

All of the tetracylcines cross the placenta and if given to the mother from the fifth month of gestation onward can result in staining of the deciduous teeth in some of the exposed fetuses and in a much smaller proportion of cases cause enamel hypoplasia. In a carefully designed prospective study of 99 women who underwent prolonged therapy with tetracylines during different periods of pregnancy, 13 children were found with discolored teeth (Toaff and Ravid, 1968); four of them had enamel hypoplasia. Of 58 fetuses exposed only before the twenty-fourth week of gestation, none showed any staining. The staining is apparently the result of chemically unaltered drug that has chelated calcium during the process of mineralization and is laid down in the teeth or bone. The tetracycline calcium complex is fluorescent and can be identified in this manner.

IV. Pharmacology of the Neonate

A. General Principles

1. PHYSIOLOGICAL

The transition from intrauterine to extrauterine life involves a number of major changes in function of the organism. While many of these are physiological changes of a functional nature, the cardiopulmonary changes also involve gross anatomic alterations as well.

Thus it is that the expansion of the lungs (*in utero* the placenta acts as a "fetal lung" to exchange oxygen and carbon dioxide) permits appropriate air exchange in the newborn. The lung is also available now for purposes of drug administration by inhalation and for clearance from the body via exhalation. *In utero*, however, the placenta has functioned not only as a "lung" but in addition has functioned to clear and metabolize many substances from the fetus to the mother, a role which must now be assumed by the organism itself. As to the lung itself, not only passive exchange of oxygen and carbon dioxide is involved in successful adaptation, synthesis of surfactant, which can be demonstrated as early as 20 to 24 weeks *in utero* but which becomes metabolically competent only about the thirty-fifth week with the incorporation of phosphatidylethanolamine and phosphatidylcholine into the molecule, needs to be successfully continued in postnatal life at an appropriate rate to ensure adequate alveolar stability. In the absence of effective synthesis and an adequate turnover rate of the material, alveolar collapse occurs progressively during expiration. This phenomenon underlies the respiratory distress syndrome (hyaline membrane disease) where inadequate or insufficient surfactant has been demonstrated as the mechanism of causation of the disease. The possibility of inducing surfactant synthesis in the human *in vivo* has been investigated with corticosteroids as the inducing agent. It has been suggested that immature infants less than 32-weeks gestational age show a lesser incidence of both occurrence of and mortality from hyaline membrane disease when β-methazone is given to their mothers during premature labor (Liggins and Howie, 1972). However, postnatal administration of hydrocortisone to affected infants (Baden *et al.*, 1972) appears to be of no avail. Glass *et al.* (1971) have suggested that there is a lower incidence of the disease in infants born to heroin-addicted mothers, but the nature of this agent precludes its voluntary experimental use. An additional agent, thyroxine, has been shown to induce surfactant experimentally in the rat lung (Redding *et al.*, 1972), but there are as yet no studies available regarding its efficacy in human subjects.

The fetal circulation converts through a transitional phase (the perinatal circulation) to its adult counterpart (Stern and Lind, 1960). This requires removal of the placenta and closure of the umbilical vessels, closure of the ductus venosus thus eliminating the fetal shunt around the liver, and final closure of both the foramen ovale and the ductus arteriosus which will convert the intrauterine right to left shunting of blood (e.g., the ventricles work in parallel) to the normal adult situation where the ventricles are arranged so their output is in series. These changes in the circulation have important implications for the relative distribution of drugs to different tissues. It must be remembered that all of the fetal channels may reopen in postanatal life under adverse conditions (hypoxia, alterations in pulmonary–systemic arterial pressure relationships). Indeed final anatomic closure of the foramen ovale does not occur until at least 2 weeks, and of the ductus arteriosus not until 6 weeks of postnatal age (Lind *et al.*, 1964).

Body composition in the newborn, especially the premature, may influence drug distribution particularly with respect to lipid-soluble agents. There is a relative lack of fatty tissue in the newborn (infants of diabetic mothers are a notable exception), which is more pronounced in the premature. In relative terms, therefore, there is probably a higher proportion of the total body lipid mass in the central nervous system of the newborn than of its adult counterpart. Considerations of metabolic activity are additionally complicated in the infant who is inappropriately small for his gestational age (fetal malnutrition, intrauterine growth retardation). In such infants oxygen consumption levels estimated on a milliliter/kilogram/minute basis tend to be much higher than for infants appropriately grown, suggesting relative preservation of metabolically active tissue at the expense of relatively inactive muscle and connective tissue mass. In such infants dosages calculated on a weight basis may be inadequate in some cases and result in toxicity at dose levels close to the therapeutic range for others. An example of the latter effect can be seen in the report of digitalis intoxication in premature infants (Levine and Blumenthal, 1962), in whom toxic effects were most noticeable for those whose weight was inappropriate for their gestational age. There are, in addition, differences in the partition of total body water with a higher extracellular portion in the newborn as opposed to the adult. This difference is of considerable importance in the calculation of bicarbonate therapy for the correction of acidemia. Thus, whereas an extracellular volume (ECV) factor of 0.3 is commonly used in the adult and older child, similar correction effectively requires a factor closer to 0.6 in the neonate.

The neonatal gastrointestinal tract shows a number of important differences *vis-à-vis* its older counterpart. In addition to obvious differences in mobility and absorptive capacity, a number of other differences may influence the ability to effectively handle orally administered agents. Thus, although stomach acidity is present from about 12 hours of life onward, the gastric contents are highly alkaline in the immediate neonatal period. This alkalinity may, however, have a highly protective effect in destroying bacteria ingested *in utero* and peripartum from infected amniotic fluid (Ramos and Stern, 1969). The lack of intestinal flora in the immediate postnatal period provides for a different intraluminal environment than encountered later on. Moreover, the oral intake of the neonate is for all practical purposes limited to milk at relatively frequent intervals so that absorptive and binding interactions in the neonatal gut need to be considered with both of these factors in mind. Finally, the possibilities for enterohepatic circulatory reabsorption of substances, especially glucuronides, are markedly enhanced by the presence of a more than adequate amount of β-glucuronidase in the neonatal gut (it is absent in the adult), capable of converting glucuronides excreted into the gastro-intestinal tract from the bile to their unconjugated and hence enterohepatically reabsorbable form (see below under bilirubin).

It is generally accepted that both renal gomerular and tubular functions are reduced in the newborn. This delay in renal excretion permits the administration of crystalline penicillin to the newborn with a dosage interval of 12 hours basis with adequate blood levels obtained without the necessity of resorting to the procaine preparation. On the other hand, the propensity for achievement of toxicity via this mechanism is obviously great. There is also evidence for end organ unresponsiveness of the tubule (e.g., to parathormone), a mechanism which has been held to be responsible for the hypocalcemic tetany of the newborn (Connelly et al., 1963). The premature infant is additionally hampered by diminished renal ability to conserve base with a lower renal bicarbonate threshold resulting in a relatively easy tendency to systemic acidosis. This can usually be overcome by the addition of bicarbonate to the feedings but may on occasion require parenteral correction. If uncorrected, the resultant acidemia may seriously impair weight gain of the infant in the long term. Acidosis also dissociates the binding of anions to albumin (cf. bilirubin) and may thus result in important changes in the ratio of the bound-to-free (available) fractions of therapeutic agents.

Hepatic biotransformation has two opposing functions with respect to substances handled by the liver, e.g., conversion to a biologically active form and/or detoxification with subsequent preparation for total inactivation or excretion from the organism. Detailed consideration of a number of the mechanisms involved using an endogenous substance (bilirubin) follows elsewhere in this section. The maturational delay in hepatic activity in the neonate results in the same dualism seen with the reduced renal capacity of the newborn (e.g., augmented, prolonged therapeutic levels versus easier toxicity). The tragedy of neonatal chloramphenicol intoxication with the subsequent lethal "gray syndrome" thus resulted from a combination of the reduced hepatic capacity to conjugate the drug coupled with the limited renal ability to excrete it (Weiss et al., 1960).

Not all aspects of hepatic function are, however, immature at birth. A recent study (Räihä, 1973) has shown that phenylalanine hydroxylase activity is present in human liver after the eighth week of gestation and that at about the thirteenth week it reaches the level found in adult liver. Despite this, hyperphenylalaninemia and/or a reduced tolerance to phenylalanine is found in some low-birth-weight infants. This would suggest a reduced efficiency of some other component of the phenylalanine-hydroxylating system. Thus, it appears likely that varying rates of maturation may exist within the same system or chain of biological reactions responsible for the hepatic biotransformation of an agent and that maturational delays in such biological end probuct activity need not always reflect the same intermediary defect. Finally, the factors which enhance or retard the appearance of specific hepatic activity may vary widely. In many instances the substrate itself is suspected of being the responsible agent in inducing enzyme activity (cf. bilirubin and glucuronyltransferase), while in other situations both enhancing and retarding factors may be operative. Thus pyruvate kinase activity may be induced earlier in rat liver after weaning by feeding a high carbohydrate diet, and inhibited when a high fat one is offered instead (Hahn and Skala, 1971).

The recent demonstration of excessive serum hexachlorophene levels after topical application to neonatal skin and the presence of characteristic spongioform lesions in the central nervous system (Hall and Reid, 1972; Lockhart, 1972) of affected infants has focused attention on the potential hazards of this agent. Systemic absorption with measurable blood concentrations has been demonstrated following its use as a soap or cream (Curley et al., 1971) and as a powder (Adler et al., 1972). Its application to excoriated skin, particularly in the diaper area, is reminiscent of similar central nervous system toxicity seen and identified a number of years ago wth boric acid (Goldbloom and Goldbloom, 1953). It must be pointed out, however, that the passage of pharmacological active chemicals across the skin is not specific for hexachlorophene. Thus the suggestion to substitute soap and water for hexachloraphene washing in the newborn may be equally as dangerous to the organism, since the resultant absorption of free fatty acids carries serious implications vis-à-vis the competitive binding with bilirubin on the albumin molecule (Chan et al., 1971). In addition to skin and mucous membranes, enhanced absorption via the conjunctiva of the eye may also occur. Bauer et al. (1973) have demonstrated severe atropinelike gastrointestinal toxicity with ileus and systemic levels from cyclogyl (cyclopentolate) mydriatic drops in a set of premature twins. The usual topical adult doses of such agents are here clearly toxic and should be lowered if systemic toxicity is to be avoided.

The thermal instability of the newborn, which is more marked in the premature, may have a number of adverse pharmacological results. Thus, hypothermia both directly and through the medium of responsive vasoconstriction increases the tendency to acidosis, with subsequent effects both on biological system functions and albumin binding of agents. Even prior to a fall in body temperature, a lowered *environmental* temperature below the "neutral zone" (in a newborn 32°–34°C) calls forth a compensatory rise in metabolic heat production manifested as an increase in oxygen consumption (Stern *et al.*, 1965). Its accompanying increase in serum nonesterified fatty acids (NEFA) (Schiff *et al.*, 1966) will result in a reciprocal fall in blood glucose. The hypoglycemia carries serious implications for the oxidative phosphorylation processes which are both glucose and oxygen dependent, while the rise in serum NEFA provides a competitive binder with other anions for the albumin molecule.

2. Pharmacological

The important mechanism for drug disposition which exists during intrauterine life, namely, the maternal organism, is no longer available after delivery occurs and the umbilical cord is severed. The newborn infant is truly on his own, adapting to extrauterine existence. The presence of drugs may add to an already complex situation and may compromise successful adjustment on the part of the neonate. More often than not the presence of drugs in the neonate is not due to direct administration but is the consequence of medications administered to the mother prior to or during delivery. Another source of drug, considered only recently, is the intake of foreign compounds with breast milk (see Section IV,B). Any drug, independent of the age of the host, will exert an effect contingent upon its concentration at the site of action and its interaction with specific receptor sites. Processes of absorption, distribution, metabolism, and excretion influence such concentration and will be discussed for this restricted age group together with a review of basic principles.

a. Absorption. The route by which the drug is administered is important since it determines the rate at which the drug will enter the circulation. Few studies have been published regarding the absorption of drugs from the oral route in the newborn, although drugs are commonly administered by mouth at this age. An early study demonstrated that a triple sulfonamide preparation was absorbed more slowly in premature infants than in the full-term neonate (Fichter and Curtis, 1956). Chloramphenicol, which has been extensively studied, is well absorbed by the gastrointestinal tract and similar conclusions were drawn from studies of other antibiotics such as erythromycin and tetracycline. The absorption and secretion of riboflavin, a vitamin which is absorbed by a saturable transport process in the proximal small intestine, were found to be strikingly different than that noted in older infants and children (Jusko *et al.*, 1970). The maximum urinary excretion rate in the older subject was fivefold higher than in the neonate, but the duration of the maximum rate achieved in the neonate persisted for a much longer period of time. Consequently, the total amount of riboflavin excreted in the urine was quite similar for both age groups when expressed as a percent of administered dose. Additional studies demonstrated that the slow and prolonged excretion of riboflavin in the neonate was not due to a limited renal excretory capacity since, when administered parenterally, the maximum excretion rate of the vitamin was similar in the newborn and in the older subject (seven times higher than that noted after oral administration). It was therefore concluded in this investigation that the slow and prolonged excretion was due to prolonged absorption from the gastrointestinal tract. Many reasons may exist for this difference in oral absorption and these include: a much lower activity of the specialized intestinal transport process, diffusion over a much longer segment of the gastrointestinal tract, and limited enzymatic hydrolysis of riboflavin in the neonate. These results obtained with riboflavin serve to emphasize the differences which may exist for drug absorption between the newborn infant and the adult.

The parenteral route is frequently used to administer drugs in the neonate when medications are prescribed because of more serious illness. The results with riboflavin demonstrate that this substance is absorbed as well in the newborn as in the older patient following parenteral administration. Comparative studies between sites are not available with respect to drug absorption and many concepts are extrapolated from animal research. An interesting experimental design demonstrated no difference in the absorption of morphine after subcutaneous injection in young versus adult rats. In this investigation, the remaining free morphine at injection sites was measured directly. Peripheral vasomotor instability in the newborn has raised the question regarding the deficiency of drug absorption from intramuscular or subcutaneous sites. Current practices of keeping sick neonates requiring medications in a neutral temperature environment provided by incubators eliminates cold stress in these babies. Administered intramuscularly, adequate concentrations of antibiotics, such as colistin, kanamycin, penicillin, polymyxin B, streptomycin, ampicillin, and oxacillin, are achieved in plasma of both premature and full-term infants. When speed of absorption by oral and intramuscular routes was compared, after the administration of labeled digoxin to infants with severe congenital cardiac malformation who required digitalization, absorption was rapid and of the same magnitude as that in adults (Hernandez *et al.*, 1969). Digoxin could be detected in the blood 5 minutes after oral administration, reaching a peak concentration in 1–3 hours, whereas by the intramuscular route the drug was delivered into the circulation 1 minute after injection and peak levels were achieved 15–30 minutes later. Comparable observations have been reported in neonates receiving nonisotopic digoxin therapy (Larese and Mirkin, 1974).

While systematic studies of the absorption of drugs in newborn infants have not been carried out, there have been several recent investigations contrasting antibiotic absorption following either parenteral or oral administration. Disposition data concerning antibiotics are more plentiful because of their frequent usage in the newborn infant. Silverio and Poole (1973) have recently compared ampicillin absorption in newborn infants with that in adults. The area under the serum concentration curve was approximately three times greater in the newborn infant. This is primarily due to decreased renal excretion but there is no question that the absorptive process from the gastrointestinal tract is functioning at a greater rate in infants than in adults. Jusko (1972) has analyzed the availability of ampicillin in the newborn infant when administered by mouth or by intramuscular injection. About two-thirds of the oral dose was absorbed in the newborn, and this can be compared with about 30% bioavailability of ampicillin from capsules in adult subjects.

b. Distribution.   Through this process, the drug which has entered the circulatory system is delivered to tissues of appropriate body compartments producing an effect when the necessary concentration at the receptor site is reached. The volume of distribution is regulated by several factors which include the rate of transport across biological membranes and the extent of binding to plasma proteins. The newborn infant has a much higher extracellular volume than the adult. Total body water also is much greater in the newborn and varies from 85% of body weight in the small premature infant to 70% in the full-term infant. Fat content, on the other hand, is lower in the premature infant (1%) than in the normal full-term infant (15%). With these changes in body composition, changes in drug distribution are to be anticipated. Yet very few quantitative data are available regarding this phenomenon.

In plasma, drugs bind mostly to albumin, and this binding depends primarily upon the molecular structure of the drug and the nature of the bond formed with albumin (see Chapter 1). Investigations of the plasma protein binding of diphenylhydantoin in heparinized plasma from normal and hyperbilirubinemic newborn infants by means of an ultrafiltration technique utilizing carbon-14 labeled diphenylhydantoin, showed an unbound fraction of 11% as compared to about 7% in adults (Rane *et al.,* 1971). The range of values in individual samples was much greater in newborn plasma than in adult plasma, probably because of the presence of competing substances such as fatty acids in the newborn. Bilirubin appeared to compete with diphenylhydantoin for the binding sites on the albumin molecule. At concentrations of bilirubin greater than 20 mg per 100 ml, the unbound fraction of diphenylhydantoin was twice as high as in plasma from nonhyperbilirubinemic infants. Chignall has also shown that neonatal plasma albumin has less affinity for the sulfonamide drug, sulfaphenazole, than does adult plasma albumin (Chignall et al., 1971). They postulated that the difference was probably due to the presence in neonatal plasma of an endogenous ligand, probably bilirubin, which has a stronger affinity for plasma albumin and, therefore, competes with the sulfonamide for binding sites on the protein. The binding of salicylate to albumin fractionated from pooled neonatal cord serum was found to be quite different from that seen with adult serum (Krasner et al., 1973). The apparent association constant of 1.7×10^5 M^{-1} in the infant was approximately one-third of the adult value. Nafcillin binding to pooled cord serum was also studied by the same investigators using the technique of equilibrium dialysis. The percentage of the drug bound increased from 16% at low antibiotic concentrations (5 μg/ml) up to 28% at 200 μg/ml. This represents considerably less binding than occurs with adult serum, where 86% of the antibiotic is bound at therapeutic antibiotic concentrations. It is reasonable to expect that similar differences in plasma protein binding between adults and newborn infants may be found with other drugs.

It is possible that this difference in binding is one of the many reasons why drugs have been reported to have greater effects and more often to result in side effects in neonates than in adults when the dose is calculated on the basis of body weight or body surface. The difference in binding may be due not only to lower concentrations of plasma proteins (particularly albumin), but there may also be qualitative differences in the binding proteins. In addition, endogenous substances during the first few days of life, especialy hormones, transferred in utero may occupy binding sites and thus reduce binding capacity. It should be borne in mind that it is only the unbound fraction of the drug which is free to cross membranes and reach receptor sites to exert drug action. Furthermore, when one considers that multiple drugs are administered to sick infants, the possibility of drug interaction is very great. As a result, the full clinical significance of plasma protein binding may unfortunately make itself apparent with the appearance of unexpected side effects or different effects from those anticipated by the prescribing physician. Just such a tragic occurrence was noted during a controlled trial of two prophylactic antibacterial regimens (Silverman et al., 1956). Two groups of premature infants were assigned to receive either penicillin and sulfisoxazole or oxytetracycline. A higher mortality rate, begining at age 3 days with an increased incidence of bilirubin encephalopathy, was recorded for the first group. Serum bilirubin concentrations in this group were consistently lower than those in the oxytetracycline-treated prematures. Studies *in vitro* demonstrated that sulfisoxazole displaced bilirubin from its albumin binding sites permitting it to pass into the brain. The competition for binding with albumin is not unique for this drug and should be considered when one or more drugs are to be given to sick infants as there may be mutual displacement. Pediatricians have become sensitized to interference with bilirubin binding because of the tragedy which occurred with sulfisoxazole. Recently, two drugs commonly used in the newborn, caffeine sodium benzoate and valium injectable, were shown to displace bilirubin from its binding to albumin (Schiff *et al.*, 1971). This displacement was noted *in vitro* using either Sephadex gel filtration or bilirubin spectral curves to assess bilirubin–albumin binding. It is of interest that in both of these fixed drug combinations, the sodium benzoate, which was used as a solubilizer or a preservative, was incriminated as the displacing agent. Thus, the recommendation has been made that when evaluating a drug for use in the neonatal period, its potential for displacement of bilirubin be assessed in advance in all of its dosage forms.

c. Metabolism.   As a general rule, the rate at which a drug is eliminated is much lower than its rate of absorption and distribution and thus constitutes the rate-limiting step in the pharmacokinetic process. Drug elimination consists of several processes that operate to remove drugs from their site of action. Renal excretory mechanisms are of importance, but other routes, such as the intestinal tract, biliary system, and lungs, may participate to a lesser degree. Lipid-soluble drugs may also be stored in body fat and in this manner removed from the receptor site, whereas other agents may accumulate in bone and teeth and thus cannot exert their pharmacological effect. The most important process by which drugs are eliminated, however, is through their biotransformation into nonactive compounds. Although some drugs may be excreted to a varying degree unchanged, most undergo metabolic transformations which serve to increase thir polarity and make them more readily available for excretion by the kidney. Most metabolic transformations occur in the liver mediated by a group of enzymes located in the microsomal faction, but other tissues may have some measurable activity when examined *in vitro*. Experimental evidence has accumulated during the last two decades that in several animal species the activity of many of these enzymes in the young is low and that achievement of adult values takes varying periods of time after birth. There are only a few *in vitro* studies employing human newborn material, and these have supported the animal studies in that liver homogenate from the neonate was unable to glucuronidate p-nitrophenol or liver slices to conjugate bilirubin. One study has examined the components of the mixed-function oxidase system in human neonatal hepatic microsomes and found that the properties of NADPH-cytochrome c reductase were identical to the enzyme isolated from rat liver (Soyka, 1970). On the other hand, a number of studies have been undertaken in vivo in which drug metabolic capacity is determined by measuring plasma half-lives of exogenous compounds administered to the infant. A comprehensive study of the elimination of sulfobromophthalein, which must be conjugated with several amino acids and with glutathione, was undertaken by Wichman in newborn infants and older children (Wichman et al., 1968). The plasma half-life decreased from 9.6 minutes in infants less than 10 days of age to 5.5 minutes in older infants and children. Half-lives were longer in premature infants than in the full-term infant during the first several days of life. The precise reason for the delay in the elimination of sulfobromophthalein in newborn infants is, of course, unknown. Deficient metabolism is suggested but it is also possible that the secretion of sulfobromophthalein into bile after conjugation is delayed. In vitro studies of the conjugating system for sulfobromophthalein have shown that activity was approximately 20% of adult values during the neonatal period in mouse liver homogenates (Krasner and Yaffe, 1968).

Other substances such as bilirubin, which undergoes glucuronidation, and p-aminobenzoic acid, which is glucuronidated and also coupled with glycine, have prolonged metabolism when evaluated in vivo in newborn infants. With p-aminobenzoic acid there is also a qualitative difference in the pattern of metabolites found in the newborn infant. The newborn excretes p-aminobenzoic acid mainly in the form of the acetylated derivative, which is not found in older children. Drug substrates, such as acetanilid, phenylbutazone, aminopyrine, and diazepam, have prolonged plasma half-lives in the neonatal period with successive increase with age in their elimination rate from plasma. While it would appear that the in vivo studies confirm the observations in animals in vitro, there are a few conflicting results. Sjöqvist et al., investigated the pharmacokinetics of nortriptyline in a newborn infant whose mother had taken an overdose of this compound for suicidal purposes just prior to delivery (Sjöqvist et al., 1972). The disappearance of the drug, which is almost completely metabolized under normal circumstances, was followed in plasma samples in both mother and infant for several days after birth, and the appearance of the hydroxylated metabolites of the drug was also determined in urine samples. The concentration of drug in maternal plasma was five times higher than that seen in newborn plasma, probably because of lower plasma protein binding in the newborn. The plasma concentrations of nortriptyline declined exponentially in both subjects with a half-life of 17 hours in the mother and 56 hours in the infant. It should be emphasized, however, that half-lives above 60 hours can also be seen normally in the adult. The main hydroxylated metabolite of nortriptyline was found in high concentrations in the infant's urine, suggesting that this metabolite is formed in the infant without difficulty. In addition, the same group of investigators has found that the steady-state plasma concentrations of diphenylhydantoin in newborn infants treated with a dose of 10 mg/kg/day were half of those noted in adults treated with 5 mg/kg/day. Perhaps the decrease in protein binding of dipheylhydantoin in newborn plasma may increase the volume of distribution of the drug and its rate of metabolism by making a larger amount of unbound drug available to the metabolizing liver cell.

Deficient drug metabolism appears to have been the basis for many of the adverse effects found when drugs were prescribed to newborn infants in a dosage based on body size. Adverse effects are often unanticipated and may be serious, such as the sequence of events which occurred following the use of chloramphenicol in newborn and premature infants. The cardiovascular collapse following drug administration was named the "gray syndrome" and was subsequently found to be associated with a prolonged and high concentration of chloramphenicol in the blood. The pharmacokinetics of the drug were investigated only after the adverse effects occurred and the half-life in plasma was found to be 26 hours in contrast to 4 hours obtained in older children. These results should have been anticipated since 90% of chloramphenicol is metabolized via glucuronidation prior to excretion from the organism. Pediatricians have recognized for years that mechanisms for glucuronidation are limited in the human newborn and premature infant; a finding used to explain the elevation of unconjugated bilirubin in the neonatal period. *In vitro* studies in several different animal species using slices and homogenates have supported this *in vivo* observation with respect to bilirubin metabolism. Few studies, however, have been done with fetal or neonatal human liver tissue *in vitro*. Glucuronyltransferase activity was found to be virtually absent in fetal life and reduced at birth in liver suspensions (Lathe and Walker, 1958b). A study of the ability of human newborn infants to conjugate via the glucuronide pathway was carried out by measuring the percentage of salicylamide glucoronide found in the urine following the oral administration of salicylamide in a single dose of 20 mg/kg of body weight. The amount of salicylamide recovered as the glucuronide was determined quantitatively and showed a large variation among the 14 infants in whom this parameter was investigated on the fifth day of life (Stern et al., 1970). The variation ranged from 45% of the dose excreted of the glucornide to as little as 8% of the dose. Furthermore, there was an inverse relationship between the serum indirect bilirubin concentration found on the fifth day of life and the urinary percentage of the dose of salicylamide appearing as the glucuronide. In the normal adult, approximately 40 to 50% of a single oral dose of salicylamide appears as a glucuronide. Thus, several of the newborn infants were glucuronidating at rates comparable to those found in the adult. This wide variation in the ability to form the glucuronide for salicylamide among newborn infants is probably genetically determined. The five- to sixfold differences between infants would suggest that there would be great difficulty in arriving at a uniform dosage schedule other than on the basis of individual assessment.

It should not be concluded that all drug metabolic pathways are deficient in activity in the newborn infant. In vitro studies in the mouse using liver suspensions have shown that the process of sulfation functions at the same level of activity as in suspensions derived from adult animal liver (Percy and Yaffe, 1964). It is important to point out that many sulfated derivatives are found in the human organism during the perinatal period as the product of metabolism of both drugs and endogenous compounds during fetal and early neonatal life. Acetylation appears to be active in the newborn infant as mentioned previously in the discussion of glycine conjugation following administration of benzoic acid or p-aminobenzoic acid. On the other hand, it has been reported that the capacity of the liver to acetylate sulfonamide is limited in the newborn period when compared to adults, resulting in high protracted blood levels after comparatively small doses (Fichter and Curtis, 1956). Rane and co-workers (1974) in Stockholm studied seven newborn infants of epileptic mothers treated with diphenylhydantoin throughout pregnancy. The rate of plasma disappearance of diphenylhydantoin in the newborns was of the same order of magnitude as previously reported in adults. Similar findings were noted with the anticonvulsant carbamazepine following transplacental transmission to the newborn when the drug was used for the management of epilepsy in the mother. Half-lives of 8.2–27.7 hours were found (Rane et al., 1975). These are comparable or even shorter than those found in adults after a single oral dose but are in the same range as those found in adults after multiple oral doses. Since both diphenylhydantoin and carbamazepine have the capability of inducing their own metabolism, it is possible that the results noted in these two studies are the consequences of induction by the continuous treatment of the pregnant women with diphenylhydantoin or carbamazepine. Other studies, however, suggest that the neonatal metabolism of diphenylhydantoin and benzodiazepine derivatives was not enhanced when investigated under similar clinical conditions. (See Chapter 1 for further discussion.)

Discussion of drug metabolism would be incomplete without mention of the possibility of increasing the activity of a deficient enzyme system, particularly in patients of the neonatal age group. The phenomenon of pharmacological induction has been found in a wide variety of animal species and can be produced by the administration *in vivo* of any one of a long list of drugs and chemicals that are commonly consumed by man. Barbiturates represent the prototype of the pharmacological inducer, and their effects, when administered *in vivo*, have been extensively studied. Administration is associated with an increase in liver weight and an augmentation of microsomal protein synthesis. Most inducing agents are capable of accelerating their own metabolism as well as that of many other compounds by stimulation of hepatic drug-metabolizing enzymes. Barbiturate administration to the neonatal mouse or rabbit has been associated with a dose-related increase in bilirubin glucuronide formation as determined *in vitro* (Catz and Yaffe, 1968). Administration of the drug shortly before term to the pregnant animal was also associated with a marked increase in bilirubin glucuronide-forming capacity in the neonate. This approach has been applied to the human newborn infant following the successful demonstration that phenobarbital was capable of inducing glucuronide formation in an older infant with congenital unconjugated hyperbilirubinemia. Administration to the human newborn, either commencing at birth or to the mother prior to delivery, is followed by a significant reduction in the degree of hyperbilirubinemia during the neonatal period. The beneficial effect of phenobarbital upon neonatal hyperbilirubinemia probably involves several mechanisms which are impaired in the neonate. Included among these, in addition to enhanced glucuronidation, are facilitated transport and uptake by the liver cell and increased biliary flow. It should be emphasized, however, that this phenomenon of enzyme induction following administration of drugs, such as phenobarbital, is a nonspecific event. Inductive effects are not limited to one enzyme system, and this approach should be used with caution and only after full consideration of the benefit to be gained against the risk of nonspecific induction of a variety of enzymes whose effects may not be noted for many years after birth. Recently the phenomenon of induction has been demonstrated in tissue culture. Foreskins from newborn infants obtained at circumcision were shown to contain an enzyme system that hydroxylates the carcinogen benzpyrene (Levin *et al.*, 1972). When the foreskins were cultured in the presence of benzanthracene, a two- to fivefold increase in the activity of benzpyrene hydroxylase was obtained. The tissue culture technique has important implications for the study of drug metabolic processes in the human neonate where availability of tissue samples is greatly limited.

d. Excretion. While the most important factor in determining drug dosage is that of drug metabolism, urinary excretion is the final route by which the drug, either unchanged or metabolized, is eliminated from the organism. In the newborn infant, the traditional parameters of kidney function, glomerular filtration rate, and renal plasma flow are approximately 30–40% of adult values. Tubular mechanisms are also important for the excretion of some drugs and although this phenomenon has not been studied in depth at this age, it is known that the infant cannot excrete hydrogen ions as well as the older child. On the other hand, the reabsorption of sodium, chloride, amino acids, and glucose via the renal tubule is very efficient in the newborn infant. Antibiotics have been extensively investigated in the newborn infant, probably because they are used frequently in this age group for therapeutic reasons. They furnish an excellent example of the mechanisms of renal excretion of drugs because they are usually eliminated from the organism without prior metabolism. Earlier studies have demonstrated that the clearance of penicillin G in premature infants was only 17% of that obtained in older children when values were corrected for surface area. Pharmacokinetic studies of ampicillin showed that following an intramuscular injection of 10 mg/kg of body weight the serum half-life was prolonged during the first 2 weeks of postnatal life but rapidly decreased with a less gradual change at 2–4 weeks of postnatal age and no further change beyond 1 month of age (Axline *et al.*, 1967). To determine if the postnatal age-related changes in serum half-life, which appeared to approach adult values of 1.6 hours by 3 weeks of age, were independent of birth weight and thus of prenatal age, multiple dose response determinations were made in infants of widely varying birth weights. The serum half-life always appeared to decline with increasing postnatal age, and the rate of change was nearly identical in all infants despite marked weight differences at birth. Since a direct correlation exists between gestational age and the birth weight of a premature infant, these data suggested that the maturation in serum half-life values was actually a postnatal phenomenon. The apparent volumes of distribution of ampicillin were similar in all age groups. Urinary excretion, however, increased with increased postnatal age, so that premature infants older than 2 weeks excreted 32% of the dose in 12 hours in contrast to 40% of the dose excreted by adults during the same time period. These data suggest that maturation of renal mechanisms alters elimination rates and thus the serum half-life of ampicillin. The same results were found with other penicillins, including methicillin and oxacillin. Several aminoglycoside antibiotics, which in contrast to penicillin are eliminated mainly by glomerular filtration, were also investigated. Patterns of elimination into the urine and the serum half-lives for kanamycin, neomycin, and streptomycin were very similar qualitatively to that found with penicillin. For kanamycin, infants less than 48 hours old excreted 20% of the injected dose in the first 12 hours. The amount appearing in the urine increased to adult values of 60% by 1 week of age. Serum half-life was 18 hours during the first 2 days of life but decreased to 6 hours between 5 and 22 days of age. The half-life in adults is 2 hours. The recovery of streptomycin in the urine of premature infants 1–3 days of age was 29% during the first 12 hours following injection, whereas in adults 70% was excreted during this time period. Of extreme interest in this investigation was the finding that another drug, colistin, a member of the aminoglycoside group, which is also eliminated by glomerular filtration, gave a distinctly different pattern following intramuscular injection of a single dose of 5 mg/kg of body weight. No differences were found in serum half-life among the very young infants, older infants, and adults. If glomerular filtration, the principle excretory route for colistin in adults, is the mechanism for elimination in the small infant, the serum half-life should have been prolonged as it was for other antibiotics excreted primarily by this mechanism. These unexpected observations with colistin suggest that perhaps the drug is handled differently by the neonatal kidney. Most importantly, they do not permit generalization about drug excretion in the young infant. It therefore becomes necessary to evaluate each drug administered in this age group when elimination is mainly via renal excretion.

e. *Receptor Function.*   The pharmacodynamic effect of a drug is a result of an interaction between the drug molecule and tissue receptor sites. It is important to determine whether receptor sites are functional during the perinatal period since drug administration may be to no avail if there is no receptor. Investigations in dogs have shown that the cardiovascular system of the newborn pup and adult respond similarly to the pressor effects of catecholamines (Privitera *et al.*, 1969). In addition, since norepinephrine increased heart rate equally in both groups, the β-adrenergic receptor system must have also been functional. Human data for adrenergic β receptors have already been well discussed for the fetus. In the premature and full-term infant, a very well-designed investigation has recently been reported, in which the intensity of the mydriatic effect of drugs was determined by comparing photographs taken in a rigidly controlled and reproducible manner. The mydriatic action of sympathomimetic substances occurs through adrenergic α receptors in the iris. In 70 premature and full-term infants, α adrenergic receptors were demonstrated to be present since the eyes of all infants responded to the instillation of phenylephrine hydrochloride (Lind et al., 1971). The degree of mydriasis correlated with birth weight. To ascertain whether catecholamines could be released in response to a drug, tyramine was instilled. The eyes of small premature infants did not respond, and there was positive correlation between the percent mydriasis and gestational age as well as birth weight. These data suggest that in the small premature infant, the sympathetic storage mechanism was not totally developed in the eye and possibly a similar situation may exist in other organs. Of fundamental importance is the demonstration that receptor sites are present and able to respond to a drug administered at early stages of development.

B. Drugs in Breast Milk

In the previous sections of this chapter, the problem of injury to the fetus by drugs administered to the mother has been discussed at some length. The passage and excretion of drugs and chemical substances into breast milk have received very little attention by pharmacologists and consequently our knowledge regarding mechanisms and kinetics of transport is extremely limited. With a resurgence of interest in this method of nourishing newborn infants, it is appropriate to discuss the presence of foreign compounds in breast milk and their effects upon the nursing neonate.

1. PHYSIOLOGY OF LACTATION

Milk is synthesized in the mammary gland, a compound tubuloalveolar endocrine organ, in which the secretory cells discharge their product into the alveoli. The myoepithelial cells surrounding the alveolar cells contract and force the milk from the alveoli into the ductile system. In the alveolar cells, milk proteins are synthesized by the ribosomes of the rough endoplasmic reticulum and then transferred to the Golgi apparatus where they receive their carbohydrate complement. The resultant glycoproteins are contained within vacuoles in the cell, which migrate toward the apical portion of the cell where they are transferred across the cell membrane into the lumen. Lactose, the predominant carbohydrate in milk, is synthesized within the Golgi apparatus by lactose synthetase. This enzyme consists of two different proteins, A and B. The B protein is an α-lactoglobulin which appears to be an important regulator of lactose synthesis since it is eliminated into milk together with lactose by way of secretory vesicles

(Brew, 1969). Lipids, which are synthesized within the mammary gland, are extruded into the ductile system by a process which has been termed "reverse pinocytosis." During this process the fat globule becomes surrounded by the cellular membrane at the apex of the cell, and this becomes pinched off to allow the droplet to slide into the lumen. The synthesis and secretion of milk are a result of a highly complex hormonal interaction which involves the combined effect of estrogen and progesterone, the secretion of which is regulated by both pituitary and placental follicle stimulating hormone (FSH) and luteotropic hormone (LH). At the end of gestation and just prior to parturition, the levels of estrogen and progesterone fall, and the inhibitory effect of prolactin release is diminished. This pituitary hormone stimulates the alveolar cells to produce and secrete milk. Just at parturition, the vascular network within the gland is greatly dilated because of glycoprotein storage and increased cellularity. As a consequence of the vasodilatation, there is an increase in capillary permeability and ready passage of plasma proteins, particularly immunoglobulins, into colostrum. Following the stimulation which results from infant suckling, oxytocin is released by the pituitary. This results in the contraction of the myoepithelial cells and milk flow is established.

In several animal studies, hormones have been shown to influence milk production. Thyroid hormone, for example, will increase milk yield when given systemically. Today, hormone supplements are banned in the cow because of their potential adverse effects for the human consumer. There are many reports regarding the inhibition of human lactation by administration of estrogens or androgens, either independently or in combination (Llewelyn-Jones, 1968). Low-dosage preparations containing combinations of progestational agents and estrogens used to suppress ovulation (contraceptive therapy) may also diminish lactation (Billingsley, 1969). Combination therapy may, in addition, influence the composition of milk probably by affecting the activity of the pyridine nucleotide transhydrogenase, which regulates the flow of molecular energy within the mammary gland cell (Villee, 1963). Intranasal oxytocin has been employed to overcome the inhibition of milk secretion in women with inadequate lactation due to psychological reasons. The results have not been too encouraging (Luhman, 1963). On the other hand, Lyons has shown that administration of human growth hormone preparations significantly increases the yield of milk as evidenced by a doubling in the weight gain of the suckled infant as compared to control periods in which placebo was administered (Loyns et al., 1968). The phenothiazines have been shown to affect the mammary gland, probably as a result of suppression of the prolactin inhibitory factor in the hypothalmus (Danon et al., 1963). Galactorrhea is a well-known side effect in female patients receiving chlorpromazine for psychiatric disorders. Development of a drug with mammotropic action without sedative effect would be of importance in the management of women with insufficient lactation.

2. EXCRETION OF DRUGS INTO MILK

Study of the excretion of drugs and chemicals into human breast milk has been hampered because of the difficulty in collecting adequate and representative samples. It is clear that any drug in the maternal organism must traverse the endothelium of capillaries into the alveolar cells and then be secreted into the lumen along with the milk. The route of administration of the drug to the mother will only be important with regard to the concentration the drug might achieve in maternal plasma as well as the appearance time with respect to administration. Blood flow to the mammary gland is of the utmost importance since it will determine the rate of presentation of the drug for elimination into milk. Indeed, animal studies suggest that there is marked increase in mammary blood flow during lactation perhaps facilitated by a decrease in intramammary pressure which occurs when alveolar secretions are removed via the sucking mechanism. Rasmussen (1961) has systematically studied the passage of a number of drug substances from plasma to milk in cows where constant plasma levels were maintained by continuous intravenous infusion. The general conclusions derived from these experiments are presented below since they probably are operative in humans as well. Each of the drugs tested, sulfonamide, antibiotics, barbiturates, antipyrine, ethanol, and urea, exhibited a constant ratio between the concentration in an ultrafiltrate of milk and an ultrafiltrate of plasma. This ratio was found to be independent of both plasma concentrations and the volume of milk produced during the experimental period. The data suggested, therefore, that these small drug molecules are transported via passive diffusion. The pH of the milk is around 6.5 and as anticipated this has a marked effect upon diffusion of drugs which are ionizable. Thus, compounds such as barbiturates, organic acids, sulfonamides, diuretics, and benzylpenicillin, all weak acids, had a lower concentration in milk than in ultrafiltrates of plasma. Weak bases, such as antihistamines, lincomycin, and erythromycin, had a much higher concentration in milk than in plasma; as predicted from knowledge of their ionization. While the pH gradient in humans between plasma and milk is less marked, the same principle will apply to drug excretion.

The mere presence of drugs in milk does not imply adverse effects upon the infant as the drug may be excreted in an inactive form into milk, metabolized by the infant's gastrointestinal tract, or not absorbed by the infant's gastrointestinal tract. A comprehensive review of the literature regarding excretion of drugs in breast milk was published in 1965 by Knowles. No attempt will be made to list or review these data at this point since they are similar to those dicsussed above (Section III,C).

Current data regarding the physiology and pharmacology of drug secretion into breast milk suggest that this may be a potentially significant route of drug exposure for the neonate (Catz and Giacoia, 1972; Schou and Amdisen, 1973). The general conclusion can be made that nearly all drugs ingested by the mother are excreted into her milk either in unchanged form or as metabolites. Data regarding the qualitative as well as the quantitative content of drugs in breast milk are urgently needed as well as are studies regarding the kinetics of transport. The prescription of drugs during pregnancy for the management of maternal disease and their effect upon the intrauterine host is similar to the prescription of drugs for the nursing mother and their passage into breast milk and the effect upon the nursing infant. The thalidomide tragedy has played a role in alerting physicians and the public to the potential hazards of prescribing drugs during pregnancy. On the contrary, no such concern appears to exist with respect to prescribing drugs to the lactating mother. Until now, there has been no calamity comparable to that seen with thalidomide traceable to ingestion of compounds present in milk. Porphyria, following the ingestion of the fungicide, hexachlorobenzene, by the lactating mother has been seen in nursing infants. Similarly, the devastating effects of mercury upon the central nervous system have been described in nursing infants whose mother ate seafood contaminated with methylmercury (Minamata disease). There are also reports of hemolysis and kernicterus in glucose-6-phosphate dehydrogenase deficient nursing infants who received sulfonamides from breast milk. Other compounds such as atropine, anticoagulants, antithyroid drugs, antimetabolites, cathartics, dihydrotachysterol, iodides, narcotics, radioactive preparations, bromides, ergot, tetracyclines, and metromidazole have resulted in adverse effects in the nursing infant. Their administration to the lactating mother is contraindicated. Some compounds, while appearing in breast milk, have not been shown to be associated with adverse effects. It should be emphasized, however, that only short-term effects have been looked for. It may very well be that long-term effects are present but have been overlooked. Breast feeding should be contraindicated in mothers with illnesses which require large doses of any drug. Continued surveillance of those infants who have been exposed to pharmacological agents in breast milk is of importance if meaningful data regarding effects of drugs in breast milk upon the infant are to be obtained. Awareness on the part of the physician treating the lactating mother of the nursing infant as a drug recipient will serve to minimize adverse effects since drugs will only be prescribed when actually needed.

C. Metabolism of Bilirubin in the Fetus and Newborn

Approximately 30% of all newborns show some degree of visible jaundice (serum bilirubin greater than 5 mg %) in the neonatal period. Bilirubin is a nonpolar organic anion catabolic product of heme degradation that does nobody any good and has the propensity under appropriate circumstances of resulting in damage to the central nervous system (cf. kernicterus). In blood, bilirubin is bound to albumin and rapidly transferred to the liver where its uptake is governed by at least two cytoplasmic acceptor proteins (Y and Z). It is subsequently conjugated with glucuronic acid involving an endoplasmic reticulum enzyme, uridine diphosphate-glucuronic acid (UDPGA) transferase (cf. glucuronyltransferase). The product is bilirubin glucuronide which is rapidly excreted into the bile cannaliculus probably by an energy-dependent mechanism, and thence normally eliminated via the gut.

Bilirubin affords an excellent illustrative model and vehicle for the understanding of drug metabolism in the newborn because many of the mechanisms involved are shared by other biologically important endogenous and exogenous anions (e.g., drugs and steroids). This community of interest raises such questions as: How are steroids, drugs, dye, radiographic agents, and other organic anions transferred from placenta into the liver cell? How does the regulation of bilirubin glucuronide biosynthesis affect the formation of glucuronides of other anionic compounds? What is the excretory and possible reabsorptive (enterohepatic) mechanism that these anions share with bilirubin and bile pigments, etc. In addition, bilirubin metabolism, disposition, and distribution in the body is frequently influenced (in both beneficial and detrimental directions) by a variety of exogenously administered and endogenously active pharmacological agents. Thus from both points of view an examination of the bilirubin pathway and the factors which influence it afford a decided insight into the pharmacology of the perinatal period.

1. THE MEASUREMENT OF BILIRUBIN

In 1916 van den Bergh and Müller recorded the observation that serum from patients with hemolytic jaundice did not react promptly with diazotized sulfanilic acid except in the presence of alcohol, whereas serum from patients with obstructive jaundice reacted immediately in aqueous solution, thus establishing the concept of "direct"- and "indirect"-reacting bilirubin. Current methods which record these two fractions are basically modifications of the methodology of Malloy and Evelyn (1937) which determines "direct"-acting, and total bilirubin, with the subtraction product serving as the "indirect"-acting fraction. The "indirect"-acting fraction represents unconjugated bilirubin while the "direct"-acting fraction is conjugated bilirubin diglucuronide.

Clinically the differences in toxicity with respect to the brain (i.e., kernicterus) of the two fractions is a function of their different physical properties. Bilirubin itself (indirect-acting, unconjugated) is insoluble in water, but highly soluble in lipids accounting for its ready entry into the lipid-rich central nervous system. By contrast glucuronidated bilirubin (direct-acting, unconjugated) is soluble in aqueous solution and relatively insoluble in lipids. Thus the elevation of the indirect fraction represents a distinct hazard for kernicterus while even extreme elevations of the direct-acting fraction do not. In addition, direct-acting (conjugated) bilirubin may be found in urine in the presence of an elevated serum bilirubin level, while indirect (unconjugated) bilirubin will not appear even in the fact of extreme serum elevations (cf. acholuric jaundice).

2. NEONATAL JAUNDICE

The hyperbilirubinemia of the newborn is an elevation of the unconjugated (indirect-acting) fraction of serum bilirubin. It is the result of the inability of an immature hepatic system to cope with the load of bilirubin presented to it. Although a number of etiologic mechanisms (i.e., hemolysis, extravascular bleeding, polycythemia) may involve excessive red cell production and breakdown; the hyperbilirubinemia *itself* is an expression of the adequacy or inadequacy of hepatic function under those particular circumstances. Viewed in this light, therefore, the degree of hyperbilirubinemia, or number of exchange transfusions, is not an accurate assessment of the severity of neonatal hemolytic disease (Rh or ABO incompatibility). This needs to be assessed on the basis of its hemolytic or isoimmune components (i.e., anemia, antibody formation), since for a given degree of hemolysis the amount of unconjugated bilirubin retained in serum will depend on the efficacy of the liver in handling the presented load.

The principal source of bilirubin is the normal daily destruction of circulating red cells resulting in the degradation of about 1% of the total hemoglobin mass per day. There is the possibility of some bilirubin arising directly from degradation of hemoglobin within the bone marrow in very immature red cells, but this is normally not a major component to the bilirubin pool.

In man, there is effectively quantitative conversion of the prosthetic heme group to bilirubin so that 1 gm hemoglobin yields 34 mg of bili-rubin. Thus a newborn infant weighing 3 kg with a theoretical blood volume of 300 ml and a total Hb mass of 54 gm would destroy Hb at the rate of 0.5 gm/day and yield 17 mg of bilirubin to be handled by the liver (Brown, 1962). By contrast the normal adult degrades 6–7 gm Hb per day with the production of the order of 250 mg bilirubin but possesses sufficient hepatic reserve to clear 7 times this amount before becoming jaundiced. The newborn liver is, however, already at its maxi-mal ability to clear the pigment, and possesses little if any reserve ca-pacity to cope with even slight increases in the amount of bilirubin it may be required to handle. It is, therefore, not surprising that about 30% of all newborns show some degree of clinical icterus. Moreover, the con-cept of a hepatic reserve in the adult in distinction to the near maximal functioning capacity in the newborn offers a ready explanation for the severe hyperbilirubinemia seen in the newborn under hemolytic condi-tions, contrasted with its almost total absence, even under massive hemolytic circumstances, in the adult.

The hepatic conjugation of bilirubin is the result of a series of en-zymatic steps terminating in the enzymatic transfer of glucuronic acid to the acceptor substance bilirubin in the following end reaction system:

2 UDP-Glucuronic acid + bilirubin

$$\downarrow \text{glucuronyltransferase}$$

Bilirubin diglucuronide + UDP

The limiting factor in this reaction is the adequacy and availability of the enzyme glucuronyltransferase, which has been identified in the micro-somal fraction of the liver cells (Schmid *et al.*, 1957). The enzymatic system is oxygen dependent and subject to regulation by optimal condi-tions of pH, temperature, etc. It is, therefore, not surprising that infants with perinatal problems who are acidotic, hypoxic, or cold tend to show higher levels of serum bilirubin than do their relatively unstressed normal counterparts.

3. FETAL BILIRUBIN METABOLISM

Bilirubin has been identified in amniotic fluid as early as the twelfth week of gestation. Its normal disappearance at about 36 weeks (an event which may be used as an index of fetal maturity) probably reflects both the dilutional effect of increased amniotic fluid as well as the maturation of fetal placental function.

Normally, unconjugated bilirubin resulting from the breakdown of fetal red cells is cleared through the placenta into the maternal circulation. For bilirubin to be transported across the placenta, it is necessary for it to remain in the unconjugated form since the conjugated pigment is less readily transferred across the placental barrier (Schenker *et al.*, 1967). Thus, whereas in the adult, bilirubin clearance requires conversion to the conjugated form, the precise opposite applies to the fetus. Several factors limit the ability of the fetus to conjugate bilirubin. These include deficient glucuronidation due to limited activity of glucuronyltransferase, as well as reduced capacity for excretion of the conjugated bilirubin glucuronide from the hepatic cell. In addition, unlike the adult, the fetus (and infant at birth) shows significant amounts of β-glucuronidase in the intestinal tract which can hydrolyze any bilirubin glucuronide formed back to its unconjugated form, in which it can be reabsorbed via the enterohepatic circulation (Section IV,C,4,e).

An interesting and possibly important biological phenomenon occurs in the case of infants who have undergone intrauterine transfusion for the management of severe hemolytic disease, and in whom large quantities of adult hemoglobin have been instilled into the peritoneal cavity. These infants characteristically show high direct-acting (i.e., conjugated bilirubin levels in cord blood and subsequent bilirubin determinations in the newborn period have yielded a partition ratio almost entirely comprised of the direct-acting component with levels reaching as high as 45 to 50 mg%. In keeping with the physical properties of conjugated versus unconjugated bilirubin, these infants show no evidence for kernicterus and exchange transfusion for control of hyperbilirubinemia is, under such circumstances, not indicated. Moreover, the presence of such high levels of direct-acting bilirubin at birth suggests an enhanced ability of the fetal conjugating system leading to the possibility that bilirubin itself, in this instance, derived from both adult cells intraperitoneally and largely hemolyzed fetal cells secondary to severe hemolytic disease, may be a powerful inducer of activity of the hepatic conjugation system *in vivo*.

4. The Mechanisms of Neonatal Hyperbilirubinemia

We may now consider the etiology of hyperbilirubinemia in the newborn on the basis of single or combined effects of the following mechanisms: (a) formation of bilirubin from heme, (b) the uptake of bilirubin by the liver, (c) hepatic conjugation, (d) excretion of conjugated bilirubin from liver to gut, (e) reabsorption of bilirubin from the gastrointestinal tract. The interrelationships of these mechanisms and their sequential role in the metabolism of bilirubin are shown in Fig. 1.

BILIRUBIN METABOLISM

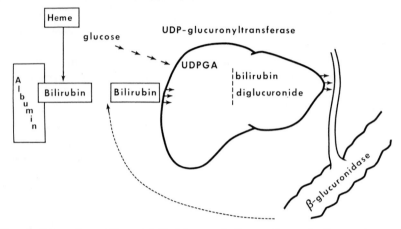

FIG. 1. Schematic outline of bilirubin metabolism pathway in the newborn.

An approach to the clinical course of neonatal jaundice in such terms provides a more readily physiological understanding of the underlying mechanisms involved rather than a simple listing of etiologic causes.

a. Increased Formation of Bilirubin. Polycythemia, either occurring spontaneously or as a result of accidental or purposeful placental transfusion, will result in an increased bilirubin load. Infants of diabetic mothers tend to be polycythemic, although the precise reason is unknown. The occurrence of polycythemia unexpectedly at birth has been ascribed to overstimulation of hematopoietic activity by erythropoietin secondary to intrauterine and perinatal hypoxia, but clear evidence for this is lacking. The situation also occurs in cyanotic congenital heart disease and in some infants who demonstrate intrauterine growth retardation (possibly on the basis of intrauterine hypoxia). The twin-to-twin transfusion syndrome represents a situation where one twin may be profoundly polycythemic at the expense of his anemic cohort. Since as much as an addition one-third of the total circulating blood volume may be sequestered in the placenta at birth, accidental (i.e., delayed cord clamping with the baby held below the placenta) or purposeful cord stripping placental transfusion can seriously augment the total bilirubin pool.

Hemolytic disease with its augmented breakdown of red cells provides an increase in bilirubin reflected in hyperbilirubinemia in the newborn much more readily than in the adult because of the limited ability of the newborn liver to cope with the load (see above). With the increasingly common use of Rh immune globulin, we may anticipate a continuing reduction in the number of cases of anti-D isoimmunization. Since Rh immunization is D specific, there should be an ever increasing proportion of so-called "atypical" Rh situations (anti-c, -E, etc.). In addition, the rarer causes (Kell, Duffy, Lewis, etc.) may on occasion also be involved.

Isoimmunization due to incompatibility in the ABO system may also result in hemolytic disease (Mollison and Cutbush, 1959). Although it has been suggested that the hemolysis is generally milder in nature, the bilirubin produced is in no way different from that resulting from Rh incompatibility. Moreover, it shares with all hemolytic situations the increased propensity for production of kernicterus (see below) and should be managed accordingly.

Among the nonimmune hemolytic causes of neonatal hyperbilirubinemia, considerable interest has been evoked by the problem on glucose-6-phosphate dehydrogenase (G-6-PD) deficiency. Here the deficiency of the enzyme results, through a series of intermediary steps, in an ultimate lack of reduced glutathione within the red cell. This results in a reduced stability of the cell and increased sensitivity to its oxidative destruction both from hydrogen peroxide (H_2O_2) generated within the cell, as well as from a variety of drugs and other substances which act as oxidizing agents. Among the latter are included the antimalarial drugs, sulfonamides, the Italian broad bean (*Vicia faba* L.), mothballs (naphthalene), salicylates, vitamin K, and nitrofurantoin. The disease is transmitted as a sex-linked recessive with males predominantly affected although carrier females may also be symptomatic on occasion. Although there are many subvariants of the enzyme involved, two basic form groupings are generally recognized—the Negro and the Mediterranean–Oriental group. As with sickle cell disease, its geographical distribution bears an inverse relationship to the occurrence of malaria (presumably the G-6-PD deficient red cell is an inappropriate place for survival of the malarial parasite). Although the North American Negro population carries the defect with an estimated gene frequency of 13%, sensitivity is almost entirely restricted to the antimalarial preparations and possibly the sulfonamides. Except for a suggestive report of a higher incidence of jaundice in G-6-PD deficient Negro prematures than in their nondeficient controls, it does not appear to be a major problem in this population group. By contrast, the disease may cause severe symptoms in the Mediterranean and Oriental groups. Two forms of presentation in the newborn have been recognized. The first presenting as hyperbilirubinemia with or without some anemia in the first few days of life is difficult to distinguish clinically from mild Rh or ABO incompatibility. A negative Coombs test and appropriate G-6-PD study, especially in a suspicious population group, should allow for an exact diagnosis. It has been suggested that the G-6-PD deficient red cell in the newborn is sufficiently unstable to undergo spontaneous hemolysis, although it must be remembered that the almost universal prophylactic administration of vitamin K in the newborn does provide a potential oxidizing agent to this group.

The second and much more vicious form of clinical presentation occurs on exposure of a previously unrecognized infant to a powerful oxidizing agent. The commonly implicated one in this group in naphthalene, usually from diapers or bedclothes stored in mothballs which have been kept, awaiting the baby's return from hospital. Sudden massive and severe hemolysis, with bilirubin levels reaching 40 to 50 mg% and higher and the tragic occurrence of kernicterus were reported in such a group of North American born, Greek, Italian, and Chinese infants by Naiman and Kosoy (1964), in whom hemolysis and kernicterus occurred following such exposure between 10 days and 1 month of age. The occurrence of kernicterus beyond the first week of life, a finding supported by reports of the condition in Greece (Doxiadis et al., 1961), supports the view that there is no such thing as increased protection from the CNS dangers of bilirubin as the baby gets older. There is no evidence to support the concept of maturation of the "blood–brain" barrier for bilirubin, nor indeed is there any concrete evidence for the existence of any such barrier other than that governed by the solubility characteristics of the bilirubin fractions and the capacity for protein binding of the unconjugated fraction. The fact that with increased maturation of the liver, bilirubin levels will *usually* decrease should not be confused with an increased resistance to toxicity since elevations to a dangerous degree, if they do occur as in the case of G-6-PD dependent hemolysis, may result in kernicterus well beyond the first week of life (see also below under Crigler–Najar syndrome). Increasing population mobility and a tendency to homogenization of the ethnic origins of population groups, may increase the importance of the condition in North America. In addition to those population groups already reported, examples of its neonatal expression have been seen in families from the Middle East (Sephardic Jews), India, and Portugal. Moreover, its identification as a cause of familial "idiopathic" hyperbilirubinemia in several families of Anglo-Saxon and Western European origin suggests the possibility of its rarer but nevertheless possible occurrence in "nonsuspect" groups as well. Although the defect is common in the south of France, Corsica, and Sardinia, it has yet to be identified in French-Canadian families, reflecting the origin of this population group from the northern portion of the European continent. In view of its potentially serious effects and implications for future health of the individual, it is recommended that routine screening policies be considered for the known "high risk" ethnic population groups. This can be accomplished by screening maternal blood for the carrier state in such groups. Moreover, it should be borne in mind as a possible cause of unexplained neonatal jaundice especially when the latter is associated with a degree of hemolysis.

Other forms of hemolytic disease may occasionally express themselves in the neonatal period. These include pyruvate kinase deficiency, and some of the hemoglobinopathies (Oski and Naiman, 1966). In congenital (spherocytic) hemolytic anemia, hyperbilirubinemia in the newborn may occasionally be the presenting sign although the increase in osmotic fragility of the red cells which will confirm the diagnosis is usually difficult to demonstrate before 6 weeks to 3 months of life.

i. Hemorrhagic reabsorption. Reabsorption of extravasated hemoglobin constitutes an important mechanism for augmenting the bilirubin load. Unlike the intravascular situation in which red cells of different ages break down in a given proportion per day, extravasated blood does so all at the same time and is thus capable of providing a sudden "bolus" of bilirubin into the system. The hemorrhage may be obvious as in tissue bruising following birth trauma or "concealed" in which case no signs of discoloration will be present. Among the latter causes, large cephalohematomas and intracranial hemorrhages are important sources of such hyperbilirubinemia. In addition, adrenal hemorrhages which may be bilateral and are often associated with birth asphyxia can also serve as sources of excess bilirubin production.

ii. Sepsis. The role of sepsis in hyperbilirubinemia is worthy of both comment and in need of reevaluation. Although it is generally listed in most texts high in the differential diagnosis, hyperbilirubinemia is rarely the sole sign of infection. Moreover, it is also unlikely that sepsis is responsible for otherwise asymptomatic hyperbilirubinemia. The mechanism of any hyperbilirubinemia which may result from infection is not clear. There is little evidence to support hemolysis during systemic neonatal infection as a common occurrence, nor are the organisms involved usually hemolytic *in vivo*. In the absence of any direct hepatic involvement (i.e., hepatitis) it is more likely that the augmentation of bilirubin levels seen during the course of systemic infections reflects local metabolic alterations (i.e., pH, temperature, oxygen supply) which may have an adverse effect on the integrity of liver enzyme systems (see below).

b. Hepatic Uptake of Bilirubin. Although a defect in the hepatic uptake of bilirubin has been postulated as being at least in part responsible for one of the familial hyperbilirubinemic syndromes (Gilbert's disease), the precise nature of any such defect and its role in neonatal hyperbiliruinemia has only recently received investigative attention. Levi, Gatmaitan, and Arias (1969a) have proposed the existence of two hepatic cytoplasmic factors acting as organic anion-binding proteins which bind bilirubin and prevent its rediffusion into the plasma once it has entered the liver cell. These have been designated as the Y and Z proteins. They have proposed (Levi et al., 1969b) that in the newborn infant a relative deficiency of the Y protein may be responsible for neonatal hyperbilirubinemia as a reflection of a decreased ability of the liver to transfer unconjugated bilirubin from plasma secondary to insufficient intracellular bilirubin binding. Acceptance of the potential role of this mechanism indicates an additional factor capable of contributing to the failure of the newborn infant's inability to cope efficiently with his bilirubin load.

c. *Conjugation of Bilirubin.* A congenital familial defect due to deficiency of glucuronyltransferase in humans has been identified. Individuals so affected show progressive increases in unconjugated bilirubin which ultimately results in kernicterus from bilirubin deposition in the brain (Crigler and Najar, 1952). The condition, appropriately named Crigler–Najar's disease, while fortunately rare has allowed for the delineation of some important aspects of bilirubin handling and toxicity, among which is the demonstration that under appropriate circumstances kernicterus can occur beyond the neonatal period. The animal analog of this situation is the Gunn rat, in whom the heterozygote shows partial deficiency of the enzyme with the homozygous form resulting in severe neurological symptoms and subsequent early death. The Gunn rat strain has been used extensively for experimental purposes relating to bilirubin metabolism and toxicity. An *in vitro* system (Lathe and Walker, 1958b) using rat liver microsomes as a source of hepatic enzymes, has also been used extensively to study the enhancement and depression of glucuronyltransferase activity which may occur in the presence of a number of substances (see below).

Prematurity itself with its maturational delay in the enzyme system thus emerges as a factor in the hyperbilirubinemia of the newborn. Similarly, the variations in levels of bilirubin in normal full-term infants can be related to differences in the levels of, and maturational rate of improvement in, the transferase system (Stern et al., 1970). Sepsis, acidosis, and asphyxia are associated with increased levels of bilirubin, presumably by altering local metabolic conditions of pH, temperature, and oxygen tension which are necessary for optimal enzyme function (see above).

i. Breast milk jaundice. Clinical observation has led to the conclusion that breast-fed infants tend to higher bilirubin levels than do their bottle-fed counterparts. The relationship appears to be valid even if one corrects for any increase in hematocrit in the breast-fed group which may in some instances receive less fluid intake. Experimentally some breast milks show marked inhibition of an *in vitro* conjugating system suggesting the presence of a factor which can depress glucuronyltransferase activity. Arias *et al.* (1964) have suggested that the factor responsible is pregnane-$3\alpha,20\beta$-diol. Others (Ramos *et al.*, 1966; Adlard and Lathe, 1970) have questioned the role of this particular steroid. There is general agreement both on the presence of the factor in breast milk and also on the likelihood that it is a steroid derivative. Clinically, however, what is required for its expression as hyperbilirubinemia are both the presence of the inhibitor and the existence of a sufficiently inadequate conjugating system. As there is a variation in conjugating capacity of normal infants, with differences ranging up to a sixfold factor (Stern *et al.*, 1970), a breast milk containing a given degree of inhibiting substance may or may not produce hyperbilirubinemia depending upon the initial conjugating capacity of the hepatic system of the paticular infant in question. Similar reasoning can be applied to the fact that often discontinuance of breast feeding results in a fall in serum bilirubin, which does not become elevated again when breast feeding is reinstituted. Since the liver is maturing progressively in the immediate neonatal period, time will permit the enzyme system to cope with a partial inhibitor which a day or two earlier might have resulted in a bilirubin rise. Although this is usually the case, a small number of infants will show continued reelevation of bilirubin with breast milk feeding for several months, suggesting in them the presence of a much more powerful type or a greater amount of inhibiting substance in the particular milk.

ii. Other inhibiting substances. Arias *et al.* (1965) have described the occurrence of familial transient neonatal hyperbilirubinemia associated with an inhibiting factor present in the plasma. In addition, a number of other endogenous and exogenous substances have been implicated as capable of *in vitro* and *in vivo* suppression of glucuronyltransferase activity. In addition to one or more of the steroids of the estrogen–progesterone group (Hsia *et al.*, 1960; Sas and Herczeg, 1970), experimental evidence exists to support the ability of novobiocin to reduce enzyme activity (Lokietz *et al.*, 1963). Other agents suspected of a similar effect include the phenothiazines and their derivatives (e.g., chlorpromazine), vitamin K, and the ester propionate preparation of erythromycin.

d. Excretion of Conjugated Bilirubin. Once conjugated, the "direct-acting" bilirubin diglucuronide must be transported from the liver cells into bile cannilicules. Although little is known of the precise mechanism involved, the process presumably involves an active transport system. Should the capacity of conjugate exceed that of the cell to excrete the conjugated product, accumulation of conjugated bilirubin will occur. Infants with severe hemolytic disease, particularly those who have been subjected to intrauterine transfusions, frequently show a high "direct-acting" component to their bilirubin levels. This has in the past been attributed to "inspissated bile syndrome" and/or hepatocellular damage. The situation is a self-limited one and there is no evidence to support either hepatic tissue destruction or biliary obstruction as its cause. Indeed, it seems more likely that the elevation in the "direct-acting" fraction reflects a "pile-up" of conjugated bilirubin secondary to an imbalance between the rate of conjugation in the cell and the rate of subsequent excretion from it. If a large amount of substrate (i.e., bilirubin) floods such a system (as occurs in severe hemolytic disease), the end result will be elevation of total bilirubin in which the direct (conjugated) fraction will play a large proportionate role.

e. Reabsorption of Bilirubin from the Gut (the Enterohepatic Circulation). The contribution of bilirubin sequestered in meconium in the gut of the newborn to the total bilirubin pool has attracted considerable interest and attention. The bilirubin concentration of meconium is approximately 1 mg/gm. For an average 200-gm meconium-containing neonatal gastrointestinal tract, there is thus 200 mg of bilirubin available to the enterohepatic circulation as contrasted to an endogenous bilirubin production of 6–8 mg/kg/day. In this regard meconium differs from adult feces which contains very little if any bilirubin. The difference arises from the absence of an intestinal bacterial flora for the reduction of bilirubin to urobilirubin in the newborn and the presence of β-glucuronidase in the fetal and neonatal intestine. The latter affords the opportunity for the hydrolysis of bilirubin diglucuronide, excreted into the gut, to bilirubin, thereby making possible its reabsorption via the enterohepatic circulation into the bloodstream. In this connection it has been shown that anicteric infants have greater stool excretions of bilirubin during the first few days of life than icteric ones (Ross *et al.*, 1937). This finding has been confirmed clinically with unconjugated hyperbilirubinemia noted in high intestinal obstruction (Boggs and Bishop, 1965) and in situations of delayed passage of meconium (Rosta *et al.*, 1968) in the newborn period.

5. The Binding of Bilirubin to Albumin

Unconjugated bilirubin is bound in plasma to albumin. The resulting complex is a nondiffusable one, and the binding to albumin thus plays a vital role in the prevention of egress of bilirubin from serum into the tissues, especially the lipid-rich brain. The amount of "free" and "bound" bilirubin at any given time is thus a function both of the quantitative amount of albumin in the circulation, as well as of the capacity of the albumin to bind any bilirubin present.

The binding process is pH dependent and tends to dissociation of the complex with acidosis. Moreover, the presence of one or more anions which may compete with bilirubin for common binding sites on the albumin molecule may result in large amounts of "free" unconjugated bilirubin despite the presence of sufficient albumin to theoretically bind all the bilirubin in the system. Thus, by displacing bilirubin from its binding site these anions will promote the occurrence of kernicterus at relatively low levels of bilirubin (see below).

Since the clinical demonstration by Silverman et al. (1956) of the association between the administration of sulfisoxazole to premature infants and the occurrence of kernicterus at low levels of serum bilirubin, a number of endogenous and exogenous substances have been identified as competitors with bilirubin for one or more albumin binding sites. These include hematin and the nonesterified fatty acids. Hematin is present in increased amounts in hemolytic conditions. Its presence affords a ready explanation for the higher risk for kernicterus in hemolytic as compared to nonhemolytic hyperbilirubinemias. The nonesterified fatty acids are elevated in plasma under conditions of both hypothermia and hypoglycemia. In addition to sulfisoxazole, salicylates and caffeine sodium benzoate will displace bilirubin from its albumin binding sites, and it is likely that other drugs, singly or in combination, may share this capacity (Schiff et al., 1971). Not only should these agents be avoided in the newborn who is jaundiced, they should also be withheld from a nursing mother who is capable of transmitting them via the breast milk route.

6. Kernicterus

In its strictest sense the term "kernicterus" is an anatomic one referring to the bilirubin staining of the brain, most noticeable in the basal ganglia, seen in infants who die of the condition. The term is a historic classic one, but it requires the death of the patient and autopsy demonstration for its confirmation. It would seem preferable to use the term "bilirubin encephalopathy" to describe the occurrence of the syndrome in the neonate and the unfortunately disastrous late neurological sequelas in the survivors.

Although Zetterström and Ernstner (1956) have attributed the toxicity of bilirubin to the uncoupling of oxidative phosphorylation in brain mitochondria, this view has been challenged (Diamond and Schmid, 1967) and the precise mechanism of the brain damage is still in dispute. It follows, however, that the propensity to develop CNS damage reflects not only the serum bilirubin level, but the other associated factors which facilitate both the availability of free bilirubin and its entry into the brain (see Fig. 2).

The occurrence of kernicterus at low levels of bilirubin in infants with previous asphyxia, respiratory distress, sepsis, hypothermia, and hypoglycemia has been documented by several authors (Stern and Denton, 1965; Stern and Doray, 1968; Gartner et al., 1970; Ackerman et al., 1970). Moreover, the premature infant with his easier tendency to these metabolic disturbances is in added jeopardy as a result of a lower serum albamin level with which to bind the accumulated bilirubin. Because of these relationships rigid quantitative interpretations of serum bilirubin levels should be avoided. Not only are the available techniques not sufficiently sensitive to warrant therapeutic decisions based on 1 or 2 mg%

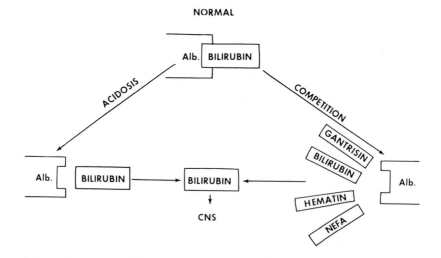

FIG. 2. Schematic representation of bilirubin-albumin binding relationship. Note possibilities of either dissociating bilirubin from albumin or displacing it by the introduction of competing anions. The end result is similar in providing more free, potentially CNS available bilirubin.

changes, they do not realistically reflect the basic clinical problem which can be stated as follows: What is important is not how much bilirubin is present, but how much is potentially available for passage into the brain.

Attempts to provide this information have led to a number of methodological approaches, both direct and indirect, to the estimation of the extent of bilirubin albumin binding in any individual clinical situation. Measurements of reserve albumin binding capacity by estimating the capacity of the serum to bind an inorganic dye (Waters and Porter, 1961) have been proposed for this purpose. A number of such agents have been used, e.g., phenosulfopthalien (PSP), 2-(4'-hydroxybenzeneazo)benzoic acid (HBABA), and brom cresol green. These, however, do not directly estimate the amount of "free" versus "bound" bilirubin and have been shown to yield spurious results both in clinical situations (Lucey et al., 1967) as well as in the laboratory, probably as a result of their failure to indicate the relative ability of any competing anions to actually displace bilirubin from its binding sites (Chan et al., 1971). An alternative methodology which separates free and bound bilirubin (Kaufman et al., 1969) using Sephadex columns appears to be much more promising and also affords the possibility of quantitatively estimating the actual amount of free bilirubin present.

7. TREATMENT OF HYPERBILIRUBINEMIA

Exchange transfusion remains the most rapid, certain, and effective way to lower serum bilirubin. The contribution of this technique to the prevention of kernicterus is now a matter of historical record (Allen et al., 1950). Recently, several new approaches toward control of and reduction in serum bilirubin have afforded a good deal of insight into the mechanisms of bilirubin handling *in vivo*, in addition to providing options where the transfusion procedure is either impossible or undesirable. While these mechanisms may be effective in reducing bilirubin levels, their greater potential lies in the possibility of preventing the hyperbilirubinemia before threatening levels are approached.

a. Enzyme Induction. A number of agents have been demonstrated as effective in reducing bilirubin levels by inducing the hepatic enzyme systems involved in bilirubin clearance. Morphologically these are reflected as an increase in microsomal appearance and activity in the liver. Phenobarbital has been the most widely used of these agents and has been shown to reduce bilirubin levels both when administered to the infants themselves (Trolle, 1968) or to their mothers in the latter stages of gestation (Maurer *et al.*, 1968). There is also evidence that the administration of phenobarbital will enhance glucuronidating activity *in vivo* (Stern *et al.*, 1970). A number of other substances have been shown to be similarly effective in experimental situations. These include dicophene (DDT) as well as several other pesticides, alcohol, diethylnicotinamide (Coramine), and diphenylhydantoin. Waltman *et al.* (1969) have effectively administered ethanol to women near term with resultant lowering of serum bilirubin levels in their offspring. Since ethanol has also been used to delay the onset of labor, there exists a possibility of a combined beneficial independent effect from the use of this agent, both in the prevention of prematurity and the control of one of its potentially hazardous consequences.

b. Phototherapy. The North American Indians were apparently aware of the beneficial effects of the sun in reducing the yellow color of a baby exposed to its light. The effect on bilirubin can also be demonstrated *in vitro* and, it is well known to laboratory personnel in that a sample left in the light will show a fall-off in measurable serum bilirubin levels as opposed to one stored in a dark cupboard. Biochemically the result is a partial breakdown of bilirubin with a resultant shift in the absorption spectrum of the serum (Blondheim *et al.*, 1692).

The therapeutic application of phototherapy for neonatal hyperbilirubinemia first proposed by Cremer *et al.* (1958) in England has been used extensively in South America (Obes-Polleri, 1967), and more recently on this continent (Lucey *et al.*, 1968) both for the reduction of an elevated serum bilirubin and for the "prophylactic" prevention of its occurrence in prematures. The photodecomposition of bilirubin is theoretically most effective in the presence of blue light whose peak emission at 480 nm is close to the absorption maximum of bilirubin in serum (460–465 nm). Clinically, however, both blue and white light appear to be effective in excess of an illumination level of 200 footcandles (see below). *In vitro,* the by-products comprise biliverdin with an absorption maximum at 650 nm, resulting from the loss of two hydrogen atoms from bilirubin (photooxidation) and at least two dipyrroles with absorption maxima at 380 and 280 nm. The latter are water soluble and therefore much less diffusible into the central nervous system. They have additionally been identified as being readily excretable into both bile and urine. *In vivo,* however, photodecomposition yields little or no biliverdin but only the dipyrroles. This is presumably a reflection of the fact that whereas the *in vitro* studies simulate a plasmalike environment, the *in vivo* effect is within the skin, on bilirubin which is virtually completely protein bound and therefore resists photooxidation. The by-products themselves show no neurotoxicity in brain tissue culture media or *in vivo* in animal experiments. Moreover, their absorption maxima are well below that of bilirubin making it exceedingly unlikely that they would displace bilirubin from its albumin binding sites. The failure to adequately quantitatively relate the fall in serum bilirubin *in vivo* to the dipyrroles recovered has led to a lingering suspicion that the *in vitro* and *in vivo* effects of phototherapy are entirely different. Ostrow *et al.* (1974) have suggested that the action of light in some way either alters the bilirubin molecule itself, or the necessity for it to be conjugated prior to its passage through the liver.

In clinical practice it appears that 200–400 footcandles of the wavelength spectrum between 300 and 600 nm are effective in reducing serum bilirubin *in vivo*. Although theory favors blue light, both white and daylight lamps are also effective, with daylight possibly being safer. Giunta and Rath (1969) have reported a difference in serum bilirubin levels in infants kept in a brighter nursery as opposed to those in a darker one in the same hospital. Studies of the natural variations in environmental lighting depending both on the amount of sunlight, time of day, and location of the infants within the nursery reveal a wide range of variability in illumination intensity for all three of these parameters (Stern *et al.*, 1971). These variations suggest an environmental explanation both for the seasonal variations in bilirubin levels within any given geographical area and for the reported lower incidence of hyperbilirubinemia in areas with more sunny climatic conditions. Moreover, within any nursery the position of the baby in relation to the sources of external light into the room may play a major role in determining the amount of illumination received.

c. Intestinal Binding and Excretion of Bilirubin.   Attempts to block the reentry of bilirubin from the intestinal tract by absorbing bilirubin in the gut using both medicinal charcoal (Ulstrom and Eisenklam, 1964) and cholestyramine (Lester *et al.*, 1962) have met with only minimal success. More recently however, Poland and Odell (1971) have employed orally administered agar for this purpose. Their results show both a reduction in serum bilirubin levels as well as enhancement of bilirubin excretion in the meconium of agar-fed versus control infants. Agar stabilizes bilirubin in aqueous solution and prevents its bacterial conversion. It also possesses the properties of a colloid laxative. Their work suggests a further method of reducing serum bilirubin level by "immobilizing" and removing bilirubin from the gut, thus preventing its reentry into the enterohepatic circulation. In this connection it would appear reasonable to assume that the reported beneficial effects of early versus delayed feeding in lowering serum bilirubin in the newborn reflect an increase in bacterial flora as well as earlier expulsion of meconium in the earlier fed infants, both resulting in a reduction of the available intestinal content of reabsorbable bilirubin.

8. IMPLICATIONS FOR DRUG METABOLISM

The circumstances which operate both to cause the accumulation of bilirubin and to heighten the risk for its neurotoxicity have important implications for the metabolism and handling of drugs by the newborn. Conjugation in the liver is an important mechanism for detoxification and clearance of many drugs. The limited capacity of the conjugation mechanism is held to be largely reponsible for the so-called "gray syndrome" of chloramphenicol intoxication in which a dosage schedule on a milligrams/kilogram body weight basis appropriate for older children resulted in dangerously excessive levels in premature infants.

The binding of bilirubin to albumin can be adversely affected by a number of exogenous drugs (i.e., sulfisoxazole, acetylsalicytic acid, caffeine sodium benzoate) which act as competing anions with bilirubin for one or more common binding sites on the albumin molecule. Their administration will thus result in an increase of "free" unconjugated bilirubin with its potential for ready passage into the CNS. Not only the active drug, but any additive preservative or stabilizing chemicals used in any particular formulation may be responsible for altering the bilirubin albumin binding relationship (Schiff et al., 1971).

Agents which are capable of enhancing bilirubin clearance through enzyme induction may also enhance mechanisms which will alter clearance rates for drugs similarly handled and thereby alter individual dosage requirements. Clearly, therefore, there is a need to reevaluate the basis upon which dosage of drugs are assigned for the neonatal patient. Use of proportional dosages based on weight or surface area ignores completely the pharmacokinetics of the particular agent involved. Moreover, the existence of wide individual variations in drug metabolizing ability make uniform dosages hazardous other than on the basis of the minimum capacity to handle the drug. Finally, the presence of hyperbilirubinemia combined with the ability of some drugs to displace bilirubin from its albumin binding sites imposes not only caution but also the necessity of acquiring this information before the administration of any new drug. Such knowledge of the capacity of any individual drug to affect the bilirubin albumin relationship should be a mandatory requirement in the licensing of any agent used in the newborn.

D. Biological Role of the Catecholamines

The neuroectodermal origin of the chromaffin cells of the adrenal medulla has been accepted by most investigators. The primitive sympathetic cells are probably totipotent and serve as precursers of both the sympathetic neurons and the chromaffin cells. These cells have been recognized in adrenal glands of the 27-mm human fetus and in all subsequent stages of development. Following the initial invasion of the adrenal cortex by chromaffin cells and their precursors (16- to 27-mm stage), the intraadrenal chromaffin cells develop independently and more slowly that the chromaffin tissue of the aortic region, so that in the fetus the bulk of chromaffin tissue lies outside the adrenal gland. The largest collections of cells are associated with the abdominal paravertebral sympathetic plexuses (organs of Zuckerkandl). Coupland (1952) demonstrated the presence of pressor amines in extracts of extraadrenal chromaffin bodies of a 70-mm human fetus, and in both the adrenal medulla and paraaortic bodies of 95-mm and older specimens (Coupland, 1953). The principal and almost total amine present in fetal chromaffin tissue appears to be norepinephreine (West et al., 1951), although significant amounts of epinephrine have been demonstrated in human fetal tissue obtained as early as the first trimester (Greenberg and Lind, 1961).

The catecholamines are dihydroxylated phenolic compounds, the most significant being 3,4-dihydroxyphenylethylamine (dopamine), norepinephrine, and epinephrine. The amino acid tyrosine is oxidized to 3,4-dihydrophenylalanine (dopa), which is decarboxylated by dopa decarboxylase, yielding dopamine in chromaffin tissue. Hydroxylation of the side chain of dopamine yields norepinephrine. Some of the storage granules in nerve endings and adrenal medulla contain phenylethanolamine-N-methyltransferase, the enzyme responsible for the methylation of norepinephrine to form epinephrine. This enzyme is found in the organ of Zuckerkandl but not in the adrenal medulla during fetal life (Villee, 1969). After the first year of life it is also found in the adrenal medulla. Thus the fetal adrenal medulla is probably unable to form significant quantities of epinephrine. In contrast, in the adult, the medulla is almost the exclusive source of the epinephrine fraction of total catecholamines.

What role, if any, the catecholamines play in fetal life is uncertain. The demonstrable isolation of amines with pressor activity may reflect some function in the regulation of fetal vascular tone. Dopamine (see below) is localized in the brain in the adult where it functions as a neurotransmitter, but to date any role in the regulation of CNS development is only speculative, and it appears to be absent from fetal brain at least during the first trimester (Greenberg and Lind, 1961). As in the adult, the medullary cells may have a regulatory influence on the secretion of steroid hormones by the adrenal cortex; however, it is more likely that the major component of this regulatory influence lies in the fetal pituitary through the media of the tropic hormones.

There is experimental evidence supporting both *in vitro* and *in vivo* placental transfer of catecholamines (Morgan *et al.*, 1972). In humans, urinary output of epinephrine and norepinephrine during the course of pregnancy remains within normal limits until the onset of labor. Concomitant with the onset of labor there is a marked increase in the output of both epinephrine and norepinephrine, especially the latter (Goodall and Diddle, 1971). After delivery there is also a gradual increase in both reaching the highest level at the 6- to 18-hour postpartum period and then declining. While this may indeed represent a nonspecific response to "stress," it may pose a potential hazard for the fetus in whom Adamsons *et al.* (1971) have shown experimental evidence of asphyxia following catecholamine administration to the mother secondary to a vasoconstrictive effect on the uterine circulation. Similarly, the stressed newborn infant with asphyxia shows a rise in plasma pressor activity (Holden *et al.*, 1972). Such increases, if they do occur, are unlikely to result from hypoxemia alone which is a poor stimulus to catecholamine excretion in the newborn (Stern *et al.*, 1964) but rather from the more powerful provocative combination of hypercarbia and acidemia. Experimentally the newborn infant can selectively respond to tilting (baroreceptor response) with an increase in urinary norepinephrine excretion, and to insulin-induced hypoglycemia with a marked increase in epinephrine (Greenberg *et al.*, 1960). It is interesting that despite the lesser tissue amounts of epinephrine present in the neonate, this particular stimulus (hypoglycemia) is capable of provoking a large selective increase in epinephrine excretion. Similarly, either induced or inadvertently occurring hypothermia results in increases in norepinephrine excretion in the newborn (Stern *et al.*, 1965), a finding qualitatively different from the adult in whom epinephrine represents the major metabolite provoked by cold exposure (Section IV,D,2).

1. GLUCOSE REGULATION

A possible role for epinephrine in the regulation of postnatal blood glucose levels arises from the demonstration that the hypoglycemic intrauterine growth-retarded newborn lacks the normal endogenous urinary epinephrine response to insulin-induced hypoglycemia even during normoglycemic periods (Stern *et al.*, 1967). In addition, infants of diabetic mothers show extremely low urinary catecholamine levels in both hypo-

and normoglycemic periods when compared to nondiabetic mother control infants (Stern et al., 1968). Epinephrine is, however, quantitatively not a very effective stimulus to correcting hypoglycemia compared to other such agents, e.g. glucagon, corticosteroids. Moreover, the poor catecholamine response in both the above situations could more appropriately be attributed to an adrenal medullary exhaustion phenomenon as a result of prolonged intrauterine hypoglycemia rather than a primary pathophysiological mediator of its production. In this connection it is notable that the excellent clinical results obtained in treating hypoglycemic infants of diabetic mothers with a catecholamine analog (susphrine) are more likely a result of an insulin suppression effect, rather than that of a primary effect on glucose either by enhancing glycogen breakdown in the liver or preventing glucose uptake by peripheral tissues (Schiff et al., 1973).

2. THERMOREGULATION

When exposed to a cold environment, the homeothermic organism must increase heat production in order to maintain his body temperature. There are two methods of accomplishing this: a physical method of muscular contraction and shivering, and a chemical method capable of increasing heat production in the absence of muscular activity. The latter is often referred to as nonshivering thermogenesis. Studies in adult experimental animals and man suggest that quantitatively shivering is a more important mechanism with nonshivering, chemical, thermogenesis playing a secondary reserve role in the adult. In the newborn period a reversed situation occurs. Thus the newborn of most mammalian species, man included, do not readily shiver in the cold yet they show an increase in both oxygen consumption and heat production when exposed to a cool environment.

The nature of the mediator of nonshivering thermogenesis appears to be different in newborns as opposed to adult man. Although the catecholamines are involved in both, epinephrine is the major responsible agent in the adult. By contrast, newborn infants exposed to cold (with resultant increases in oxygen consumption and metabolic activity) show large increases in norepinephrine excretion with little change in epinephrine levels (Stern et al., 1965). The exogenous infusion of norepinephrine in newborns at term by Karlberg et al. (1965) demonstrated an immediate thermogenic effect with an increase in oxygen consumption. Moreover, changes in the respiratory quotient observed during thermogenesis suggested that fat was the preferred fuel. Subsequently Schiff et al., (1966) showed an in vivo increase in urinary norepinephrine excretion simultaneous with an increase in serum nonesterified fatty acids (NEFA) following cold exposure. They confirmed the thermogenic nature of the stimulus by demonstrating both a rise in NEFA and a sustained rise in body temperature after norepinephrine infusion. It is now generally accepted that the catecholamines regulate NEFA by activation of an adipose tissue lipase. Chemical thermogenesis is largely a local phenomenon occurring almost exclusively in brown adipose tissue which is present in relative abundance in the neonate as compared to the older child and adult. Under the influence of the catecholamines (in the newborn norepinephrine), triglycerides are split into glycerol and NEFA. The NEFA is either oxidized (30%), reesterified to triglycerides (60%), or released into the circulation (10%). The oxidized fraction represents an obvious thermogenic reaction. In addition, the apparently purposeless hydrolysis and resynthesis of triglycerides is potentially highly exothermic. This would suggest that the increases in NEFA obtained after cold exposure mirrors, rather than causes, chemical thermogenesis in the cold and reflects the much greater lipolytic activity occurring within the adipose tissue itself.

The ability to respond with a norepinephrine increase to cold exposure not only governs successful heat production in the term infant, but failure to do so may in fact represent the biochemical defect in the maturational delay of thermal stability seen in premature infants who require added incubator external heat in order to maintain their body temperature. Small premature infants, unable to defend their body temperature against removal from an incubator environment (32°–34°C) to that of an average room (23°–25°C), are unable to increase urinary norepinephrine excretion on exposure to this challenge. When studied longitudinally the same infants were able to successfully limit their rectal temperature drop coincident with maturation of the ability to increase norepinephrine excretion on removal from the protective incubator environment (Stern, 1970).

The norepinephrine-induced increase in NEFA carries with it a risk for two potentially hazardous effects. As seen in Fig. 2, the nonesterified fatty acids bind competitively with bilirubin on the albumin molecule for at least one identical site (Chan et al., 1971) and hypothermia clinically can thus predispose to the occurrence of kernicterus at lower levels of serum bilirubin. Moreover, the known inverse NEFA–glucose relationship (Dole, 1956) can result in severe hypoglycemia following exposure to cold (Mann and Elliot, 1957). In this connection it is noteworthy that infants of diabetic mothers with both low epinephrine and norepinephrine levels also lack the reverse compensatory increase in NEFA which normally accompanies hypoglycemia, an occurrence which may afford them a degree of protection with respect to the risk for CNS damage from serum bilirubin elevations which do occur with greater frequency and to a higher level than in comparably gestational aged infants born to non-diabetic mothers.

Although peripheral vasoconstriction in response to hypothermia represents an additional catecholamine effect, the baroreceptor response can obviously occur irrespective of any changes in the thermal environment. It has been proposed that postneonatal closure of the ductus arteriosus under extremely hypoxemic conditions is dependent on the release of pressor amines (Dawes, 1968). Although this effect can be produced after exogenous administration, evidence that this represents an *in vivo* endogenously governed mechanism for ductus closure is lacking. Moreover, as indicated above hypoxia alone is a relatively ineffective stimulus to neonatal catecholamine excretion when compared to the response elicited by hypercapnea and acidosis. More recently Stephenson *et al.* (1970) have demonstrated a fall in arterial oxygen tension in normal newborn infants on exposure to a cool environment. They suggested their findings to be the result of a catecholamine-mediated pulmonary vasoconstrictive effect resulting in an increase in both intrapulmonary and intracardiac right to left shunting of blood from the pulmonary to the systemic circulation.

3. ROLE OF DOPAMINE

Dopamine has two functions: it serves as a precursor of norepinephrine and presumably functions as a neurotransmitter in the areas of the brain involved in coordinating motor activity, where it is localized. Circulating catecholamines do not penetrate into the central nervous system and the catecholamines present in brain are synthesized there. The brain contains noradrenergic as well as dopaminergic and serotinergic neurons. These biogenic amine-containing neurons are involved in the regulation of body temperature, ovulation, mood, behavior, and motor coordination (Axelrod and Weinshillbaum, 1972) These CNS effects have to date not been effectively studied in the newborn infant, although it is suspected that the central thermogenic effect may be a direct effect of both dopamine and norepinephrine in the thalamic region. In this connection it is interesting that Moore (1963) had suggested that in the newborn kitten dopamine is an effective, if short-lived, thermogenic stimulus.

The catecholamines are almost entirely metabolized in the body and thus only relatively small quantities of unchanged amines are found in urine. The main metabolites of norepinephrine and epinephrine are vanillymandelic acid (VMA) and 3-methoxy-4-hydroxyphenylglycol. These compounds result from the action of both monoamine oxidase and catechol-O-methyltransferase in the liver which inactivates catecholamines released from the adrenal medulla. Monoamine oxidase is also present

within neurons where it serves to inactivate excessive amounts of norepinephrine locally. The biotransformation products of dopamine found in
urine are homovanillic acid (HVA), a major metabolite, and methoxytyr-
amine. Products of brain amine metabolism can be found in cerebrospinal
fluid, including VMA, HVA, and 5-hydroxyindoleacetic acid. The major
metabolite of norepinephrine in the central nervous system is 3-methoxy-
4-hydroxyphenylglycol. The excretion of this compound in the urine may
indicate metabolism of catecholamines in the brain.

4. Catecholamine-Mediated Disorders

The finding of a marked depletion of dopamine in the corpus striatum
of patients with Parkinson's disease and its subsequent therapy with dopa
has led to renewed interest in reexamining the catecholamine pathway
in CNS disorders. In the newborn, mongolism (Down's syndrome) has
to date received the greatest attention. Rosner et al. (1965) demonstrated
low levels of serotonin in whole blood of patients with Down's syndrome.
Although substitution therapy has had no obvious effects on the degree
of mental retardation, Bazelon et al. (1967) have claimed some improvement in the degree of hypotonia after 5-hydroxytryptophan therapy.
More recently, Wetterberg et al. (1972) have reported a decrease in the
activity of plasma dopamine-β-hydroxylase, the enzyme responsible for
forming norepinephrine from dopamine, in older children and adults with
mongolism. Their data on newborn affected versus nonmongoloid controls
are also suggestive of a difference but the number of neonatal patients
reported is as yet small. If a difference between cause and effect assigna-
tion in these findings is to be made, it is critical to know whether such
defects, as they become identified, are present from birth or only appear
in later life.

In familial dysautonomia (Riley–Day syndrome) there appears to be
a defect in catecholamine synthesis at the dopamine → norepinephrine
level and children so affected show increased HVA and diminished VMA
excretion in urine (Smith et al., 1963). The disease is a rare congenital
disorder occurring primarily although not exclusively in children of east-
ern European Jewish ancestry. It is characterized by defective lacrima-
tion, recurrent vomiting, emotional lability, skin blotching, lack of pain
sensitivity and motor coordination, labile hypertension, and excessive
sweating. The children also show a hyperreactivity to infused norepinephrine (Smith and Dancis, 1964). Although the precise nature and site of
the biochemical defect remains to be elucidated, the findings to date appear to be sufficiently consistent as to warrant the use of a urinary

HVA:VMA ratio as a screening test for the early detection of infants so affected.

REFERENCES

Ackerman, B. D., Dyer, G. Y., and Leydorf, M. (1970). *Pediatrics* **45**, 917–925.
Ackermann, E., Rane, A., and Ericsson, J. L. E. (1972). *Clin. Pharmacol. Ther.* **13**, 652–662.
Adamsons, K., Mueller-Heubach, E., and Myers, R. E. (1971). *Amer. J. Obstet. Gynecol.* **109**, 248–262.
Adlard, B. P. F., and Lathe, G. H. (1970). *Arch. Dis. Childhood* **45**, 186–189.
Adler, V. G., Burman, D., Corner, B., and Gillespie, W. A. (1972). *Lancet* **2**, 384–385.
Allen, F. T., Jr., Diamond, L. D., and Vaughan, V. D., III. (1950). *Amer. J. Dis. Child.* **80**, 779–791.
Anderson, H., Barr, B., and Wedenberg, E. (1970). *Arch. Otolaryngol.* **91**, 141–147.
Arias, I. M., Gartner, L. M., Seifter, S., and Furman, M. (1964). *J. Clin. Invest.* **43**, 2037–2047.
Arias, I. M., Wolfson, S., Lucey, J. F., and McKay, R., Jr. (1965). *J. Clin. Invest.* **44**, 1442–1450.
Axelrod, J., and Weinshilbaum, R. (1972). *N. Engl. J. Med.* **287**, 237–242.
Axline, S. G., Yaffe, S. J., and Simon, H. J. (1967). *Pediatrics* **39**, 97–107.
Baden, M., Bauer, C. R., Colle, E., Klein, G., Taeusch, H. W., Jr., and Stern, L. (1972). *Pediatrics* **50**, 526–534.
Barnes, J. M., and Denz, F. A. (1954). *Pharmacol. Rev.* **6**, 191–242.
Bauer, C. R., Trepanier-Trottier, M. C., and Stern, L. (1973). *J. Pediat.* **82**, 501–505.
Bazelon, M., Paine, R. S., Cowie, V. A., Hunt, P., Houck, J. C., and Mahanand, D. (1967). *Lancet* **1**, 1130–1133.
Billingsley, F. S. (1969). *J. Fla. Med. Ass.* **56**, 95–97.
Bleyer, W. A., and Breckenridge, R. T. (1970). *J. Amer. Med. Ass.* **213**, 2049–2053.
Blondheim, S. H., Lathrup, D., and Zabriskie, J. (1962). *J. Lab. Clin. Med.* **60**, 31–39.
Bloomfield, D. K. (1970). *Amer. J. Obstet. Gynecol.* **107**, 883–888.
Boggs, T. R., and Bishop, H. (1965). *J. Pediat.* **66**, 349–356.
Bongiovanni, A. M., and McPadden, A. J. (1960). *Fert. Steril.* **11**, 181–186.
Boreus, L. O. (1967). *Biol. Neonate* **11**, 328–337.
Brazelton, B. (1970). *Amer. J. Psychiat.* **126**, 1261–1266.
Brew, K. (1969). *Nature (London)* **222**, 671–672.
Brown, A. K. (1962). *Pediat. Clin. N. Amer.* **9**, 575–603.
Catz, C. S., and Giacoia, G. P. (1972). *Pediat. Clin. N. Amer.* **19**, 151.
Catz, C. S., and Yaffe, S. J. (1968). *Pediat. Res.* **2**, 361–370.
Chan, G., Schiff, D., and Stern, L. (1971). *Clin. Biochem.* **4**, 208–214.
Chignall, C. F., Vessell, E. S., Starkweather, D. K., and Berlin, C. M. (1971). *Clin. Pharmacol. Ther.* **12**, 897–901.
Cohen, M. M., Hirschhorn, K., Verbo, S., Frosch, W. A., and Groeschel, M. M. (1968). *Pediat. Res.* **2**, 486–492.
Cohlan, S. Q. (1969). *Pharmacol. Physicians* **3**, 1–5.
Connelly, J. P., Crawford, J. D., and Watson, J. (1963). *Pediatrics* **30**, 425–432.
Conway, A., and Birt, B. D. (1965). *Brit. Med. J.* **2**, 260–263.
Corby, D. G., and Schulman, I. (1971). *J. Pediat.* **79**, 307–313.

Coupland, R. E. (1952). *J. Anat.* **86**, 357–372.
Coupland, R. E. (1953). *J. Endocrinol.* **9**, 194–203.
Cremer, R. J., Perryman, P. W., and Richards, D. H. (1958). *Lancet* **1**, 1094–1097.
Crigler, J. F., Jr., and Najar, V. A. (1952). *Pediatrics* **10**, 169–179.
Curley, A., Hawk, R. E., Kimbrough, R. D., Natheson, G., and Finberg, L. (1971). *Lancet* **2**, 296–297.
Danon, A., Dikstein, S., and Sulman, F. G. (1963). *Proc. Soc. Exp. Biol. Med.* **114**, 366–368.
Dawes, G. S. (1968). "Foetal and Neonatal Physiology." Yearbook Publ., Chicago, Illinois.
Diamond, I., and Schmid, R. (1967). *Science* **155**, 1288–1289.
Dole, V. P. (1956). *J. Clin. Invest.* **35**, 150–154.
Doxiadis, S. A., Fessas, P., Valaes, T., and Mastrokalos, N. (1961). *Lancet* **1**, 297–301.
Duhring, J. L., and Zwirek, S. J. (1971). *Amer. J. Obstet. Gynecol.* **110**, 670–671.
Ehrhardt, A. A., and Money, J. (1967). *J. Sex Res.* **3**, 83–100.
Ehrhardt, A. A., Greenberg, N., and Money, J. (1970). *Johns Hopkins Med. J.* **126**, 237–248.
Elliasson, R., and Aström, A. (1955). *Acta Pharmacol. Toxicol.* **11**, 254–263.
Emerson, D. J. (1962). *Amer. J. Obstet. Gynecol.* **84**, 356–357.
Eriksson, M. (1971). *Acta Pediat. Scand., Suppl.* **211**.
Fabro, S., and Sieber, S. M. (1969). *In* "The Foeto-Placental Unit" (A. Pecile and C. Finzi, eds.), Int. Congr. Ser. No. 183, pp. 313–320. Excerpta Med. Found., Amsterdam.
Fichter, E. G., and Curtis, J. A. (1956). *Pediatrics* **18**, 50–58.
Fillmore, S. J., and McDevitt, E. (1970). *Ann. Intern. Med.* **73**, 731–735.
Food and Drug Administration. (1956). "Guidelines for Reproductive Studies for Safety Evaluation of Drugs for Human Use." FDA, Washington, D.C.
Gartner, L. M., Snyder, R. N., Chalon, R. S., and Bernstein, J. (1970). *Pediatrics* **45**, 906–917.
Giunta, F., and Rath, J. (1969). *Pediatrics* **44**, 162–167.
Glass, L., Rajedgourda, B. K., and Evans, H. E. (1971). *Lancet* **2**, 685–686.
Goldbloom, R. B., and Goldbloom, A. (1953). *J. Pediat.* **43**, 631–643.
Goodall, McC., and Diddle, A. W. (1971). *Amer. J. Obstet. Gynecol.* **111**, 896–904.
Greenberg, R. E., and Lind, J. (1961). *Pediatrics* **27**, 904–911.
Greenberg, R. E., Lind, J., and von Euler, U. S. (1960). *Acta Pediat. Scand.* **49**, 780–785.
Gregg, N. (1941). *Trans. Ophthalmol. Soc. Aust.* **3**, 35.
Guarino, A. M., Gram, T. E., Schroeder, D. C., Call, J. B., and Gillette, J. R. (1969). *J. Pharmacol. Exp. Ther.* **168**, 224–228.
Hahn, P., and Skala, J. (1971). *Clin. Obstet. Gynecol.* **14**, 655–668.
Hall, G. A., and Reid, I. A. (1972). *Lancet* **2**, 1251.
Harley, J. D., Farrar, J. F., Gray, J. B., and Dunlop, I. C. (1964). *Lancet* **1**, 472–473.
Hart, C. W., and Naunton, R. G. (1964). *Arch. Otolaryngol.* **80**, 407–412.
Herbst, A. L., Ulfelder, H., and Poskanzer, D. C. (1971). *N. Engl. J. Med.* **284**, 878–881.
Hernandez, A., Burton, R. M., Pagtakham, R. D., and Goldring, D. (1969). *Pediatrics* **44**, 418–428.
Herxheimer, A. (1971). *Lancet* **1**, 448.
Holden, K. R., Young, R. B., Piland, J. H., and Hurt, G. W. (1972). *Pediatrics* **49**, 495–503.

Hsia, D. Y. Y., Dowben, R. M., Shaw, R., and Grossman, A. (1960). *Nature (London)* **187**, 693.

Jacobson, B. D. (1962). *Amer. J. Obstet. Gynecol.* **84**, 962–968.

Jost, A. (1961). *Harvey Lect.* **55**, 201–226.

Juchau, M. R., and Dyer, D. C. (1972). *Pediat. Clin. N. Amer.* **19**, 65–79.

Juchau, M. R., and Pedersen, M. D. (1973). *Life Sci.* **12**, 193–204.

Jusko, W. J. (1972). *Pediat. Clin. N. Amer.* **19**, 81–100.

Jusko, W. J., Khanna, N., Levy, G., Stern, L., and Yaffe, S. J. (1970). *Pediatrics* **45**, 945–949.

Kallen, B., and Winberg, J. (1969). *Pediatrics* **44**, 410–417.

Kalter, H. (1954). *Genetics* **39**, 185–196.

Karlberg, P., Moore, R. E., and Oliver, T. K., Jr. (1965). *Acta Pediat. Scand.* **54**, 225–238.

Katz, R. G., White, L. R., and Sever, J. L. (1968). *Clin. Pediat.* **7**, 323–330.

Kaufman, N. A., Kapitulnick, J., and Blondheim, S. H. (1969). *Pediatrics* **44**, 543–548.

Kenny, F. M., Preeyasombat, C., Spaulding, J. S., and Migeon, C. J. (1966). *Pediatrics* **37**, 960–966.

Knowles, J. A. (1965). *J. Pediat.* **66**, 1068–1082.

Krasner, J., and Yaffe, S. J. (1968). *Amer. J. Dis. Child.* **115**, 267–272.

Krasner, J., Giocoia, G. P., and Yaffe, S. J. (1973). *Ann. N.Y. Acad. Sci.* **226**, 101–114.

Larese, R., and Mirkin, B. L. (1974). *Clin. Pharmacol. Ther.* **15**, 387.

Larsson, K. S. (1962). *Acta Odontol Scand.* **20**, Suppl. 31.

Larsson, K. S., and Boström, H. (1965). *Acta Paediat. Scand.* **54**, 43–48.

Larsson, Y., and Sterkey, G. (1960). *Lancet* **2**, 1424–1426.

Lathe, G. H., and Walker, M. (1958a). *Quart. J. Exp. Physiol. Cog. Med. Sci.* **43**, 257.

Lathe, G. H., and Walker, M. (1958b). *Biochem. J.* **70**, 705–712.

Lenz, W., and Knapp, K. (1962). *Deut. Med. Wochenschr.* **87**, 1232.

Lester, R. L., Hammaker, L., and Schmid, R. (1962). *Lancet* **2**, 1257.

Levi, A. J., Gatmaitan, Z., and Arias, I. M. (1969a). *J. Clin. Invest.* **48**, 2156–2167.

Levi, A. J., Gatmaitan, Z., and Arias, I. M. (1969b). *Lancet* **2**, 139–140.

Levin, W., Conney, A. H., Alvares, A. P., Merkatz, I., and Kappas, A. (1972). *Science* **176**, 419–420.

Levine, O. R., and Blumenthal, S. (1962). *Pediatrics* **29**, 18–25.

Liggins, G. C., and Howie, R. N. (1972). *Pediatrics* **50**, 515–525.

Lind, J., Stern, L., and Wegelius, C. (1964). "Human Foetal and Neonatal Circulation." Thomas, Springfield, Illinois.

Lind, N., Shinebourne, E., Turner, P., and Cottom, D. (1971). *Pediatrics* **47**, 105–112.

Llewellyn-Jones, D. (1968). *Brit. Med. J.* **4**, 387.

Lockhart, J. D. (1972). *Pediatrics* **50**, 229–235.

Lokietz, H., Dowben, R. M., and Hsia, D. Y. Y. (1963). *Pediatrics* **32**, 47–51.

Lucey, J. F., Valaes, T., and Doxiadis, S. A. (1967). *Pediatrics* **39**, 876–883.

Lucey, J. F., Ferreiro, M., and Hewit, J. (1968). *Pediatrics* **41**, 1047–1054.

Luhman, L. A. (1963). *Obstet. Gynecol.* **21**, 713–717.

Lutwak-Mann, C., and Hay, M. F. (1962). *Brit. Med. J.* **2**, 944–946.

Lyons, W. R., Li, C., Ahman, N., and Rice, W. (1968). *Proc. Int. Symp. Growth Horm., 1st, 1967* p. 349.

MacAuley, M. A., Berg, S. R., and Charles, D. (1968). *Amer. J. Obstet. Gynecol.* **102**, 1162–1168.

McBride, W. G. (1961). *Lancet* **2**, 1358.

426   SUMNER J. YAFFE AND LEO STERN

McGlothlin, W. H., Sparkes, R. S., and Arnold, D. O. (1970). J. Amer. Med. Ass. 212, 1483–1487.
McMurphy, D. M., and Boréus, L. O. (1968). Biol. Neonate 13, 325–339.
Malloy, H. T., and Evelyn, K. A. (1937). J. Biol. Chem. 119, 481–490.
Mann, T. P., and Elliot, R. I. K. (1957). Lancet 1, 229–234.
Marsk, L., Theorell, M., and Larsson, K. S. (1971). Nature (London) 234, 358–359.
Matz, G. J., and Nauntan, R. F. (1968). Arch. Otolaryngol. 88, 370–372.
Maurer, H. M., Wolff, J. A., Finster, M., Poppers, P. J., Pantuk, E., Kuntzman, R., and Conney, A. H. (1968). Lancet 2, 122–124.
Mirkin, B. L. (1971). J. Pediat. 78, 329–337.
Mollison, P. L., and Cutbush, M. (1959). Progr. Hermatol. 2, 153.
Moore, R. E. (1963). Fed. Proc., Fed. Amer. Soc. Exp. Biol. 22, 920–929.
Morgan, C. D., Sandler, M., and Pangiel, M. (1972). Amer. J. Obstet. Gynecol. 112, 1068–1075.
Murphy, M. L. (1965). In "Teratology Principles and Techniques" (J. G. Wilson and G. Warkany, eds.), pp. 145–184. Univ. of Chicago Press, Chicago, Illinois.
Naiman, J. L., and Kosoy, M. H. (1964). Can. Med. Ass. J. 91, 1243–1249.
Nelson, M. M., and Forfar, J. O. (1971). Brit. Med. J. 1, 523–527.
Nishimura, H., Takano, K., Tanimura, T., and Yasuda, M. (1968). Teratology 1, 281–290.
Nora, J. J., Nora, A. H., Sommerville, R. J., Hill, R. M., and McNamara, D. G. (1967). J. Amer. Med. Ass. 202, 1065–1069.
Obes-Polleri, J. (1967). Arch. Pediat. Urug. 38, 77–100.
Oki, F., and Naiman, J. L. (1966). "Hematologic Problems in the Newborn." Saunders, Philadelphia, Pennsylvania.
Ostrow, J. D., Berry, C. S., and Zarembo, J. E. (1974). In "Phototherapy in the Newborn" (G. B. Odell, R. Schaffer, and A. P. Simopoulous, eds.), pp. 74–92. Nat. Acad. Sci., Washington, D.C.
Palmisano, P. A., and Cassady, G. (1969). J. Amer. Med. Ass. 209, 556–558.
Percy, A. K., and Yaffe, S. J. (1964). Pediatrics 33, 965–968.
Plummer, G. (1952). Pediatrics 10, 687–693.
Poland, R. L., and Odell, G. B. (1971). N. Engl. J. Med. 284, 1–6.
Privitera, P. J., Loggie, J. M. H., and Gaffney, T. E. (1969). J. Pharmacol. Exp. Ther. 166, 293–298.
Räihä, N. (1973). Pediat. Res. 7, 1–4.
Ramos, A., and Stern, L. (1969). Amer. J. Obstet. Gynecol. 105, 1247–1251.
Ramos, A., Silverberg, M., and Stern, L. (1966). Amer. J. Dis. Child. 111, 353–356.
Rane, A., and Ackermann, E. (1972). Clin. Pharmacol. Ther. 13, 663–670.
Rane, A., Lunde, P. K. M., Jalling, B., Yaffe, S. J., and Sjöqvist, F. (1971). J. Pediat. 78, 877–882.
Rane, A., Garle, M., Borga, O., and Sjöqvist, F. (1974). Clin. Pharmacol. Ther. 15, 39–45.
Rane, A., Bertilsson, L., and Palmer, L. (1975). Eur. J. Clin. Pharmacol. 8, 283–284.
Rasmussen, F. (1961). Acta Vet. Scand. 2, 151–154.
Redding, R., Douglas, W. H. J., and Stein, M. (1972). Science 175, 994–996.
Richards, I. D. (1969). Brit. J. Prev. Soc. Med. 23, 218–225.
Robinson, G. C., and Cambon, K. G. (1964). N. Engl. J. Med. 271, 949–951.
Rosner, F., Ong, B. H., Paine, R. S., and Mahanand, D. (1965). Lancet 1, 1191–1193.
Ross, S. G., Waugh, T. R., and Malloy, H. T. (1937). J. Pediat. 11, 397–448.
Rosta, A. J., Makoi, Z., and Kertesz, A. (1968). Lancet 2, 1138.

Sas, M. J., and Herczeg, J. (1970). *Arch. Pediat. Acad. Sci. Hung.* **11**, 35–40.

Schenker, S., Bashore, R. A., and Smith, F. (1967). "Bilirubin Metabolism" (I. A. D. Bouchier and B. H. Billing, eds.). Blackwell Scientific Publ., Oxford, England.

Schiff, D., Stern, L., and Leduc, J. (1966). *Pediatrics* **37**, 577–582.

Schiff, D., Aranda, J. V., and Stern, L. (1970). *J. Pediat.* **77**, 457–458.

Schiff, D., Chan, G., and Stern, L. (1971). *Pediatrics* **48**, 139–141.

Schiff, D., Colle, D., Wells, D., and Stern, L. (1973). *J. Pediat.* **82**, 258–262.

Schmid, R., Hammaker, L., and Axelrod, J. (1957). *Arch. Biochem. Biophys.* **70**, 285.

Schou, M., and Amidsen, A. (1973). *Brit. Med. J.* **2**, 138.

Shepard, J. H., Jamimura, J., and Robkin, M. (1971). In "Malformations congénitales des mammiferes" (H. Tuchmann-Duplessis, ed.). Masson, Paris.

Silverio, J., and Poole, J. W. (1973). *Pediatrics* **51**, 578–580.

Silverman, W. A., Anderson, D. H., Blanc, W. A., and Crozier, D. N. (1956). *Pediatrics* **18**, 614–625.

Sjöqvist, F., Bergfors, P. G., Borga, O., Lind, M., and Yagge, H. (1972). *J. Pediat.* **80**, 496–500.

Skakkebaek, N. E., Philip, J. and Rafaelsen, O. J. (1968). *Science* **160**, 1246–1248.

Smart, R. G., and Bateman, K. (1968). *Can. Med. Ass. J.* **99**, 805–810.

Smith, A. A., and Dancis, J. (1964). *N. Engl. J. Med.* **270**, 704–707.

Smith, A. A., Taylor, T., and Wortis, S. B. (1963). *N. Engl. J. Med.* **268**, 705–707.

Smith, D. W. (1970). "Recognizable Patterns of Human Malformation." Saunders, Philadephia, Pennsylvania.

Soyka, L. F. (1970). *Biochem. Pharmacol.* **19**, 945–951...

Stephenson, J. M., Du, J. N., and Oliver, T. K., Jr. (1970). *J. Pediat.* **76**, 848–852.

Stern, L. (1970). *Curr. Probl. Pediat.* No. 1.

Stern, L., and Denton, R. L. (1965). *Pediatrics* **35**, 483–485.

Stern, L., and Doray, B. (1968). *Proc. Int. Congr. Pediat., 12th* pp. 512–513.

Stern, L., and Lind, J. (1960). *Annu. Rev. Med.* **11**, 113–126.

Stern, L. Lind, J., and Leduc, J. (1964). *Acta Paediat. Scand.* **53**, 13–17.

Stern, L., Lees, M. H., and Leduc, J. (1965). *Pediatrics* **36**, 367–373.

Stern, L., Sourkes, T. L., and Räihä, N. (1967). *Biol. Neonatorum* **11**, 129–136.

Stern, L., Ramos, A., and Leduc, J. (1968). *Pediatrics* **42**, 598–605.

Stern, L., Khanna, N. N., Levy, G., and Yaffe, S. J. (1970). *Amer. J. Dis. Child.* **120**, 26–31.

Stern, L., Khanna, N. N., and MacLeod, P. (1971). *Union Med. Can.* **100**, 506–513.

Stutzman, L., and Sokal, J. E. (1968). *Clin. Obstet. Gynecol.* **11**, 416–427.

Thiersch, J. B. (1952). *Amer. J. Obstet. Gynecol.* **63**, 1298–1304.

Toaff, R., and Ravid, R. (1968). In "Drug Induced Diseases" (L. Meyler and H. M. Peci, eds.), pp. 117–113. Excerpta Med. Found., Amsterdam.

Trolle, E. (1968). *Lancet* **2**, 705–708.

Uchida, I. A., Holunga, R., and Lawler, C. (1968). *Lancet* **2**, 1045–1049.

Uhlig, H. (1957). *Arzenim.-Forsch.* **12**, 61.

Ulstrom, R. A., and Eisenklam, E. (1964). *J. Pediat.* **65**, 27–37.

van den Bergh, H., and Muller, P. (1916). *Biochem. Z.* **77**, 90.

Villee, C. A. (1963). In "Modern Trends in Human Reproductive Physiology" (H. M. Carey, ed.), Vol. 1. Butterworth, London.

Villee, D. B. (1969). *N. Engl. J. Med.* **281**, 473–484.

Waltman, R., Bonerra, F., Nigrin, G., and Pipat, C. (1969). *Lancet* **2**, 1265–1267.

Warrell, D. W, and Taylor, R. (1968). *Lancet* **1**, 117–119.

428   SUMNER J. YAFFE AND LEO STERN

Waters, W. J., and Porter, E. G. (1961). *Pediatrics* 33, 749–757.
Weiss, C. F., Glazko, A. J., and Weston, J. (1960). *N. Engl. J. Med.* 262, 787–794.
Welch, R. M., Harrison, Y. E., Conney, A. H., Poppers, P. J., and Finster, M. (1968). *Science* 160, 541–542.
West, G. B, Shepherd, D. M., and Hunter, R. B. (1951). *Lancet* 2, 966–969.
Wetterberg, L., Gustavason, K. H. Backström, M., Ross, S. B., and Frodin, O. (1972). *Clin. Genet.* 3, 152–153.
Wichman, H. M., Rind, H., and Gladtke, E. (1968). *Z. Kinderheilk.* 103, 262–276.
Wilkins, L. (1960). *J. Amer. Med. Ass.* 172, 1028–1032.
Wilson, J. G. (1965). *In* "Teratology Principles and Techniques" (J. G. Wilson and G. Warkany, eds.), pp. 251–277. Univ. of Chicago Press, Chicago, Illinois.
World Health Organization. (1967). *World Health Organ., Tech. Rep. Ser.* 364.
Yaffe, S. J., Rane, A., Sjöqvist, F., Boréus, L. O., and Orrenius, S. (1970) *Life Sci.* 9, 1189–1200.
Zetterström, R., and Ernstner, L. (1956). *Nature (London)* 178, 1335.
Zimmerman, E. F., Andrew, F., and Kalter, H. (1970). *Proc. Nat. Acad. Sci. U.S.* 67, 779–785.

Index